T0256740

 Thieme

Color Atlas of Dermatology

Martin Rocken, MD
Professor and Chairman
Department of Dermatology
Tübingen University
Tübingen, Germany

Martin Schaller, MD
Professor
Department of Dermatology
Tübingen University
Tübingen, Germany

Elke Sattler, MD
Staff Physician
Department of Dermatology and Allergology
Ludwig Maximilian University
Munich, Germany

Walter Burgdorf, MD
Tutzing, Germany
Former Professor and Chairman
Department of Dermatology
University of New Mexico
Albuquerque
New Mexico, USA

With 189 color plates by Professor Juergen Wirth

Thieme
Stuttgart · New York

Library of Congress Cataloging-in-Publication Data

Taschenatlas Dermatologie. English.
Color atlas of dermatology / Martin Rocken ... [et al.] ; with color plates by Juergen Wirth ; [translator, Walter Burgdorf].
p. ; cm.
ISBN 978-3-13-132341-5 (pbk.)
I. Rocken, Martin. II. Title.
[DNLM: 1. Skin Diseases--diagnosis--Atlases. 2. Skin Diseases--therapy--Atlases. WB 17]

616.50022'3--dc23
2011036883

This book is an authorized translation of the German edition published and copyrighted 2010 by Georg Thieme Verlag, Stuttgart. Title of the German edition: Taschenatlas Dermatologie. Grundlagen – Diagnostik – Klinik.

Translator: Walter Burgdorf, Tutzing, Germany

Illustrator: Professor Juergen Wirth, Dreieich-Offenthal, Germany

Important note: Medicine is an ever-changing science undergoing continual development. Research and clinical experience are continually expanding our knowledge, in particular our knowledge of proper treatment and drug therapy. Insofar as this book mentions any dosage or application, readers may rest assured that the authors, editors, and publishers have made every effort to ensure that such references are in accordance with the **state of knowledge at the time of production of the book.**

Nevertheless, this does not involve, imply, or express any guarantee or responsibility on the part of the publishers in respect to any dosage instructions and forms of applications stated in the book. **Every user is requested to examine carefully** the manufacturers' leaflets accompanying each drug and to check, if necessary in consultation with a physician or specialist, whether the dosage schedules mentioned therein or the contraindications stated by the manufacturers differ from the statements made in the present book. Such examination is particularly important with drugs that are either rarely used or have been newly released on the market. Every dosage schedule or every form of application used is entirely at the user's own risk and responsibility. The authors and publishers request every user to report to the publishers any discrepancies or inaccuracies noticed. If errors in this work are found after publication, errata will be posted at www.thieme.com on the product description page.

© 2012 Georg Thieme Verlag,
Rüdigerstrasse 14, 70469 Stuttgart, Germany
http://www.thieme.de
Thieme New York, 333 Seventh Avenue,
New York, NY 10001, USA
http://www.thieme.com

Cover design: Thieme Publishing Group
Typesetting by primustype R. Hurler,
Notzingen, Germany
Printed in China by Asia Pacific Offset Ltd.
Hongkong

ISBN 978-3-13-132341-5   1 2 3 4 5 6

Preface

No organ is as exposed to the environment as the skin. It is the interface between individuals and their surroundings. The skin protects us against a variety of potentially harmful agents—ultraviolet irradiation, thermal damage, mechanical stress, pathogenic microbes, and a variety of small and large molecules including allergens. The skin also plays an important role in maintaining a stable internal environment, regulating body temperature and water content.

Disturbances in the function of the skin can produce a broad spectrum of diseases, which often extend beyond the skin to have systemic effects. No other organ presents such a large variety of diseases, including a number which are potentially life-threatening. Skin diseases have the potential to interfere with body language—with how we see ourselves and how others react to us. Thus a number of common diseases such as eczema and psoriasis, which do not cause permanent damage and are not often fatal, still disrupt the lives of millions of affected people.

Skin diseases are very common and thus place considerable demands on health care systems. The problem is exacerbated by the fact that the incidence of several common skin diseases and tumors is on the increase. Both the aging population and environmental factors play a role in these increases, but in many instances, we do not know what is responsible.

The most deadly skin tumor is the melanoma. Its incidence has doubled every decade for the past half-century; exposure to ultraviolet irradiation seems to be the most important factor. Melanoma is about to become the fourth most common metastatic tumor among fair-skinned individuals. Basal cell carcinoma is already the most common human malignancy, with an incidence of > 1 : 140. The problems with skin cancers are made worse by the widespread use of immunosuppressive agents to treat autoimmune diseases and make organ transplantation possible. In addition, patients with HIV/AIDS and immunodeficiency are also at greater risk for many tumors.

Dermatologists have at their disposal a much wider spectrum of systemic medications than they did a generation ago. They must become skilled in using all the new medications. In addition, other specialties are also benefitting from advancements in the pharmaceutical industry, so that physicians and patients are increasingly confronted with skin reactions to new and unusual drugs. The new and expensive medications are particularly relevant for many of the common disorders—such as psoriasis and atopic dermatitis—so that one cannot ignore both their medical and economic impact. Our abilities to treat autoimmune diseases, such as lupus erythematosus, have also greatly increased, once again challenging dermatologists to work effectively with other specialties to provide maximum care for this group of patients.

A decade ago no one expected an increase in severe infectious diseases of the skin. The antibiotic armamentarium was strong and all were optimistic. Instead we have been confronted with increasing antibiotic resistance, dramatic infections, and even diseases where we are threatened with running out of possible therapeutic choices. Sexually transmitted diseases have made a modest resurgence, and patients with either HIV/AIDS or iatrogenic immunosuppression present with a bewildering array of unusual and generally severe viral, bacterial, and fungal infections.

The skin also serves as a window on many systemic diseases. One can often recognize underlying malignancies, metabolic diseases, and inflammatory disorders with obvious systemic significance based purely on the skin examination. Dermatology thus interacts with almost every other discipline, both at a diagnostic and therapeutic level.

In our view, dermatology is marked by three important characteristics. Firstly, one must be able to accurately describe skin findings; this coupled with a good visual memory and hard study makes it possible for the dermatologist to generally make a rapid diagnosis—often to the amazement of colleagues or patients. Secondly, a profound appreciation of cutaneous biology and how it relates to disease is required to plan appropriate topical and systemic therapy; in addition, considerable technical skill is also required as dermatology is both a medical and a surgical specialty. Thirdly, the dermatologist must be a caring physician, a true friend to the patient. In addition to ensuring that the best possible therapy is offered, he or she must be aware of the many psychosocial problems that accompany common skin diseases, like acne, atopic dermatitis, and psoriasis, and help the patients and their families address these issues. The rewarding feature is that although in some instances one must be satisfied with supportive or even palliative approaches, in many instances therapeutic measures can be dramatically successful or even curative.

The classic position of dermatology in medicine, coupled with the many advances of the last 20 years in understanding pathogenesis, facilitating diagnosis, and improving therapy, have encouraged us to use the classic Thieme "flexibook" format to present our specialty. The concept of brief texts facing informative and detailed color plates is an effective way to give the reader a clear and relevant introduction to dermatology. This book is in no way designed to compete with established large textbooks designed for the specialists. Instead our goal is to give students an almost painless introduction to dermatology over a short period of time, making not only the study of the skin, but all medical studies, more rewarding and pleasurable. We also hope that young dermatology residents and physicians in training in other specialties will find this book useful as a quick refresher, hopefully helpful in common clinical situations. The specialist may appreciate our work as a reminder of the intricate relationship between scientific advances and clinical dermatology.

Every book reflects the efforts of many individuals. We would like to thank the many friends and colleagues who have helped us so generously in preparing this book.

We would especially like to thank Ms. Susanne Schimmer who skillfully coordinated our efforts to produce the final texts and plates for the German edition. About one-third of the book was originally written in English, the rest in German, and the authors worked together to prepare texts in both languages. Walter Burgdorf, a native English speaker, was responsible for the final English texts. Ms. Angelika-Marie Findgott and Ms. Annie Hollins from Thieme Publishers managed the English edition of the book.

The photographers in our Tübingen clinic, Mr. Oliver Hallmaier and Ms. Marianne Kelch were extremely helpful and provided almost all the photographs; other sources are listed on page 392. Professor Juergen Wirth provided all the diagrams, helping convert our medical knowledge into instructive visual material. Dr. Gisela Metzler provided all the photomicrographs while Professor Helmut Breuninger helped with the pages on operative dermatology.

We hope that every reader enjoys this book and learns from it. In addition, if it helps our colleagues to make the correct dermatologic diagnoses and provide helpful therapy, then in the end our patients will benefit. Without them, this book would not have been possible.

Tübingen, Munich, and Tutzing

Martin Rocken
Martin Schaller
Elke Sattler
Walter Burgdorf

Contents

I Basic Principles

Contents

II Diagnosis of Dermatologic Diseases

III Treatment of Dermatologic Diseases

IV Dermatologic Diseases

Contents

Contents

XI

Contents

Contents

Contents

V Appendix

I Basic Principles

A. Dermatology

Dermatology is the medical specialty devoted to the study of the skin and its diseases, as well as their treatment.

■ Numbers

The distribution of dermatologists is highly variable:
- Germany—1:16 000
- USA—1:30 000
- UK—1:300 000
- Africa—1:many million.

Thus the daily function of a dermatologist or dermatologic service can vary from primary care of the skin, to a consultant role, to training health-care workers to treat large numbers of patients.

■ Demand

Between 15% and 25% of patients presenting to pediatricians and family doctors have skin disease, which is often one of their reasons for seeking medical care. Not all dermatologic services can be provided by dermatologists; every health-care worker must be able to identify and treat common skin diseases.

■ Costs

Dermatologic treatment can be very expensive. In some health-care budgets, the cost of topical agents is 20%–25%. Many new highly effective medications are available for diseases such as atopic dermatitis, psoriasis, and skin cancer, but it is unclear how to pay for them in an age of increasing costs and shrinking budgets.

B. Frequency of Skin Diseases

The following examples underline the medical-economic importance of dermatology:
- every teenager develops some degree of acne. Few other diseases have an incidence of almost 100%
- the most common inflammatory skin disease, atopic dermatitis, has experienced a surge in prevalence and, depending on the country studied, affects 5%–20% of the population. This surge has been coupled with an increase in asthma and allergic rhinitis
- basal cell carcinoma is the most common malignant tumor of man, affecting almost every white inhabitant of sunny climes
- melanoma is the most dangerous cutaneous tumor. It, too, has increased dramatically in incidence with a lifetime risk approaching 1:50 for Western Europe. It is the fourth most common metastatic tumor in Europe.

C. Functions of the Skin

The skin is the one organ every person sees every day. It forms the interface between an individual and their environment. It is one of the largest organs with a surface area of $1.5–2.0\,\mathrm{m}^2$. The skin also contains adnexal (skin-derived) structures such as hair, nails, and sweat glands, as well as vessels, nerves, melanocytes, and a skin-associated immune system.

■ Protection

The skin provides mechanical support, forms a barrier for the exchange of fluids and gases, protects against invasion of microorganisms, and modulates the unavoidable exposure to heat, cold, and ultraviolet (UV) light.

■ Immune Response

Innate immunity starts in the keratinocytes of the skin and may lead to antigen processing by the skin's own dendritic cells, the Langerhans cells. The skin is patrolled by memory T cells capable of responding to repeated attackers, moncytes and mast cells.

■ Sensation

The skin has a rich network of nerves with a variety of sensory receptors providing exquisite sensitivity. Try moving just one hair on your arm and see how quickly the free nerve endings warn you. Sensation and protection interact; when an arthropod bites you, the itch response may induce you to scratch your skin and eliminate the invader.

■ Temperature Control

Regulation of skin blood flow and sweating are both essential for maintaining core temperature.

■ Identification

We recognize each other by our skin and its features. The social role of the skin cannot be underestimated, as shown by great interest in cosmetic procedures and the considerable social impact of skin diseases on patients.

— Dermatology and the Skin —

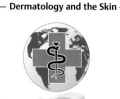

Percentage of family
practice patients

25%

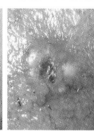

Skin diseases

Costs

A. Dermatology

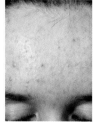

Acne
Almost all adolescents affected

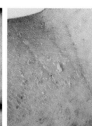

Atopic dermatitis
5%–20% prevalence

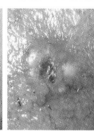

Basal cell carcinoma
Most common tumor in humans

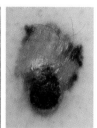

Melanoma
Lifetime risk 1:50
Incidence increasing worldwide

B. Frequency of Skin Diseases

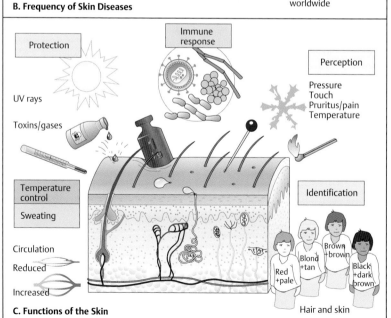

Protection

Immune response

Perception

UV rays

Pressure
Touch
Pruritus/pain
Temperature

Toxins/gases

Temperature control

Sweating

Identification

Circulation

Reduced

Increased

Red +pale

Blond +tan

Brown +brown

Black +dark brown

Hair and skin

C. Functions of the Skin

1 Introduction

3

A. Embryology

The skin consists of the epidermis with layers of variously differentiated keratinocytes and an underlying dermis with adnexal structures, vessels, and nerves, as well as subcutaneous fat. The skin develops from the ectoderm and mesoderm. Initially there is a single layer of ectodermal cells, but by around 8 weeks, a flattened outer layer (periderm) appears. By birth, the complex epidermis is present. Melanocytes migrate into the skin from the neural crest, as do nerves. The dermis, with its connective tissue, derives from the mesenchyme. The adnexal structures develop from the interaction between epidermal invaginations and supporting mesenchymal structures.

B. The Epidermis

Keratinocytes. The epidermis is the outer layer of the skin. It is formed by keratinocytes which are arranged into multiple layers:
- *stratum basale*—anchors the epidermis to the dermis and contains cuboidal stem cells which continuously divide, allowing for replacement of the epidermis
- *stratum spinosum*—the bulk of the epidermis, so named because connecting desmosomes appear as "spines" under the microscope
- *stratum granulosum*—an area where the keratinization process is completed and keratohyalin granules become visible
- *stratum lucidum*—an amorphous band between the stratum granulosum and stratum corneum, only seen on the palms of the hands and soles of the feet
- *stratum corneum*—remnants of keratinocytes, consisting of keratin and cell walls without nuclei.

Other epidermal cells. Three other cells are found in the normal epidermis:
- *melanocytes*, which synthesize melanin, the main photoprotective factor (Ch. 3.2)
- *Langerhans cells*, which are the antigen-processing cells of the skin (Ch. 5.3)
- *Merkel cells*, which are neuroendocrine cells that function as mechanoreceptors. They arise from the neural crest: cytologic markers include cytokeratin 20, neuropeptides, and dense core granules. They interact with cutaneous nerves in specialized structures known as hair disks.

Clinical correlate: Merkel cell carcinoma is an uncommon but highly aggressive cutaneous malignancy.

Cell junctions. There are several types of cell junctions in the epidermis. Each plays an important pathophysiologic role:
- *desmosomes*—complex structures with many proteins holding cells together. Among the most important are the desmogleins (Ch. 14.11)

Clinical correlate: The pemphigus group features dissolution of the epidermis, mediated by autoantibodies directed primarily against desmogleins. Staphylococcal scalded skin syndrome is caused by bacterial toxins that damage desmogleins.

- *adherent junctions*—connect actin filaments and involve cadherins and catenins; they have an involvement in signaling as well as adherence
- *gap junctions*—formed by connexins, which are arranged to create hexagonal pores connecting two cells allowing rapid transport of materials or signals; defects can cause deafness and skin diseases.

C. The Basement Membrane Zone

Many different proteins interact to anchor the epidermis to the dermis. Key components of the basement membrane zone (BMZ) are *hemidesmosomes*, structures in the lower pole of basal cells sharing many features with desmosomes, and the basal membrane, made up of the lamina lucida and lamina densa. The BMZ contributes the barrier function, allowing molecules to diffuse to and from the dermis.

Clinical correlate: Mutations in proteins of the BMZ lead to epidermolysis bullosa, a family of diseases featuring easy blistering (Ch. 16.1). Antibodies against these proteins cause a variety of autoimmune bullous diseases including bullous pemphigoid (Ch. 15.1). Inflammation at the dermal–epidermal junction is a feature of many inflammatory diseases including lupus erythematosus (Ch. 17.5), lichen planus (Ch. 14.8), graft versus host disease (Ch. 14.9), and many drug reactions.

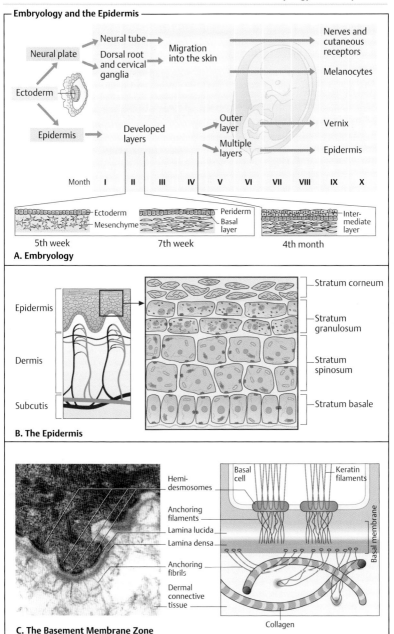

A. Embryology

B. The Epidermis

C. The Basement Membrane Zone

The adnexal structures include hair, nails, and glands; all are formed by an interaction between strands of epithelial cells which extend into the dermis and interact with mesenchymal components.

A. The Adnexal Glands

Sweat and sebaceous glands are prototypal adnexal structures, consisting of strands of epithelial cells which lie in the dermis, but retain their external connection. There are four basic types of glands.

Eccrine glands. Eccrine glands are widely distributed over the body, but are most concentrated on the palms and soles. They are not found on the lips, external ear canal, clitoris, and labia minora. Each individual has several million. They consist of a coiled secretory portion and a long duct coursing through the dermis to open onto the epidermis. Eccrine sweat is usually clear and odorless, so the eccrine glands are to some extent "the skin's kidneys." Skin contains antimicrobial peptides. Some medications are secreted through eccrine sweat.

Apocrine glands. These glands are associated with hair follicles; their secretory duct empties into the upper part of the hair follicle. They are richest in the axillae and groin. They function via "decapitation secretion," where the free luminal end of the cell is shed with the secretory products. Apocrine sweat is odoriferous; the glands are known as *Duftdrüsen* (smell glands) in German. Their function may be to produce pheromones for sexual attraction and other messaging. In some species they have antibacterial effects. The lactiferous glands of the breasts are closely related to apocrine glands.

Apoeccrine glands. These glands are found in the axillae of adults and have overlap features of eccrine and apocrine glands, with both types of secretory cells found in the coiled gland. They open directly on the skin surface, not via hair follicles.

Sebaceous glands. These glands also are intimately associated with hair follicles, as their oily secretion lubricates the follicle to allow the hair shaft to grow outwards against less resistance. Sebaceous glands are very androgen sensitive. When they function to excess, the skin becomes oily (*seborrhea*). They play a key role in acne (Ch. 26.1).

B. Temperature Control

Resting state. Eccrine glands are intimately involved in temperature control. In a resting state, evaporative loss of water through the skin is approximately 900 mL daily. This *insensitive water loss* provides about 20% of the cooling effect of the skin.

Core temperature. The body maintains a central temperature at 37 °C. By varying skin blood flow, the heat lost by convection and radiation (dry heat loss) can be manipulated over a wide range. For example, digital blood flow can change 500-fold between warm and cold temperatures. Shunts in the digital circulation controlled by contractile glomus cells (*Sucquet–Hoyer anastomosis*) make this variation possible.

> **Clinical correlate:** Glomus cell tumors are painful tumors (Ch. 22.4) derived from the regulatory contractile glomus cells.

Sweating. When the ambient temperature rises, less dry heat loss can occur, so sweating assumes a major role. Sweating is an active process controlled by cholinergic sympathetic fibers. With increased temperature and physical activity, sweat volumes of 1–4 L/hour are possible. Because the eccrine sweat is rich in electrolytes, attention must be paid to replacing not only fluids but also sodium chloride and other ingredients.

> **Clinical correlate:** When one lives in a warm climate, acclimatization occurs, so that baseline sweating increases, electrolyte concentration in sweat decreases, and thirst increases. No such adjustments are possible in cold climates, so humans are dependent on heating and clothing. Furred and feathered animals can increase their insulation by fluffing their outer coats. "Goose bumps" in humans are residual ineffective attempts to fluff the hairs to provide protection.

Adnexal Structures

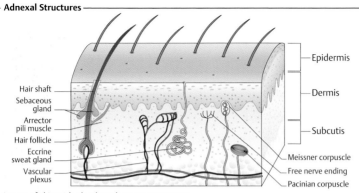

Epidermis

Dermis

Subcutis

Hair shaft
Sebaceous gland
Arrector pili muscle
Hair follicle
Eccrine sweat gland
Vascular plexus

Meissner corpuscle
Free nerve ending
Pacinian corpuscle

Layers of skin with glands and sensory structures

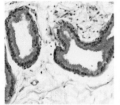
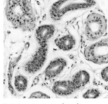
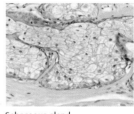

Apocrine sweat gland   Eccrine sweat gland   Sebaceous gland

A. The Adnexal Glands

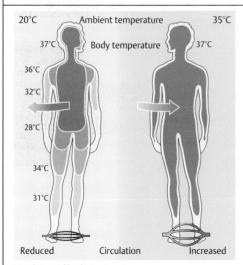

20°C   Ambient temperature   35°C
37°C   Body temperature   37°C
36°C
32°C
28°C
34°C
31°C

Reduced   Circulation   Increased

Regulation of body temperature

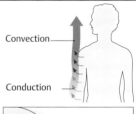

Convection

Conduction

Diffusion

H_2O

Sweat gland

Cooling through evaporation

B. Temperature Control

A. The Dermis

The dermis is the major structural component of the skin. It is known in German as *Lederhaut* (leather skin), because it is what remains when hides are tanned. The dermis is derived from mesenchyme; the predominant cells are fibroblasts, which are responsible for the synthesis of collagen and elastin, the main dermal fibers. The dermis has two main compartments:

- superficial or *papillary* dermis
- deeper or *reticular* dermis.

B. Extracellular Matrix Components

Collagen. Collagen is an ubiquitous structural protein, which accounts for 70% of the dry weight of the dermis. The basic structure is triple helix rich in glycine, proline, and hydroxyproline, formed in fibroblasts and secreted as procollagen. Extracellular modifications include cleavage of amino and carboxy terminal extensions, and fiber formation involving cross-links. Tropocollagen molecules are formed into microfibrils, which are twisted into collagen fibrils.

Major collagen types include:

- *type I*—the main structural protein
- *type III*—blood vessels, skin
- *type IV*—an essential component of the BMZ
- *type VII*—anchoring fibrils in the upper dermis
- *type XVII*—hemidesmosomes.

Clinical correlate:
- Mutations in structural collagens lead to Ehlers–Danlos syndrome (Ch. 19.1) with joint hypermotility and skin extensibility, and also blood vessel instability, if type III collagen is affected.
- Mutations in Type VII collagen are responsible for dystrophic epidermolysis bullosa (Ch. 16.1).
- Type XVII collagen is abnormal in one form of junctional epidermolysis bullosa and a target for antibodies in bullous pemphigoid and pemphigoid gestationis.
- Vitamin C is essential for collagen cross-linking.

Elastic fibers. Elastic fibers account for only 2%–3% of the dry weight of skin, but are predominant in the aorta and ligamentum nuchae. They impart a resilience and stretchability to the skin. Smooth muscle cells can also synthesize elastin.

Elastic fibers consist of:

- *elastin*—a central amorphous mass composed of cross-linked tropoelastin monomers; the main linkage enzyme is lysyl oxidase, which is copper dependent. Desmosine and isodesmosine form bridges between the monomers
- *microfibrils*—consist of a wide variety of 10–12-nm proteins surrounding an elastin core; the best known are fibrillin 1 and 2
- *microfibrillin-associated glycoprotein* (MAGP)—essential to tropoelastin linkages.

The papillary dermis has a fine network of microfibrils (oxytalan fibrils) sometimes with small amounts of elastin (elaunin), while in the reticular dermis, complete elastic fibers are present.

Clinical correlate:
- Abnormalities in elastin lead to saggy skin (cutis laxa) (Ch. 19.1).
- Disorders in copper metabolism for example Menkes syndrome (Ch. 38.1) also have elastic fiber defects.
- Marfan syndrome (aortic dilation, arachnodactyly, subluxed lens) is the best known fibrillin defect.
- Ultraviolet (UV) light induces changes in elastic fibers, which play a major role in cutaneous aging.

Extrafibrillary matrix. The main constituents are proteoglycans, composed of core proteins and glycosaminoglycans (GAGs), which are also known as mucopolysaccharides because of their slimy, tenacious nature. The main GAGs in the skin are hyaluronic acid, heparin sulfate, chondroitin sulfate and keratin sulfate. All except hyaluronic acid are arranged along linear core proteins forming proteoglycans. Hyaluronic acid is the major component and binds covalently. Proteoglycans are active in signal transduction and are by no means an inert substance, as suggested by the old name *ground substance*.

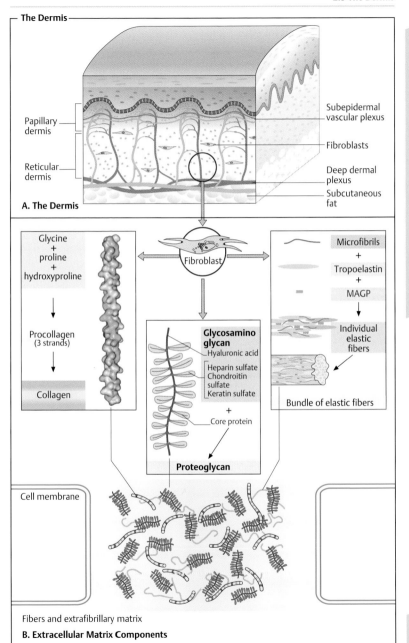

The Dermis

Papillary dermis

Reticular dermis

Subepidermal vascular plexus

Fibroblasts

Deep dermal plexus

Subcutaneous fat

A. The Dermis

Glycine
+
proline
+
hydroxyproline

Procollagen
(3 strands)

Collagen

Fibroblast

Microfibrils
+
Tropoelastin
+
MAGP

Individual elastic fibers

Bundle of elastic fibers

Glycosamino glycan
Hyaluronic acid
Heparin sulfate
Chondroitin sulfate
Keratin sulfate
+
Core protein

Proteoglycan

Cell membrane

Fibers and extrafibrillary matrix

B. Extracellular Matrix Components

2 Embryology and Anatomy

9

A. Hair Development and Structure

Human hair plays a major role in forming one's image and also has biological functions. Scalp hairs provide sun protection, as skin cancers are more common on bald scalps. The density varies from 615/cm² at age 25 to 425/cm² after 70 years of age. The eyelashes, eyebrows, and hairs in the anterior nares help to protect these orifices from airborne particles.

The first hair follicles appear in the 10th week of embryonic life, resulting from an interaction between the epithelial hair germ and the underlying mesenchymal cells. Further follicular epithelial regions differentiate into the sebaceous glands, apocrine glands, and the bulge or regenerating region of the hair follicle. The hair papilla determines the size of the hair bulb and thus the hair thickness. The papillae contain a vascular coil and nerves. The hair bulb envelops the hair matrix and hair matrix cells, which differentiate into the cells of the hair shaft and inner root sheath. The activity of the melanocytes within the matrix determines the hair color. The outer root sheath surrounds the hair follicle.

The infundibulum starts where the sebaceous duct enters the follicle. Just below this, the outer root sheath thickens at the site of attachment of the arrector pili muscle into the bulge region, which contains epithelial stem cells. It also blends with the epidermis at the distal end of the follicle (isthmus).

The hair shaft consists of a medulla, cortex, and cuticle. The cortex is the main component of hair; it contains cornified hair matrix cells analogous to the striatum corneum but formed into a cylindrical mass. The outer layer of the hair shaft is the cuticle, whose overlapping shingle-like cells interdigitate with the cuticle of the inner root sheath, anchoring the hair in the follicle.

B. The Hair Cycle

Hair growth occurs in repetitive cycles. The 3–6-year period with stable hair growth and maximal follicular size, with high mitotic activity in the matrix, is known as the *anagen phase*. Next, the hair follicle enters a short 2-week transitory period known as the *catagen phase*, with apoptosis of the hair bulb region and regression to about one-third of its previous length as the hair papilla condenses and moves upward. At the now-elevated base of the hair shaft, the hypopigmented keratinized club hair forms. After 2–4 months of the *telogen* or resting phase, the club hair is pushed aside by the next anagen hair developing from the interaction between the bulge region and the papilla, and then shed. Normally more than 80% of hairs are anagen and less than 20% telogen, with only a fraction of a percent catagen.

C. Types of Hair

Lanugo hairs are fetal hairs and only seen in premature infants. They are long, thin, nonmedullated, soft, and usually without pigment.

> **Clinical correlate:** Numerous lanugo hairs in adults may be a sign of an underlying carcinoma.

Vellus hairs are the normal body hairs, usually <2 cm, thin, nonmedullated and colorless. *Terminal hairs* are long, thick, pigmented hairs with a medulla. They are present at birth on the scalp, as well as forming eyelashes and eyebrows. *Sexual hairs* are specialized terminal hairs which appear during puberty as androgens influence vellus hairs in certain body areas, such as the axilla, genitalia, and beard area of men.

I Basic Principles

The Hair, Nails, and Subcutaneous Fat

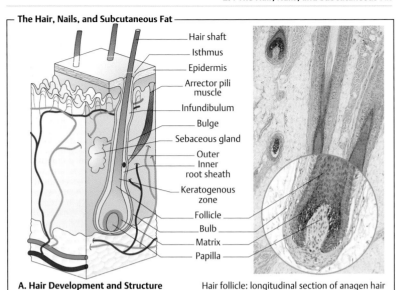

- Hair shaft
- Isthmus
- Epidermis
- Arrector pili muscle
- Infundibulum
- Bulge
- Sebaceous gland
- Outer
- Inner root sheath
- Keratogenous zone
- Follicle
- Bulb
- Matrix
- Papilla

A. Hair Development and Structure

Hair follicle: longitudinal section of anagen hair

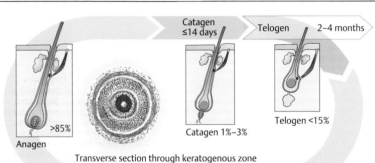

Catagen ≤14 days

Telogen 2–4 months

Anagen >85%

Catagen 1%–3%

Telogen <15%

Transverse section through keratogenous zone

Anagen 2–6 years

B. The Hair Cycle

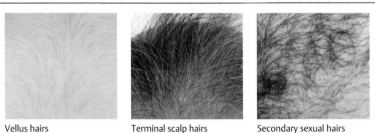

Vellus hairs

Terminal scalp hairs

Secondary sexual hairs

C. Types of Hair

2 Embryology and Anatomy

11

D. Nail Development and Structure

The nail unit develops between the 9th and 20th embryonal week as pocketlike invagination of the epidermis at the distal end of the digits. It consists of the nail matrix, nail plate, nail bed and periungual skin or paronychium. The nail stabilizes and projects the fingers and toes, serves as an important tool, and has significant cosmetic effects. In many animals and some humans it is an effective weapon.

The *nail matrix* is the growth zone of the nail; it extends for 3–6 mm beneath the proximal nail fold. The proximal part of the nail fold forms the superficial third of the nail plate, while the more distal part forms the rest of the plate. The nail plate thus consists of a hard outer layer of flat, closely packed, corneocytes and a thicker, more elastic, less cellular deeper layer.

The nail plate is sealed proximally by the *cuticle (eponychium)* and laterally by the nail folds. At its distal end, the 0.5–1.0 mm yellow–brown *onychodermal band* marks the site where the nail plate loses its adherence to the nail bed. Distal to this attachment, the free nail appears white because of the underlying air, and covers the *hyponychium*, a thin stripe of skin without dermatoglyphics or adnexal structures. The lunula is a half-moon-shaped white zone covering the distal matrix at the base of the thumbnails and sometimes other nails.

The size and thickness of the nails is highly variable. Most nails are more convex in the transverse view than along their long axis. The shape of the distal phalanx influences that of the overlying nail. Nails grow slowly; a finger nail requires 4–6 months to replace itself, while a toenail needs 12–18 months. Nails grow faster at night than during the day, in summer than in winter, in young individuals than in the elderly, and in men than women. Skin diseases may be associated with more rapid nail growth (psoriasis) or slowed nail growth (atopic dermatitis). Both longitudinal ridges and a shingle-like surface pattern are more common in the nails of older adults.

The capillaries are visible through the transparent nail plate and cuticle. Using capillary microscopy, vessel changes can be visualized in the nail fold, helping diagnose collagen–vascular diseases such as systemic sclerosis and dermatomyositis. Anemia (pale), methemoglobulinemia (blue–gray) and pigmented disorders (melanin deposits, melanocytic nevus, or melanoma) can be seen through the nail, as can subungual tumors such as glomus tumors. About 10%–20% of visible light, 5%–10% of UVA and 1%–3% of UVB pass through a normal nail plate and reach the nail bed.

Clinical correlate: Phototoxic drug reactions may result in onycholysis (loosening of the nail), as the light can pass through the nail and cause a toxic reaction.

E. Subcutaneous Fat

The subcutaneous fat or subcutis lies between the dermis and the muscle fascia, tendons, or ligaments. The fat layer varies greatly in thickness, because of regional differences, with normal padding on the buttocks to make sitting comfortable but almost no fat on the dorsal aspects of the digits for flexibility. In addition, age and sex, as well as genetic, endocrine, and metabolic factors influence of the amount of subcutaneous fat.

Clinical correlate: Measuring the thickness of skin folds at predetermined sites is the traditional way of assessing the amount of body fat.

The subcutis contains numerous connective-tissue septae which carry lymphatics, blood vessels, and nerves. The network of septae keeps the lobules of fat in place and provides support. The smallest functional unit is the microlobule which is nourished by an arteriole. *Adipocytes* are metabolically active, and a variety of noxious stimuli (toxins, metabolic by-products, enzymes, or microbes) can reach them via the circulation, initiating an inflammatory response.

The vast majority of fat is known as white fat. It serves as a site for energy storage, as well as providing thermal insulation and padding. Newborns have about 5% brown fat, which is more rapidly metabolized producing heat directly. Brown fat is usually located on the back and along large vessels. Adults have only rudimentary deposits. Brown fat has smaller lipid droplets and is rich in mitochondria. The rapid production of heat is necessary for infants, who cannot shiver as adults do routinely when exposed to cold.

Clinical correlate: A rare adult tumor is a *hibernoma*, tumor of brown fat. It was given its unusual name because hibernating animals also store brown fat.

— The Hair, Nails, and Subcutaneous Fat —

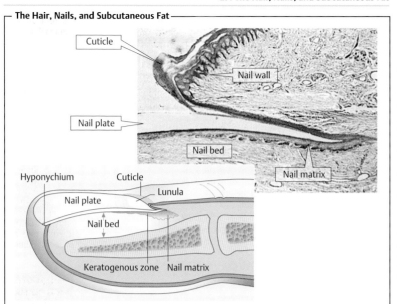

D. Nail Development and Structure

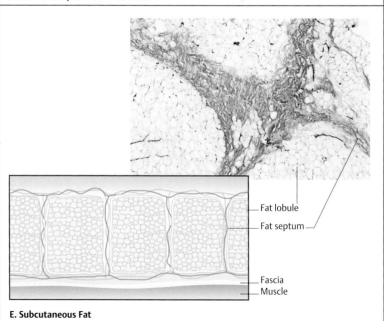

E. Subcutaneous Fat

A. Keratinization

The epidermis is a self-renewing structure.

The transition from the cuboidal cells of the basal layer to the scales of the stratum corneum is a complex one. The change from a basal layer keratinocyte to a corneocyte takes 14 days and then the loss of this cell remnant as scale occurs after another 14 days. The stratum corneum is the thinnest part of the epidermis but is crucial for the epidermal barrier function.

The main component of the epidermis is keratin—one of the intermediate filaments, a family of 8–11-nm structural proteins. Two cytokeratins—one basic and one acidic—combine to form a keratin filament (tonofilament), a hallmark of epithelial cells. Different pairs of keratin are transcribed and expressed at different levels of the epidermis:
- keratins 5 and 14 in the basal layer
- keratins 1 and 10 in the spinous layer
- keratins 4 and 13 in the mucosa
- keratins 6a, 6b, 16, and 17 in the hair and nails
- keratins 31–40 and 81–86 in hair.

Mutations in keratins 5 and 14 lead not only to separation in the basal layer but also to pigmentary abnormalities (epidermolysis bullosa simplex with mottled pigmentation), showing that keratins are not only structural proteins but are also active in the formation and transfer of melanosomes. Keratin 17 stimulates hair growth by inhibiting apoptosis. Nail keratins are affected in pachyonychia congenita, a genetic disorder affecting the oral mucosa and nails.

Other participants in keratinization include:
- *Odland bodies* (keratinosomes), which discharge epidermal lipids into the intercellular spaces of the stratum corneum
- profilaggrin, which is synthesized by keratinocytes in the stratum spinosum; it is the precursor of *filaggrin*, which binds together with keratin to form *keratohyalin granules*

Clinical correlate: Mutations in filaggrin are important in both atopic dermatitis and ichthyosis vulgaris.

- involucrin, which is the main component of the *cornified envelope*; it is complexly linked by a transglutaminase.

B. Structural Correlates of the Epidermis

The histological picture of the stratum corneum can be compared to a brick wall. The keratinized cells are the bricks, while the mortar is provided by epidermal lipids and adhesion molecules. The lipids stabilize the epidermis and help seal the barrier but also allow the passage of substances through the epidermis in both directions. In contrast to a brick wall, however, both the keratinocytes and the intercellular space undergo metamorphosis as they are dynamic and move outward.

Clinical correlate: Ichthyosis refers to a variety of inherited scaling disorders of the skin. Some are caused by structural mutations in keratin genes; others by mutations in enzymes that are important for lipid metabolism, underscoring the fundamental importance of the steadily changing intercellular environment. Defects in transglutaminase causing an abnormal cornified envelope are also a factor.

C. Patterns of Keratinization

There are many ways in which the epidermal differentiation can go astray:
- *orthokeratosis*—normal stratum corneum, often with a basket-weave pattern because of loss of lipids during fixation
- *hyperkeratosis*—thickening of the stratum corneum. This is normal on the palms of the hand and soles of the feet. It is abnormal in ichthyosis with retention hyperkeratosis or delayed shedding. It is also secondary to mechanical stress in calluses or with inflammatory hyperproliferation in psoriasis
- *parakeratosis*—retention of nuclei in the stratum corneum, usually because of increased epidermal turnover, as in psoriasis
- *dyskeratosis*—individual cell keratinization producing pink condensed cells rather than sheets of keratin, typically seen in actinic keratoses and squamous cell carcinomas, as well as some genetic disorders of keratinization
- *porokeratosis*: columns of parakeratosis producing cornoid lamellae; the histological finding defines the disease porokeratosis (Ch. 20.1).

Keratin

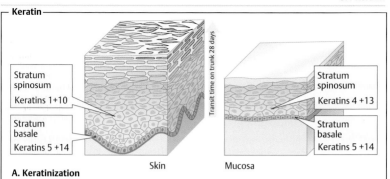

Stratum spinosum
Keratins 1+10

Stratum basale
Keratins 5 +14

Skin

Transit time on trunk 28 days

Stratum spinosum
Keratins 4 +13

Stratum basale
Keratins 5 +14

Mucosa

A. Keratinization

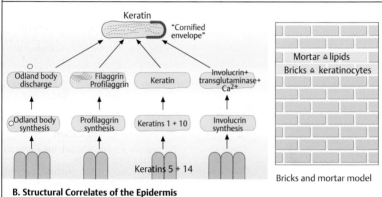

Keratin

"Cornified envelope"

Odland body discharge

Filaggrin Profilaggrin

Keratin

Involucrin+ transglutaminase+ Ca^{2+}

Odland body synthesis

Profilaggrin synthesis

Keratins 1 + 10

Involucrin synthesis

Keratins 5 + 14

Mortar ≙ lipids
Bricks ≙ keratinocytes

Bricks and mortar model

B. Structural Correlates of the Epidermis

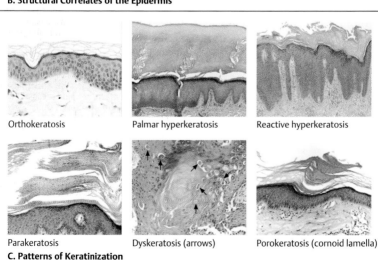

Orthokeratosis

Palmar hyperkeratosis

Reactive hyperkeratosis

Parakeratosis

Dyskeratosis (arrows)

Porokeratosis (cornoid lamella)

C. Patterns of Keratinization

3 Biochemistry

A. Melanocytes

Melanocytes are derived from the neural crest and migrate into the epidermis. On light microscopy, they are clear cells located in the basal layer. About every 10th basal layer cell is a melanocyte.

> **Clinical correlate:** Melanocytes are responsible for two common tumors—benign melanocytic nevi (moles) and melanoma.

B. Melanogenesis

Melanocytes manufacture melanin, the key pigment of the skin. The synthesis of melanin is complex starting with tyrosine; the most important enzyme is tyrosinase. An important intermediate is DOPA (a precursor of dopamine). Two major forms of melanin are made:
- eumelanin (brown–black)
- pheomelanin (red–yellow; copper).

The melanin is packaged into melanosomes in the Golgi apparatus and then transferred to keratinocytes. Melanocytes have long cell extensions (dendrites) and can provide 30–40 keratinocytes with melanin. In white individuals, a group of melanosomes is surrounded by a membrane creating a melanosome complex. In dark-skinned individuals, there are larger single melanosomes.

> **Clinical correlate:** Melanin is also important in other neural crest structures such as the retina, cochlea, and substantia nigra.

C. Defects in Melanocytes

A variety of defects lead to abnormalities of pigmentation, including:
- *albinism*—lack or reduced function of tyrosinase or other enzymes leading to defective production of melanin; often associated with visual problems
- *piebaldism*—congenital absence of melanocytes because of aberrant cell migration secondary to loss of function mutations in the tyrosine kinase (Kit) receptor; this often causes white streaks of hair (poliosis) or hypopigmented patches of skin; it may be coupled with deafness (Waardenburg syndrome)

- *transfer defects*—"ash-leaf" macules of tuberous sclerosis result from abnormal transfer of melanosomes
- *vitiligo*—an autoimmune disease with localized destruction of melanocytes.

D. Skin Color and Type

Very minor differences in melanogenesis lead to major variations in skin color. Skin color is determined by the type of melanin and by the nature of the melanosomes, not by the number of melanocytes. In black skin, the melanosomes are larger, more highly pigmented, and more slowly degraded; they primarily contain eumelanin. Brown or black hairs have eumelanin, while blond or red hairs contain more pheomelanin. Red hair also contains trichrome melanin.

Melanin provides protection against ultraviolet (UV) irradiation (Ch. 38.2). It functions as a free-radical scavenger and also has somewhat of an umbrella effect, mechanically shielding against the sun's rays. Fitzpatrick identified four different *skin types*, based on tendency to burn or tan. Type I individuals burn easily, never tan, and are at increased risk for both melanoma and other skin cancers, as shown dramatically by the Celtic population of Australia exposed to far more sun than their ancestors in the UK and Ireland.

E. Approach to Pigmented Lesions

A series of simple questions can guide one toward a better understanding of the problem, a more precise diagnosis, and even direct therapy.
- *hyperpigmented lesions*—increased melanin or increased melanocytes? Pigment in the epidermis or dermis?
- *hypopigmented lesions*—absent melanocytes or defects in melanin production and transfer?

> **Clinical correlate:** The melanocytes in the basal layer are easily damaged by inflammation. They may release melanin into the dermis, where it is taken up by macrophages (*postinflammatory hyperpigmentation*). This process is especially prominent in black skin, where, paradoxically, there may also be postinflammatory hypopigmentation.

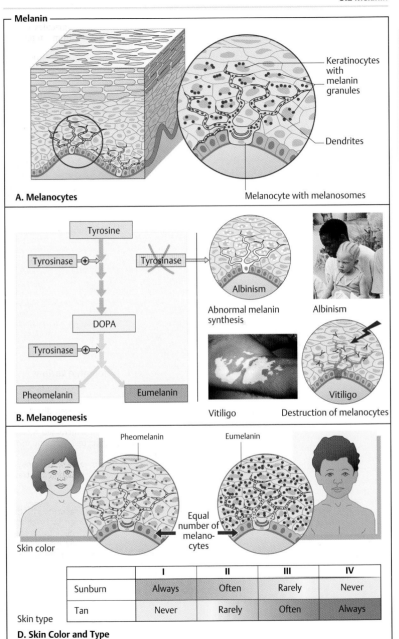

A. Melanocytes

Keratinocytes with melanin granules

Dendrites

Melanocyte with melanosomes

B. Melanogenesis

Tyrosine

Tyrosinase ⊕→

Tyrosinase

DOPA

Tyrosinase ⊕→

Pheomelanin

Eumelanin

Albinism

Abnormal melanin synthesis

Albinism

Vitiligo

Vitiligo

Destruction of melanocytes

D. Skin Color and Type

Pheomelanin

Eumelanin

Equal number of melanocytes

Skin color

	I	II	III	IV
Sunburn	Always	Often	Rarely	Never
Tan	Never	Rarely	Often	Always

Skin type

3 Biochemistry

A. Cutaneous Innervation

The skin is the largest sensory organ; it is served by a variety of nerves, including somatic sensory nerves and autonomic sympathetic fibers. The autonomic nerves help control vessel and sweat gland function. The sensory nerves transmit information about the periphery (skin) to the central nervous system (CNS).

Dermatomes. Sensory nerves follow a dermatomal pattern, best seen in zoster (Ch. 32.2). Sympathetic fibers run in a similar fashion.

Nerve fibers. *C fibers* are slow polymodal unmyelinated fibers that can sense and transmit pain, itch, touch, heat, cold, and movement.

A fibers are myelinated and have a higher conduction velocity. They interact with a variety of receptors:

- *free nerve endings* are widespread, found extending into the epidermis and around hair follicles. Known as *nocireceptors*, they sense pain, motion, touch, heat, and cold, usually by a complex pattern of reporting rather than single nerves for single messages. Try moving just a single hair to see how sensitive this system is to touch
- *Meissnerian corpuscles*—superficial mechanoreceptors, most common on the digits
- *Pacinian corpuscles*—deep mechanoreceptors with a "cut onion" pattern
- *hair disks*—complexes of Merkel cells and free nerve endings, most common on the face; they are not seen on ordinary histology but stain with cytokeratin 20.

B. The Neuronal Basis of Pruritus

Pruritus or itch is a sensory phenomenon unique to the skin. Pruritus is a poorly localized, unpleasant sensation which elicits the desire to scratch.

Neuronal basis. Many mediators trigger nocireceptors, leading to central stimulation and then the mechanical itch response. Histamine is the best known mediator for transmitting pruritus after mast cell degranulation. Interleukin (IL)-31 from T cells also mediates a relatively specific pruritus. Vanillin receptors also play a role; they transmit the burning caused by capsaicin, a substance isolated from chili peppers. Overstimulation with capsaicin can block the transmission of pruritus.

Pruritus is a distinct phenomenon, not low-level pain. The impulses are transmitted by slow C fibers to the posterior horn of the spinal cord and via two additional neurons through the hypothalamus to the sensorimotor cortex.

Note: Pruritus requires the presence of an intact epidermis and does not trigger spinal reflexes. A second-degree burn is painful but never itches, as this layer of the skin is destroyed.

Cofactors. Pruritus is not absolute but is frequently modified. Cold can suppress pruritus, while warmth tends to exacerbate it. Similarly, pain often suppresses pruritus, while the use of opiates then leads to renewed itching. *Alloknesis* is the property of inflamed or damaged skin to respond to touch or pressure with an itch response.

Causes. Many skin diseases are pruritic. When lesions are present, as with lichen planus, arthropod assault, or urticaria (most common causes), the diagnosis is easy. Pruritus may also appear without any skin findings (pruritus sine materia), either as a result of an underlying disease or without explanation. Causes include:

- hepatic disease, especially primary biliary cirrhosis
- end-stage renal disease
- diabetes mellitus
- malignancies, especially Hodgkin lymphoma and polycythemia vera.

C. Sympathetic Nerves

Sympathetic nerves transfer a variety of stimuli:

- *cholinergic fibers* innervate the arteriovenous anastomoses and sweat glands
- *adrenergic fibers* control the vessels and erector pili muscles.

Note: Patients with atopic dermatitis have an altered sympathetic response with facial pallor and blanching rather than erythema when scratched; this is known as white dermatographism (Ch. 14.4).

Cutaneous Sensation

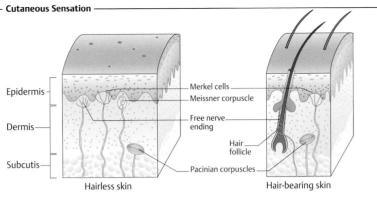

Epidermis
Dermis
Subcutis

Merkel cells
Meissner corpuscle
Free nerve ending
Hair follicle
Pacinian corpuscles

Hairless skin

Hair-bearing skin

A. Cutaneous Innervation

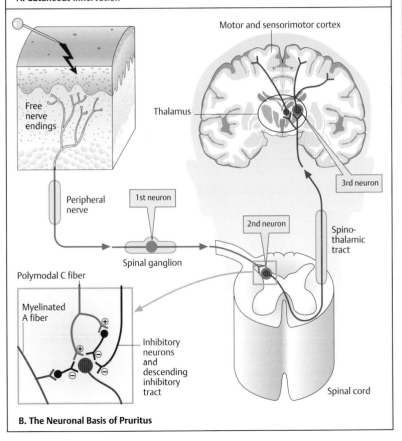

Motor and sensorimotor cortex

Thalamus

3rd neuron

Free nerve endings

Peripheral nerve

1st neuron

2nd neuron

Spino-thalamic tract

Spinal ganglion

Polymodal C fiber

Myelinated A fiber

Inhibitory neurons and descending inhibitory tract

Spinal cord

B. The Neuronal Basis of Pruritus

A. Mechanical Barriers

The purpose of the immune system is to protect the body against potentially dangerous materials such as microbes or toxins. This role is accomplished in a cascade of events. The first steps are mechanical and biologic barriers, which prevent entry of the noxious agents into the body. In nontoxic concentrations, such substances tend to induce tolerance. When harmful amounts of pathogens or toxins overcome these barriers and directly attack various cells or organs, the immune system is activated.

B. Innate Immunity

Some immune cells can phagocytose and destroy damaged cells or microorganisms. To accomplish this, they must coordinate with the somatic cells. Cell damage appears to release alarm signals, which trigger the immune response and later also enhance the effector functions of the defense. All cells that can be attacked by exogenous agents contribute to the innate response. In the skin it is keratinocytes; in the mucosa, epithelial cells; and in the liver, hepatocytes; in addition, fibroblasts and glial cells can also raise an alarm. The cells react to the stress signals by releasing a group of alarm cytokines, mainly interleukin (IL)-1. Already in the outmost cellular barrier, the keratinocytes, inflammation starts with the activation of the inflammasome. This activation leads to the transcription, processing and cleavage of IL-1 α and β. Both IL-1 forms are then the driving forces to produce and release other interleukins (IL-6, IL-18), tumor necrosis factor (TNF) and chemokines (Ch. 5.7), which attract and activate antigen-presenting cells (APCs) (Ch. 5.3). Thus, the specific or adaptive immune response is set into motion.

C. Specific Immunity

Activated APCs carrying foreign antigen migrate to the regional lymph nodes, where they use chemokines to attract naive CD4$^+$ helper T cells and CD8$^+$ cytotoxic T cells (Ch. 5.4, 5.5), presenting their antigens or haptens to these cells. The naive T cells that recognize the antigens on the basis of their receptor structure are then activated to blast forms.

An important function of activated T cells is clonal proliferation to produce a sufficient number of specific T cells to efficiently control the harmful toxin or invading microbe. With the help of the cytokine IL-2, these activated T cells can increase by a factor of 10 000 within a few days (Ch. 5.4). In the lymph nodes, activated T cells interact with B cells and signal them to start producing immunoglobulin (Ch. 5.6).

The T cells then leave the lymph nodes and return via the bloodstream to the site of initial injury, guided by a variety of cell messengers. As part of the innate response, an inflammatory reaction is initiated, which leads to the production of adhesion molecules. These enable the activated T cells to attach to vessel walls, migrate through the walls, and move into the inflamed tissue. There they are further stimulated by antigen-carrying macrophages and monocytes, to produce a group of proinflammatory mediators.

Interferon-γ (IFN-γ) plays a central role, as it induces macrophages to produce important inflammatory mediators, cranking up the entire response process by stimulating the tissue cells to produce vast amounts of free oxygen radicals, TNF, and all the other factors with which they initially signaled alarm. In contrast to the initiation phase, both the number and quantity of cytokines are now much greater (Ch. 5.7).

The initially nonspecific defense mechanisms are so effectively enhanced by the appearance of immune cells specifically directed against the triggering antigen or hapten, that the process of cleaning up can begin, with the killing and phagocytosis of the invading substances. This is dominated by either lymphocytes and macrophages or neutrophils.

— Interaction between Innate and Specific Immunity —

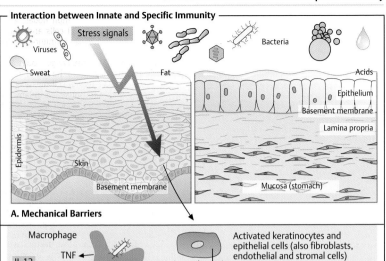

Stress signals

Viruses

Bacteria

Sweat

Fat

Acids

Epithelium
Basement membrane
Lamina propria

Epidermis

Skin

Basement membrane

Mucosa (stomach)

A. Mechanical Barriers

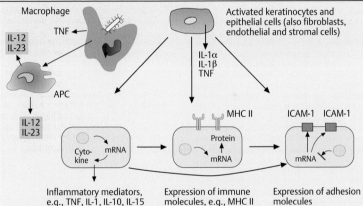

Macrophage

TNF

IL-12
IL-23

APC

IL-12
IL-23

Activated keratinocytes and
epithelial cells (also fibroblasts,
endothelial and stromal cells)

IL-1α
IL-1β
TNF

MHC II

ICAM-1   ICAM-1

Cyto-kine ↔ mRNA

Protein
mRNA

mRNA

Inflammatory mediators,
e.g., TNF, IL-1, IL-10, IL-15

Expression of immune
molecules, e.g., MHC II

Expression of adhesion
molecules

B. Innate Immunity

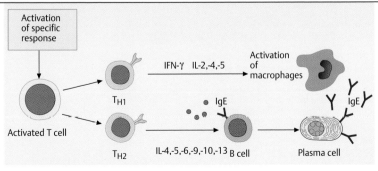

Activation
of specific
response

Activated T cell

T_H1

IFN-γ   IL-2,-4,-5

Activation
of
macrophages

T_H2

IgE

IL-4,-5,-6,-9,-10,-13   B cell

Plasma cell

IgE

C. Specific Immunity

5 Immunology

21

A. Organs of the Immune System

In contrast to most other organs, the specialized immune cells do not form solid groups of cells but are instead mobile. This does not mean uncoordinated wandering; immune cells travel between specific functional areas such as the bone marrow (primary lymphatic organ), lymph nodes, and spleen (secondary lymphatic organs); blood and lymph; or in solid organs such as the skin, central nervous system (CNS), and liver, There is usually a pattern of movement, as in the skin where cells move to the lymph nodes, blood, and then back to the skin. This circuit is also termed skin-associated lymphoid tissue (SALT).

The bone marrow. The source of all specialized immune cells is the bone marrow and, during embryonal life, the liver. Here, multipotential precursor cells develop into the various cells of the hematopoietic system; once they have acquired a certain degree of maturity, they then move into the peripheral blood or other tissues. A group of cells, including monocytes, macrophages, and B cells, leave the bone marrow very early and assume their peripheral function as naive, not-yet-activated cells. Other cells, in contrast, especially T cells, move as immature precursor cells from the bone marrow to the thymus, where they then differentiate into mature cells.

The thymus. The thymus is in the anterior mediastinum behind the superior part of the sternum. It is a loose tissue whose cortex contains dense accumulations of lymphocytes. The thymus reaches its maximum size of 40 g at around 10 years of age and then begins to regress. It is the main organ in which precursor T cells develop into immunocompetent cells. In the thymus, they mature, expressing in successive steps first the α-, and then the β-chains of the wide spectrum of T-cell receptors (TCRs), and finally CD4 und CD8 molecules.

A strict selection process occurs next, in which only those T cells that can really help the body are chosen. Via negative selection, about 90% of T cells are eliminated, primarily those with too high an affinity for self-antigens, which could potentially damage the host tissues. All the T cells whose TCR receptors cannot be stimulated by the APCs of the host, and are thus biologically useless, die through a process of neglect (lack of positive signals). Through these steps, the only mature cells to reach the peripheral blood are those that are potentially useful, around 10^9 T cells with different TCR structures.

The spleen and lymph nodes. These organs are the reservoir for B and T cells, as well as the macrophage/monocyte series and dendritic cells (DCs—"professional" APCs) (Ch. 5.3). They are the most important relay stations for the initiation and coordination of the immune response, as well as the reservoir for immune memory. Via different functional pathways, APCs stimulate T cells to differentiate and proliferate. The migratory capacity of the T cells is changed so that they can move via the blood to specific peripheral organs. Simultaneously T–B-cell interactions occur in the lymph organs, which initiate the production of immunoglobulins (Igs) by B cells, and then the isotype switch from IgM to IgA, IgD, IgE or IgG (Ch. 5.6).

BALT, GALT, MALT, and SALT. These abbreviations stand for *b*ronchus-, *g*ut-, *m*ucosa-, or *s*kin-*a*ssociated *l*ymphoid *t*issue, and describe pathways in which lymphocytes move between solid organs and secondary lymphatic organs. While the lymphocytes are preferentially assigned to a pathway, they can be directed to other sites depending on the antigens to which they are exposed.

Organs of the Immune System

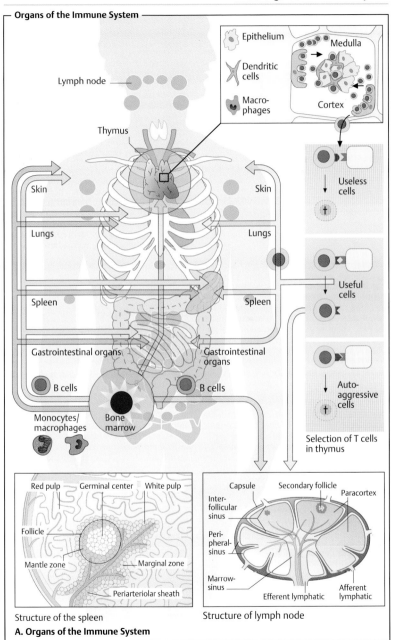

Lymph node

Epithelium

Dendritic cells

Macro-phages

Medulla

Cortex

Thymus

Skin

Skin

Lungs

Lungs

Useless cells

Spleen

Spleen

Useful cells

Gastrointestinal organs

Gastrointestinal organs

Auto-aggressive cells

B cells

B cells

Monocytes/ macrophages

Bone marrow

Selection of T cells in thymus

Red pulp   Germinal center   White pulp

Follicle

Mantle zone

Marginal zone

Periarteriolar sheath

Structure of the spleen

Capsule   Secondary follicle   Paracortex

Inter-follicular sinus

Peri-pheral-sinus

Marrow-sinus

Efferent lymphatic   Afferent lymphatic

Structure of lymph node

A. Organs of the Immune System

A. Development of Immune Cells

The cells of the immune response arise in the bone marrow. They include neutrophilic, eosinophilic, and basophilic granulocytes, mast cells, T cells, B cells, and natural killer (NK) cells, as well as the monocyte/macrophage series. These interact with one another and also control the behavior of connective-tissue cells and somatic cells.

Via surface molecules such as adhesion factors, soluble mediators, and receptors (Ch.5.7), they exchange information and influence numerous functions such as the cell cycle, activation, and migration. By means of cytokines and chemokines, the immune cells can direct the somatic cells to enhance an inflammatory reaction. The T and B cells are responsible for the specific immune response (Ch.5.4–5.6).

B. Antigen-presenting Cells

To initiate a specific immune response, APCs must recognize a potential antigen (usually a glycoprotein, less often a lipid), then phagocytose it and at the same time receive a signal identifying this antigen as potentially dangerous. Antigens are first taken up (engulfed) and then digested and modified (processed) inside the APC. Then they are presented on the surface of the APC by either the MHC Class I or Class II molecules. Recognition sequences in the processed antigen are presented to T cells on the surface of the APC by molecules of the major histocompatibility complex (MHC) (also known as human leukocyte antigen or HLA).

APCs are usually specialized cells of the monocyte/macrophage series, which form the most important bridge to specific immunity. Dendritic cells (DCs) are "professional" APCs, highly specialized macrophages. Immature DC are phagocytic cells. When stimulated they become less successful phagocytes but skilled at presenting antigen to T cells and then stimulating them. When stimulated by innate signals in the peripheral organs, laden with antigen, they migrate into the T-cell zones of lymph nodes to stimulate naive T cells there (Ch.5.4).

In the skin, Langerhans cells (LCs) in the epidermis, and dermal DCs in the dermis, are most successful at antigen presentation. Weaker APCs are macrophages and B cells.

C. Granulocytes and Mast Cells

Granulocytes. These are primarily effector cells, which effectively phagocytose pathogenic microbes and necrotic cells. Thus they are an essential component of the initial inflammatory reaction. Via cytokines and chemokines, they also help to modulate the immune response. Neutrophils are primarily responsible for cleaning up after bacterial and fungal infections as well as mechanical injuries (wound, foreign body); in contrast, basophils and eosinophils are more important in extracellular parasitic infections and allergies.

Clinical correlate: TNF-antagonists inhibit neutrophil migration into tissue. This causes susceptibility to bacterial infections.

Mast cells. This is a group of variably differentiated, often tissue-specific, immune cells, which are rich in inflammatory mediators, such as enzymes, cytokines, chemokines, proteoglycans, prostaglandins, and leukotrienes. They are capable of storing or rapidly synthesizing these mediators, which they can then quickly release if triggered. Thus they are important in both the induction and effector phases of the immune response, especially in immediate-type allergies.

D. Natural Killer Cells

Natural killer (NK) cells are a type of lymphocyte essential to nonspecific or innate response, in contrast to the role of T and B cells in specific immunity. They recognize and lyse cells on whose surface the expression of native HLA-A and HLA-B (MHC class I receptors) is clearly suppressed. They do not develop a memory response, in the sense of reacting more effectively or aggressively upon re-exposure. NK cells are primarily responsible for the elimination of virally infected cells and tumor cells, as these cells avoid recognition by cytotoxic T cells (Ch.5.4) by suppression of MHC-receptor expression.

NK cells should not be confused with natural killer T cells, an uncommon and heterogeneous group of cells sharing properties of T cells and NK cells. Most of these cells recognize CD1d, an antigen-presenting molecule that presents lipids and glycolipids to the T-cell receptor of NK T cells.

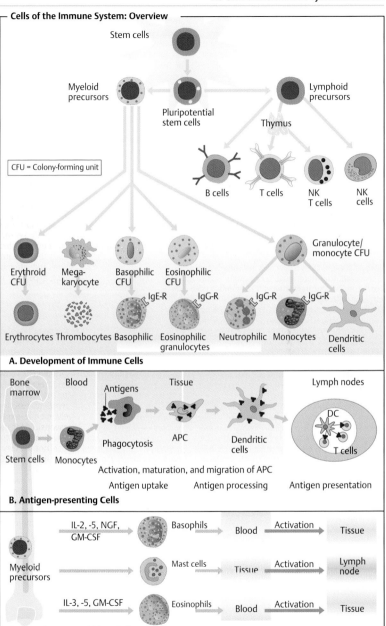

Cells of the Immune System: Overview

Stem cells

Myeloid precursors

Pluripotential stem cells

Lymphoid precursors

Thymus

CFU = Colony-forming unit

B cells   T cells   NK T cells   NK cells

Erythroid CFU   Mega-karyocyte   Basophilic CFU   Eosinophilic CFU   Granulocyte/ monocyte CFU

IgE-R   IgG-R   IgG-R   IgG-R

Erythrocytes   Thrombocytes   Basophilic   Eosinophilic granulocytes   Neutrophilic   Monocytes   Dendritic cells

A. Development of Immune Cells

Bone marrow   Blood   Antigens   Tissue   Lymph nodes

DC

Phagocytosis   APC   Dendritic cells   T cells

Stem cells   Monocytes

Activation, maturation, and migration of APC

Antigen uptake   Antigen processing   Antigen presentation

B. Antigen-presenting Cells

IL-2, -5, NGF, GM-CSF   Basophils   Blood   →Activation→   Tissue

Myeloid precursors   Mast cells   Tissue   →Activation→   Lymph node

IL-3, -5, GM-CSF   Eosinophils   Blood   →Activation→   Tissue

C. Granulocytes and Mast Cells

5 Immunology

25

A. T-cell Development and Function

T cells are the binding link between the innate and specific immune responses. They are characterized by the membrane-bound T-cell receptor (TCR).

- CD4+ or helper T cells (T_H) can induce or suppress the inflammatory immune responses via cytokines (T_{H1}, T_{H2}, T_{H17} response) or via primarily contact-dependent mechanisms (T_{reg}).
- CD8+ or cytotoxic T cells (T_C) can destroy virally infected target cells.

The TCR consists of two immunoglobulin-like glycoprotein chains, an α- and a β-chain. The TCR determines the peptide specificity of the T cell, as each T cell has only one type of TCR on its surface, limiting the range of substances with which it can interact. T cells can only be activated by APCs that present, with their MHC molecule, a peptide that fits the highly specific TCR.

The CD4 and CD8 molecules are membrane *coreceptors* that determine which MHC molecules the T cells interact with. CD4+ cells (T_H) interact with MHC class II (HLA-DR and HLA-DQ) molecules, which primarily present exogenous antigens (such as allergens or haptens) to T cells. The cytotoxic CD8+ cells (T_C) interact with MHC class I (HLA-A and HLA-B) molecules; primarily endogenous antigens such as viral and tumor peptides are presented by this route. MHC class I molecules are expressed by almost all cells, while MHC class II molecules are only expressed by APCs.

The selection of those T cells that are allowed to circulate in the body, as well as the association of a TCR with a CD4 or CD8 molecule, occurs in the thymus. Thereafter, the TCR specificity of the cell cannot be changed. The average adult has around 10^{12} T cells available, with around 10^9 different TCRs, which circulate as naive T cells until they meet their specific antigen in association with an APC and are then activated. Thus the T-cell repertoire is capable of recognizing 10^9 different peptides.

B. Interaction between Antigen-presenting Cells and T Cells

The initiation of a specific immune response requires the stimulation of naive T cells by activated APCs in the lymph nodes. The T cells circulating through the lymph node screen the antigens presented by APCs. Only those with the right TCR can recognize the antigen and then be activated by the APC. Only activated APCs can stimulate naive T cells and attract them via chemokines. The T_H cells then have the task of initiating the production of immunoglobulin by B cells in the lymph nodes, and of further activating the nonspecific effector cells, such as macrophages and monocytes, in the tissue.

Along with the trimolecular recognition complex (TCR, antigen peptide, and MHC molecule of APC), adhesion and costimulatory molecules are required for T-cell activation. Adhesion molecules are essential for cell affinity; they include intracellular adhesion molecule (ICAM)-1 and lymphocyte function antigen (LFA)-1. Costimulatory molecules are then required for T-cell activation. Important representatives are CD28 and CTLA-4 on T cells, and their partners CD80 and CD86 on APCs. Since these molecules are only expressed in quantity on APCs, only APCs can effectively stimulate naive T cells.

> **Note:** CTLA-4 is an important target molecule in treating melanoma. Blocking it with the monoclonal antibody ipilimumab leads to continued activation of T cells. This broad T-cell activation makes it possible for the first time to induce long-term remissions in about 10% of patients with metastatic melanoma. As a side effect, the agent may cause autoimmune inflammatory disease.

Another important signaling group is the cytokines. For adequate activation and clonal expansion of T cells, both IL-2 and IL-15 are required. In addition, cytokines direct the differentiation of T cells. IL-12 promotes the development of naive T_C cells into cytotoxic T_{C1} cells, and naive T_H cells into proinflammatory T_{H1} cells. IL-1, IL-6, and IL-23 induce IL-17-secreting T_{H17} cells. IL-4 induces in T_H cells the T_{H2} phenotype, the alternative to T_C, T_{H1}, and T_{H17}. T_{H2} cells induce IgE production by B cells, and activate and attract eosinophils, playing an essential role in all forms of immediate allergy.

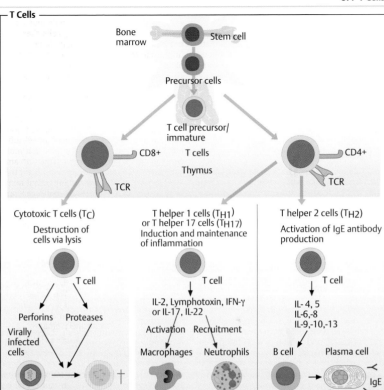

Bone marrow — Stem cell

Precursor cells

T cell precursor/immature

CD8+   T cells   CD4+

Thymus

TCR   TCR

Cytotoxic T cells (T_C)

Destruction of cells via lysis

T cell

Perforins   Proteases

Virally infected cells   †

T helper 1 cells (T_H1) or T helper 17 cells (T_H17)
Induction and maintenance of inflammation

T cell

IL-2, Lymphotoxin, IFN-γ or IL-17, IL-22

Activation   Recruitment

Macrophages   Neutrophils

T helper 2 cells (T_H2)

Activation of IgE antibody production

T cell

IL-4, 5
IL-6,-8
IL-9,-10,-13

B cell   Plasma cell

IgE

1. CD8+ T cells   2. CD4+ T cells

A. T-cell Development and Function

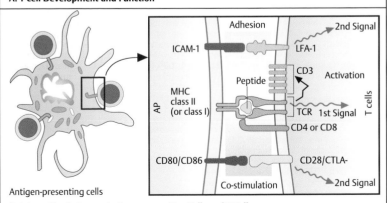

Adhesion   2nd Signal

ICAM-1   LFA-1

Peptide   CD3   Activation

MHC class II (or class I)   TCR   1st Signal   T cells

CD4 or CD8

CD80/CD86   CD28/CTLA-

Co-stimulation   2nd Signal

Antigen-presenting cells

B. Interaction between Antigen-presenting Cells and T Cells

5 Immunology

A. T_{H17} and Regulatory T Cells

Newer studies show that naive T_H cells differentiate not only into the two classic subpopulations, T_{H1} and T_{H2} cells, but also the intermediate T_{H0} stage. The two most important newly defined T_H-cell populations include the T_{H17} cells and the regulatory T cells (T_{reg}). These are two functionally well-defined groups of cells that play important roles in maintaining and limiting inflammation.

B. T_{H17} Cells

T_{H17} cells are a subpopulation of cells that are functionally similar to T_{H1} cells, but have several special features making them distinct. They do not produce IFN-γ, but instead produce interleukin 17A, the IL-17 cytokine that is generally called IL-17. In inflammatory processes, T_{H17} cells develop parallel to the T_{H1} cells, but are induced by completely different cytokines. IL-12 is crucial for the differentiation of naive CD4+ T cells into a T_{H1} phenotype. In contrast, IL-1, IL-6, and IL-23 are required for the induction of TH_{17} cells, while IL-23 (a relative of IL-12) is needed for their expansion. Another key factor is that IFN-γ suppresses the differentiation of T_{H17} cells. The importance of T_{H17} cells was recognized with the observation that both IL-17 and IL-23 play a central role in the development of autoimmune inflammatory diseases. Both cytokines are specifically activated in chronic autoimmune inflammatory diseases such as psoriasis and multiple sclerosis; according to experimental data, they play an essential role in determining the manifestations of these diseases. An especially important difference from the T_{H1} cells is that IFN-γ suppresses angiogenesis, while IL-17 stimulates it. In addition, T_{H17} cells seem to recruit neutrophils. Recent data suggest that T_{H17} cells cooperate with T_{H1} cells in delayed-type hypersensitivity reactions, such as allergic contact dermatitis, multiple sclerosis and many other inflammatory diseases.

C. Regulatory T Cells

The most important counterbalance to the T_{H1}, T_{H2} and T_{H17} cells is the CD4+ regulatory T cells, known as T_{reg}. These are activated CD4+ T cells, which express the IL-2 receptor CD25 on their surface. In addition, expression of the transcription factor FOXp3 (forkhead box p3) is essential for their development. T_{reg} cells are distinguished by their ability to paralyze the functions of T_{H1}, T_{H2}, and T_{H17} cells. While this was initially observed in vitro, it has since been confirmed in vivo. The mechanisms of both induction and action remain difficult to fully understand. In vitro, it is difficult to expand T_{reg} cells as a paralyzing T-cell population. This is in contrast to the in-vivo situation, where CD25+ T_{reg} cells routinely appear in the late phase of immune responses. In vitro, the mechanism of action appears to be dependent on cell-cell contact. In vivo, inhibition may result from contact-dependent inhibition and from soluble mediators like IL-10 and TGF-β. It remains a mystery why T_{reg} cells proliferate easily in vivo, while they are difficult to propagate in vitro.

In allergology, T_{reg} cells are of great interest as they may suppress asthma-associated phenomena in diseases that serve as models for asthma. It is generally agreed that T_{reg} cells hinder excessive damaging immune responses in vivo. Since it is not possible to grow adequate numbers of T_{reg} cells in vitro, and since there is no mechanism of targeted in-vivo induction of T_{reg} cells available, their clinical use remains speculative.

If it becomes possible to induce T_{reg} cells in therapeutically effective numbers, they may offer promise for treating various forms of inflammation, like asthma, a classic type I allergy, allergic alveolitis, and even severe forms of allergic rhinoconjunctivitis, to arrest the progression to asthma, the "atopic march." There is good evidence that hyposensitization therapy or allergen-specific immunotherapy against type I allergies involves the induction of specific Treg cells. The exact immunological modification is not fully understood and many different effects may be responsible including a shift from IgE to allergen-specific IgG.

Patients receive increasingly higher doses of substances to which they are allergic, with the aim of inducing immunologic tolerance. The allergen can be delivered subcutaneously (allergy shots) or sublingually. Hyposensitization is the only therapy that can provide long-term relief from allergic disease. There is a slight risk of adverse reactions including life-threatening anaphylaxis with subcutaneous therapy, so careful monitoring is required. Sublingual therapy seems safer, but also less efficient. Subcutaneous therapy still remains the reference therapy.

T-cell Differentiation: T$_{H17}$ and Regulatory T Cells

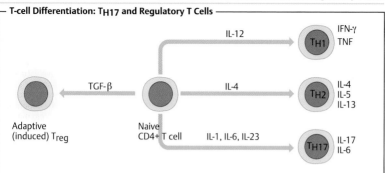

A. T$_{H17}$ and Regulatory T Cells

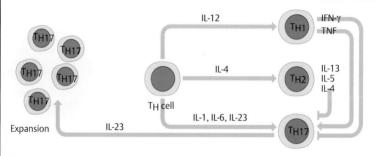

B. T$_{H17}$ Cells

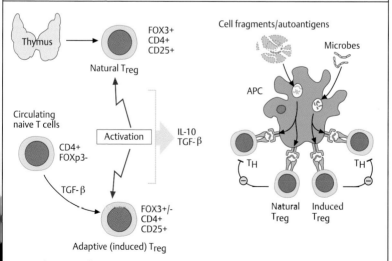

C. Regulatory T Cells

A. Development and Function of B Cells

B cells are responsible for the production of antibodies or the humoral pathway of the specific immune response. Antibodies are immunoglobulins (Igs), which consist of:
• a long ("heavy," H) chain
• a short ("light," L) chain (1).

The *H-chain* is made up of a variable region (V_H) and three or four constant regions (C_H 1–4), each of which is around 100 amino acids in length. The *L-chain* has a variable region (V_L) and a single constant region (C_L) of similar lengths. The variable regions of Igs bind to the antigen and thus determine the specificity of the antibody. The constant regions define the isotype and thus the function of the Ig. In humans there are the following isotypes:
• IgD and IgM are expressed on the surface of naive B cells. IgM is also the first Ig to be made in most immune responses, before a switch to IgG or IgA occurs
• IgG1, IgG2, IgG3, and IgG4 account for the bulk of the Igs
• IgE is crucial for immediate-type allergic reaction but makes up < 0.01 % of the total Ig quantity
• IgA is the second most common Ig and the predominant Ig on mucosal surfaces.

Antibodies recognize their antigens directly, in contrast to the TCR, which only recognizes antigens presented by MHC molecules. For each of the 10^6–10^8 receptor sequences, there is a single B cell which produces this specific Ig. In contrast to T cells, which always have a single fixed TCR, B cells can switch their isotype and the type of Ig (isotype or class switch) that they manufacture, maintaining the same antigen specificity. In addition, throughout the immune response they can slightly alter the receptor structure, producing Igs with even higher affinity for the specific antigen (affinity maturation).

Selected gene sequences in the switch region of the B-cell genome are activated to induce isotype switching. Although this process is not completely understood, T-cell cytokines regulate the encoding of a certain isotope. They activate the genes of various isotypes via membrane receptors that interact with a specific set of Janus kinases (JAK) and signal transducers and activators of transcription (STAT). For example, the production of IgG4 or IgE requires the binding of IL-4 or IL-13 on the membrane receptor, which transfers the signal via JAK1 and JAK3 to intracellular STAT6, which

then translocates to the nucleus and initiates to isotype switch to IgE in the nucleus (2).

Activation of B cells. To differentiate into Ig-secreting plasma cells, B cells must be stimulated by T_H cells, usually in the lymph-node follicles. This stimulation requires antigen, appropriate TCR, and several cofactors:
• CD4 molecule
• costimulatory CD40–CD40L interaction
• T-cell cytokines, which determine the isotype (3).

Effector function of immunoglobulins. The function of Ig is determined by the Fc portion of the constant regions. An important example is IgE, which can bind in two ways via Fc_ε:
• via the low-affinity IgE receptor ($Fc_\varepsilon RII$, CD23) to B cells, macrophages, and eosinophils
• via the high-affinity IgE receptor ($Fc_\varepsilon RI$) to mast cells and basophils.

If the correct antigen then links two bound IgE molecules, the effector cells receive activation signals. In mast cells, eosinophils, and basophils, one response to the signaling is degranulation, with the release of a variety of mediators triggering an immediate hypersensitivity reaction (Ch. 5.8).

With their ability to present peptide antigens with MHC class II molecules, and to produce cytokines for the innate immune response, B cells also function as weak APCs in the regulation of the T-cell response. They appear to suppress cell-mediated immune reactions and facilitate the differentiation of T cells into T_{H2} cells or regulatory T_{reg} cells.

B Cells

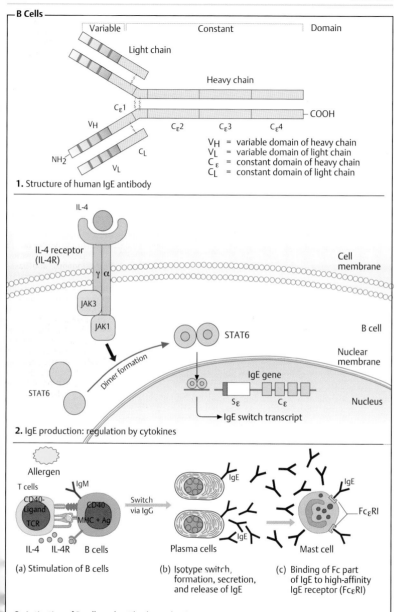

1. Structure of human IgE antibody

V_H = variable domain of heavy chain
V_L = variable domain of light chain
C_ε = constant domain of heavy chain
C_L = constant domain of light chain

2. IgE production: regulation by cytokines

(a) Stimulation of B cells

(b) Isotype switch, formation, secretion, and release of IgE

(c) Binding of Fc part of IgE to high-affinity IgE receptor ($Fc_\varepsilon RI$)

3. Activation of B cells and antibody production

A. Development and Function of B Cells

Immune cells interact via both direct cell–cell contacts and soluble molecules known as mediators. They include a broad spectrum of different molecular classes and are a crucial component of the signaling system that leads to an effective immune response.

Important mediators include:
- cytokines
- chemokines
- soluble receptors
- soluble surface molecules.

These glycoproteins represent only a portion of the many messengers; hormones, vitamins, and prostaglandins are other examples. All mediators transfer their message by binding to specific membrane-bound receptors on the surface of their target cells. Most receptors are heterodimers. After interacting with a specific mediator molecule, the two receptor molecules and the mediator form a trimolecular complex. This in turn triggers a signaling cascade, which usually reaches the nucleus of the cell, altering nucleic acid expression and protein synthesis. Factors such as binding time, affinity, and mediator or receptor concentration considerably influence the signal.

Their importance can best be shown with the example of the interferons. IFN-α and IFN-β bind to the same receptor, but transmit in part different signals, so IFN-α is used for immunostimulation and IFN-β for immunosuppression.

> **Clinical correlate:** IFN-α is used to treat both malignancies and viral diseases (melanoma, Kaposi sarcoma). Both forms of IFN seem to suppress IL-1.

A. Cytokines

The cytokines are a large family of soluble mediators which include interleukins (ILs), growth factors (GFs) and IFNs. Clinically important cytokines include the basic mediators of inflammation such as tumor necrosis factor (TNF), IL-1, and IL-6, which are rapidly released by macrophages in all forms of inflammation. Blocking IL-1 or TNF inhibits many aspects of inflammation.

A second important group is the T-cell cytokines, which confusingly can also be secreted by other cells, but regulate the course of the immune response via T cells. IL-2 is the most important T-cell growth factor. The function of T cells is determined by the cytokine pattern.

IL-2 and IFN-γ are T_{H1} cytokines that have the following effects:
- formation of TNF and free radicals in macrophages
- development of CD8+ T cells into cytotoxic cells
- driving B cells to isotype switch (Ch. 5.6) to produce complement-binding immunoglobulins.

T_{H1} cytokines and IL-17, the main cytokine of the T_{H17} cells, initiate the cell-mediated or delayed-type immune response (Ch. 5.8).

In contrast, the T_{H2} cytokines are IL-4, IL-9, and IL-13. They act differently, and:
- suppress the proinflammatory properties of macrophages
- drive B cells to isotype switch producing IgG4 and IgE
- support immediate-type allergies or type I reactions, including airway hypersecretion and increased smooth muscle tone (Ch. 5.9).

Additional important cytokines are IL-10, IL-12, and IL-23, which are made by APCs. IL-10 can block immune responses, while IL-12 and IL-23 can induce strong delayed-type hypersensitivity reactions (Ch. 5.11). IL-31 seems to induce itch.

B. Chemokines

Chemokines steer migration and homing of different immune cells, in close cooperation with IL-1 and TNF, which induce the expression of adhesion molecules by endothelial cells. This facilitates the attachment of immune cells to the vessel wall and then migration through the wall. The chemokines guide the successful migrants to the site of inflammation. The chemokine pattern determines the type of infiltrate. For example, eotaxin binds to chemokine receptor 3 (CCR3), thus attracting eosinophils and T_{H2} cells.

C. Surface Molecules

In addition to the classic soluble mediators, cell-surface molecules and receptors can have a similar function when they are separated. For example, in severe inflammation, the soluble TNF receptor is released into serum and has an anti-inflammatory effect by binding to TNF.

Important Mediators of the Immune System

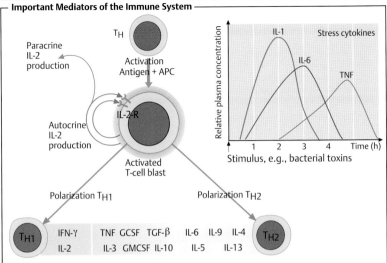

A. Cytokines

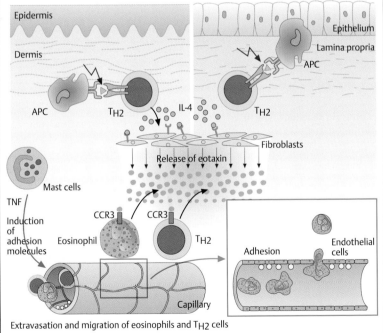

Extravasation and migration of eosinophils and T$_{H}$2 cells

B. Chemokines

5 Immunology

In the 1960s, Gell and Coombs classified adverse immune responses or intolerance reactions into four groups. Their basic classification is still useful:
- *type I*—immediate
- *type II*—cytotoxic
- *type III*—immune-complex mediated
- *type IV*—cell-mediated or delayed-type hypersensitivity.

Today we know that type I is mediated by IgE; Gell and Coombs spoke of "reagins." In addition, types II and III are far more complex and interconnected than they ever imagined.

A. Immediate Reaction (Type I)

This immune reaction is mediated by IgE antibodies. They are directed against soluble protein antigens (allergens); typical examples are pollen, animal dander, house dust mites, foods, and arthropod toxins. Allergen contact leads to linking of IgE molecules on the surface of mast cells or basophils, and triggers a cascade of events (Ch.5.9):
- release of immediate mediators such as histamine or TNF
- synthesis and release of leukotrienes and prostaglandins
- synthesis of proallergic cytokines like IL-4 or IL-5.

This cascade of shock fragments can trigger allergic rhinitis, asthma, or urticaria, and may progress to life-threatening anaphylaxis.

B. Cytotoxic Reaction (Type II)

Here, IgG antibodies react with antigens that sit on the cell surface. Targets can include medications (such as penicillin) bound to erythrocyte membranes, cell components like the Rhesus D antigen (RhD), or basement membrane components. The IgG mediates cytotoxic effects through complement and phagocytosis (Ch.5.10). IgG antibodies directed against surface receptors can also lead to false signaling. Examples of type II reactions include medication- or RhD-mediated hemolysis, heparin-induced thrombocytopenia (HIT), glomerulonephritis, and urticaria caused by anti-Fc_ε-receptor antibodies.

C. Immune-complex Reaction (Type III)

The responsible IgG antibodies are directed against soluble antigens. Examples include:
- injected serum
- fragments of pathogenic microbes, for example in bacterial endocarditis or viral hepatitis
- molds or components of hay or silage that are inhaled.

The resultant antigen–antibody complexes (immune complex) can cause local or systemic (via the circulatory system) reactions. Effector mechanisms include complement binding and activation, as well as activation of granulocytes and macrophages with vessel-wall and tissue damage (Ch.5.10). Clinical scenarios include serum sickness or localized Arthus reaction to injected products, vasculitis affecting the skin, joints, and kidneys, persistent viral hepatitis, and allergic alveolitis (farmer's lung).

D. Delayed Reaction (Type IV)

Antigen-specific T cells mediate the delayed-type hypersensitivity or cell-mediated reaction. Triggers include metal ions (such as nickel or chromium) or low-molecular-weight substances such as fragrances or preservatives, which can bind to body proteins to form complete antigens. Protein antigens from mycobacteria, bacteria, yeasts, and dermatophytes can also induce delayed reactions. The allergen contact is mediated by antigen-presenting dendritic cells and monocytes/macrophages, leading to stimulation of T cells. Released cytokines trigger the inflammation, with T cells returning to the site of antigen exposure (Ch.5.11).

Typical clinical pictures are allergic contact dermatis and dermal erythematous papules, as in a tuberculin reaction when the allergen bypasses the epidermis.

Intolerance Reactions

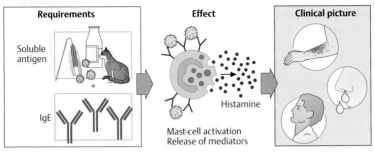

Requirements	Effect	Clinical picture

Soluble antigen

+

IgE

Histamine

Mast-cell activation
Release of mediators

A. Immediate Reaction (Type I)

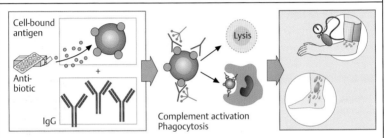

Cell-bound antigen

+

Anti-biotic

IgG

Lysis

Complement activation
Phagocytosis

B. Cytotoxic Reaction (Type II)

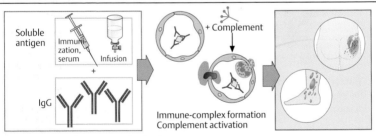

Soluble antigen

Immuni-zation, serum   Infusion

+

IgG

+ Complement

Immune-complex formation
Complement activation

C. Immune-complex Reaction (Type III)

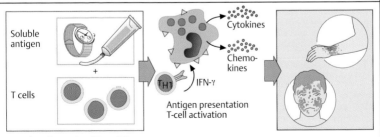

Soluble antigen

+

T cells

Cytokines

Chemo-kines

T_{H1} IFN-γ

Antigen presentation
T-cell activation

D. Delayed Reaction (Type IV)

A. IgE Production

Immediate reactions require the production of specific IgE antibodies directed against usually harmless antigens, often of animal or plant origin. Facilitated by the irritative properties or enzymatic action of the potential allergen or its carrier, these allergens penetrate the skin or mucosa in tiny amounts. There they are phagocytosed and processed by APCs, which present them via MHC class II molecules to naive T_H cells. Either an IL-12-deficient or an IL-4-rich environment induces differentiation to T_{H2} cells. Activated T_{H2} cells produce cytokines that drive an IgE isotype switch in B cells (Ch. 5.6).

The cytokines that are essential for this isotype switch are IL-4 and IL-13. The B cells require a second activation signal, for example through the interaction between CD40-ligand (CD40L) on activated T_{H2} cells and CD40 on B cells. These two signals are sufficient for the induction of IgE synthesis.

T_{H1} cells produce interferon (IFN-γ), which tends to inhibit IgE production. The coupling of IgE with membrane-bound IgE receptors on basophils and mast cells also enhances IgE production. When these cells are activated by an allergen-mediated coupling of the surface-bound IgE, they also express CD40L and secrete IL-4.

In this way, IgE sensitization is achieved. If the individual comes into contact with the allergen in the future, there is an immediate release of inflammatory mediators (histamine, prostaglandins) by the sensitized mast cells and basophils, triggering a prompt reaction.

B. Effector Mechanisms: Immediate Phase

The binding of allergen to the receptor-bound IgE on the surface of mast cells and basophils leads, via cross-linking, to three main activation phenomena:
- the rapid release of preformed substances from cytoplasmic vacuoles; the main immediate mediator is histamine
- the synthesis and subsequent release of lipid mediators like prostaglandins and leukotrienes
- the induction of cytokine production, especially IL-4 und IL-5.

Histamine, prostaglandins (especially PGD_2) and leukotrienes (primarily LTC_4) are responsible for the classic signs and symptoms of the immediate hypersensitivity reaction; these are described next.

The skin. In the skin, vasodilation and vessel leakage lead to the formation of hives or urticaria. The accompanying erythema is caused by histamine-mediated, axon-reflex-transmitted vasodilation. Deeper leakage causes angioedema.

The nose. Typical findings include nasal mucosal swelling with obstruction of the nasal airways, sneezing, and rhinorrhea.

The bronchial system. In the lungs, there is bronchial constriction, edema of the airway walls, and increased mucus production, the cardinal features of an acute asthma attack.

Other systemic findings. The most typical systemic sign of mediator release is a sharp drop in blood pressure. The maximal variant of a systemic immediate hypersensitivity reaction is anaphylactic shock.

C. Effector Mechanisms: Late Phase, Persistent Inflammation

The activation of basophils and mast cells leads to a variable combination of immediate effects and components of a prolonged allergic response. Under the influence of histamine, leukotrienes, IL-4, and, especially, TNF, vascular adhesion molecules are expressed (Ch. 5.7), which attract neutrophils and other cells. Thus, an inflammatory infiltrate can develop. Additional activation of eosinophils leads to an increase in the inflammatory response. In the IL-4-rich environment, IgE synthesis is facilitated and maintained.

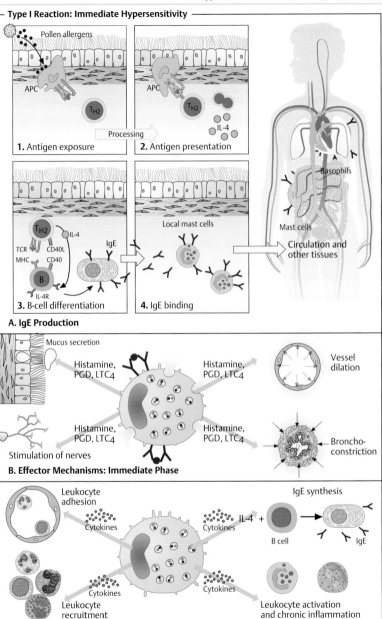

Type I Reaction: Immediate Hypersensitivity

Pollen allergens

APC

T$_{H2}$

1. Antigen exposure

Processing

APC

T$_{H2}$

IL-4

2. Antigen presentation

T$_{H2}$ — IL-4

TCR — CD40L
MHC — CD40

B

IL-4R

IgE

3. B-cell differentiation

Local mast cells

4. IgE binding

Basophils

Mast cells

Circulation and other tissues

A. IgE Production

Mucus secretion

Histamine, PGD, LTC$_4$

Histamine, PGD, LTC$_4$

Vessel dilation

Histamine, PGD, LTC$_4$

Histamine, PGD, LTC$_4$

Broncho-constriction

Stimulation of nerves

B. Effector Mechanisms: Immediate Phase

Leukocyte adhesion

Cytokines

Cytokines

Cytokines

Cytokines

IgE synthesis

IL-4 +

B cell

IgE

Leukocyte recruitment

Leukocyte activation and chronic inflammation

C. Effector Mechanisms: Late Phase, Persistent Inflammation

5 Immunology

The type II and type III reactions of Gell and Coombs are harder to put into clinical perspective, and can only be tested in vivo with difficulty. Both involve antibody-mediated processes.

A. Type II Reaction (Immunoglobulin-mediated Cytotoxicity)

The essence of a type II reaction is that an antigen bound to the surface of a cell combines with an IgG antibody. This bound antibody can then—depending on the nature of its Fc (constant) chain—activate either the complement cascade or killer cells. Either process then can proceed to lyse the antigen-laden cells. When killer cells are involved, one speaks of antibody-dependent cell-mediated cytotoxicity (ADCC).

A classic type II reaction is cytopenia—either hemolytic anemia or thrombocytopenia—caused by cell lysis. In contrast to the other three types of reactions, a type II allergy resembles an autoimmune disease. However the antibodies are not directed against genuine autoantigens, but instead against exogenous antigens which are bound to or expressed on the cell surface of hematopoietic cells. Typical allergens include medications (especially penicillin metabolites or heparins) as well as bacterial and viral antigens.

A clinically relevant thrombocytopenia typically presents as purpura on the oral mucosa and distal extremities. Tiny nonblanchable red macules (petechiae) are seen on the feet, shins, and mucosa, especially of the hard palate. Although the petechiae may become confluent, one can still usually identify tiny punctate areas.

B. Type III Reaction (Immune-complex Reaction)

Type III reactions feature disease-inducing deposition of antigen–antibody complexes (immune complexes) along the basal membrane of small vessels. Common and clinically relevant sites include the joints, renal glomeruli, and skin. Depending on the nature of the immunoglobulins and their Fc chains, the complement cascade can be activated and inflammatory cells attracted to the site of immune-complex deposition. The composition of the infiltrate is also influenced by the localization; infiltrates may be dominated by lymphocytes, macrophages, or neutrophils which migrate through the vessel walls.

Typically, the smallest vessels are affected; in the skin the usual target is the post-capillary venules. This process is referred to as immune complex vasculitis. Marked infiltrates can clinically and histologically resemble cellular type IV reactions, although the mechanisms are entirely different.

In the skin, immune-complex vasculitis presents as palpable purpura—the combination of hemorrhage and vessel-wall inflammation which produces a palpable lesion. The clinical spectrum is highly variable but can include necrosis. The Arthus phenomenon and the Schwartzman–Sanarelli reaction are the most extreme forms.

If very small proteins, such as some mold spores, are inhaled, sensitization and then a type III pulmonary reaction can occur, which is known as extrinsic allergic alveolitis or hypersensitivity pneumonitis. Here there is damage to the alveolar wall.

Since immune-complex reactions occur primarily in selected distal parts of the circulatory tree, a type III reaction can present as a systemic disorder, which resembles an acute flare of lupus erythematosus, both clinically and pathogenetically. Typical triggers include:

- bacterial infections (most common)
- extrinsic allergic alveolitis
- uncommonly, systemic therapy with penicillin or other medications
- very rarely, as a complication of hyposensitization against an allergen.

Within hours after allergen exposure, signs and symptoms such as malaise, fever, pain, and joint swelling may develop, often accompanied by an exanthem.

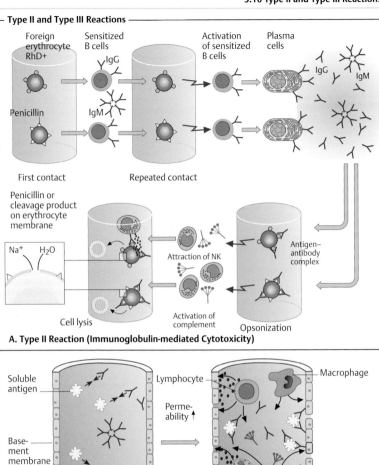

A. Type II Reaction (Immunoglobulin-mediated Cytotoxicity)

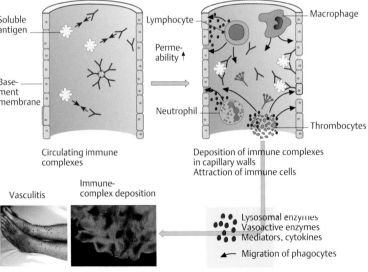

B. Type III Reaction (Immune-complex Reaction)

5 Immunology

A. Type IV Reaction

Type IV reactions are functionally best described as cell-mediated or delayed-type hypersensitivity reactions (DTHRs). This label is appropriate because in DTHR the immune response is not primarily mediated by antibodies, as in type III reactions, but instead by immune cells, which interact with the antigen or, more accurately, with antigen-laden cells.

All forms of DTHR require 1–3 days to reach their optimum strength, and are controlled by T cells. This explains the term "delayed" and also the alternate name of "T-cell-mediated immune response." However, these T cells lead to two very different forms of DTHR:
- one form is mediated by CD4$^+$ helper T cells (T_H)
- the other is mediated by CD8+ cytotoxic T cells (T_C).

Clinical forms of type IV reaction A DTHR is always directed against antigens that are not free in the blood or interstitial fluid, but instead presented on a cell surface as a peptide or hapten. Classic examples of DTHRs are the protective reactions against mycobacteria and *Trichophyton*. DTHRs can also cause less-desirable reactions, such as allergic contact dermatitis. In addition, if the triggering antigen resembles glycoproteins on normal cells, then a severe organ-specific autoimmune reaction can result.

B. CD4+ T-cell-mediated Immune Reaction

The crucial cells for the development of DTHRs are CD4+ memory T cells, of either the INF-γ-producing T_{H1} phenotype or the IL-17-producing T_{H17} phenotype. After the initial activation via APCs and antigen, the acute immune response develops after 7–10 days. When it has subsided, there always remains a population of preactivated memory cells, ready to react at the next exposure.

These cells do not express the CD45RA form of common leukocyte antigen (CLA), but instead an isoform CD45RO that characterizes memory T cells. An adult has memory cells to around 25×10^6 different antigens, suggesting exposure to about this many antigens over a lifetime.

When a second exposure occurs to an antigen for which memory T cells are present, there are two new features:
- an effective immune response can develop, even without the usual danger signals
- optimal immune responses are achieved much more quickly than in the initial activation—the average time is 3 days.

These stimulated memory cells can activate the surrounding macrophages so that they release cytotoxic substances, triggering inflammation and tissue damage. The most important mediators are IL-1 and TNF. In addition, nitrous oxide (NO) and oxygen free radicals help remove the target antigen along with the affected tissue; for example, in the skin they damage keratinocytes and produce the clinical features of contact dermatitis.

Epicutaneous provocation of a type IV allergy, such as via patch testing, shows a maximum reaction 3–5 days after application. In patch testing, it is crucial to apply the antigen in an inert vehicle, usually water or petrolatum; otherwise, during testing the patient may become sensitized to a component of the test substance. Sensitization to an allergen during patch testing is a rare but well-documented complication.

Type IV allergy directed against haptens is biologically identical to the useful type IV reaction to mycobacterial proteins, as seen in tuberculosis skin testing. The only difference is the target antigen. Type IV allergies in the skin are usually directed against haptens, substances that are too small to be recognized alone as antigens. Apparently they can bind directly to HLA molecules, modifying them enough so that they can be presented to T cells. In addition, on both the skin and mucosa, type IV allergies can also develop against proteins.

I Basic Principles

Type IV Reaction I (Delayed-type Hypersensitivity Reaction)

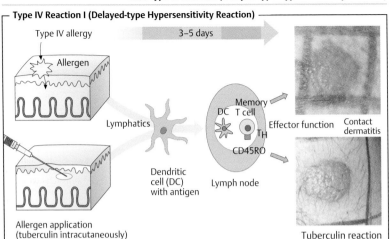

1. Effector phase of contact dermatitis and tuberculin reaction

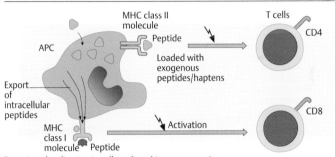

2. Antigen localization in cell-mediated immune reaction

A. Type IV Reaction

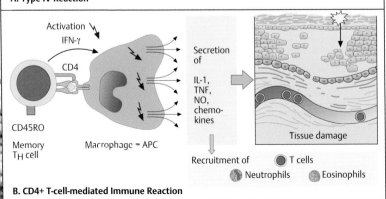

B. CD4+ T-cell-mediated Immune Reaction

5 Immunology

41

C. CD8+ Immune Reaction

Helper T cells (T_H), with rare exception, cannot directly recognize their target antigens, but instead only recognize those antigens presented to them via MHC class II molecules on antigen-presenting cells, usually macrophages. In contrast, MHC class I molecules can be expressed by all somatic cells. Thus, theoretically at least, all somatic cells can be recognized by cytotoxic CD8+ T cells (T_C). However, naive T_C cells ignore the cells that present the relevant antigen on their surface along with MHC molecules (1). To recognize their somatic target cells, T_C cells must first be activated by professional APCs (2).

If the peptides have a very high affinity for the TCR of the CD8+ cells, it appears that in vivo resting APCs can activate the T_C cells. Most peptides have only a relatively weak affinity and cannot activate their specific CD8+ cells, even when presented by APCs. Instead they require the assistance of CD4+ T_H cells to activate the T_C cells. Stimulation of the APCs, especially via the CD40–CD154 interaction and IFN-γ, make them capable of activating naive CD8+ T cells, which recognize low-affinity proteins.

The cells are then converted to cytotoxic effector T cells, also known as cytotoxic T lymphocytes (CTLs), which can then recognize peptides on somatic cells in the skin, lungs, gastrointestinal tract, liver, or other organs. The main requirement is that the activated CTLs leave the lymph nodes and move through the bloodstream to the target organs. After leaving the circulatory system, they interact directly with their target cells and then usually lyse them. The CTLs have two different mechanisms for lysis:

- one mechanism is the secretion of pore-forming proteins such as perforin and granulysin (3a). These are stored in preformed granules and, after activation of the CTL via the TCR, released into the intercellular milieu. The role of costimulatory signals in this process is unclear
- in addition, CTLs can also induce apoptosis or active cell death in the target cells via selected signaling (3b). Under numerous conditions, the cells express surface molecules such as Fas (CD95 or Apo1), which can trigger apoptosis through the enzyme cascade known as the Fas-associated death domain-like IL-1-converting enzyme cascade. If the Fas receptor of the target cell binds to the Fas ligand (CD95L) expressed on activated CTL, the apoptotic cascade proceeds, leading to nuclear fragmentation and cell death.

In almost all type IV reactions, both CD4+ and CD8+ cells are involved. CD4+ cells are almost always needed for induction of the immune response. In the effector phase, both forms of DTHR are also found together. Under most conditions under which exogenous antigens are presented—that is, in most situations where allergy develops—the T_{H1}/T_{H17} and macrophage-regulated immune response is dominant. When endogenous antigens are presented, the CTL-mediated pathway is usually primarily responsible. There are situations in which CTLs are involved in allergic reactions; this seems to be the case in drug-induced lichen planus.

Type IV Reaction (Delayed-type Hypersensitivity Reaction)

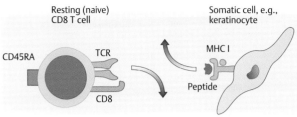

1. Ignoring a peptide-bearing target cell

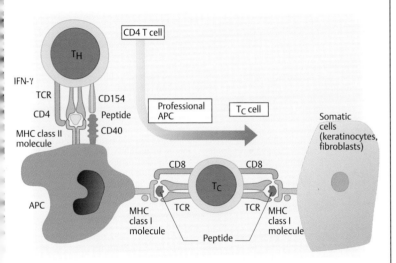

2. Activation

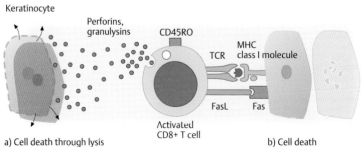

a) Cell death through lysis

b) Cell death through apoptosis

3. Destruction of somatic cells by activated T$_C$ cells

C. CD8+ Immune Reaction

5 Immunology

43

A. Genodermatoses

Cutaneous changes and diseases have long been used to identify syndromes. An inherited disorder with predominantly cutaneous findings is a *genodermatosis.* Close attention to skin findings has allowed precise identification of many disorders, and provided a pool of patients for molecular genetic analysis.

In addition, in some genodermatoses, skin findings may be a marker for potentially life-threatening internal malignancies. For example, in Muir–Torre syndrome, multiple sebaceous tumors and keratoacanthomas are a sign of an increased risk for multiple internal malignancies.

Today the causative genes, and in many instances the proteins, are known for most genetic skin disorders. The identification process has led to a deeper understanding and produced a few surprises.

One disease, several genes. Several diseases such as tuberous sclerosis (Ch. 30.1) and Carney complex (Ch. 30.3) are caused by mutations in two different genes causing almost exactly the same clinical picture.

One gene, several diseases. Mutations in the phosphate and tensin homolog gene (*PTEN*) are associated with Cowden syndrome (Ch. 30.3) as well as several other even rarer hamartoma syndromes.

Unexpected pathophysiology. The identification of calcium-channel gene defects in Darier disease and Hailey–Hailey disease (Ch. 20.1) was the first clue to the importance of calcium in keratinization.

Increased complexity. Both porphyria cutanea tarda (Ch. 30.2) and xeroderma pigmentosum (Ch. 30.2) have many more genetic twists than simple pedigree analysis ever suggested.

B. Patterns of Inheritance

Many genodermatoses are present over multiple generations because the disease is often not severe enough to influence reproduction. When a genodermatosis is suspected, a detailed family history and examination of other family members are essential. Possible patterns of inheritance are discussed next.

1. Autosomal dominant. Men and women are equally affected; 50% of all descendants of a generation are affected.

2. Autosomal recessive. Most often the parents are related. Men and women are affected for only a generation. Gene carriers are healthy.

3. X-chromosome recessive. Primarily men are affected; 50% of the sons of female carriers are affected; the female carriers are healthy but may have subtle signs of disease.

4. X-chromosome dominant. Almost all patients are women with new spontaneous mutations, as affected males are often not capable of survival. If fertile, an affected man transmits the disease to all daughters and never to sons. An affected woman transmits the disorder to 50% of her children.

C. Uses of Genetics

1. Identifying syndromes. Exact genetic testing has made the diagnosis of genodermatoses more complex and expensive but much more precise. Many new syndromes have been described.

2. Disease associations. A variety of genetic markers can be used to study disease susceptibility, especially for diseases that clearly seem multifactorial such as psoriasis. There are genetic differences between early-onset and late-onset psoriasis.

3. Prenatal diagnosis and counseling. As the precision of genetic diagnosis has increased, so has the capacity for prenatal diagnosis for rare devastating disorders, such as some forms of ichthyosis or epidermolysis bullosa. Today it is rare to be unable to provide significant advice to concerned patients or parents on the pattern of inheritance and risk to future offspring. Techniques employed include amniocentesis, chorionic villus sampling, preimplantation analysis and sophisticated imaging techniques.

4. Gene therapy. Keratinocytes can be harvested, cultured, transfected with defective or missing genes, and replaced in the patient. Thus, it is theoretically possible to restore missing enzymes and perhaps even structural proteins to the skin. In addition, stem cells can be directed to develop in an organ-specific fashion, making it possible to create skin replacements that do not induce an immune response.

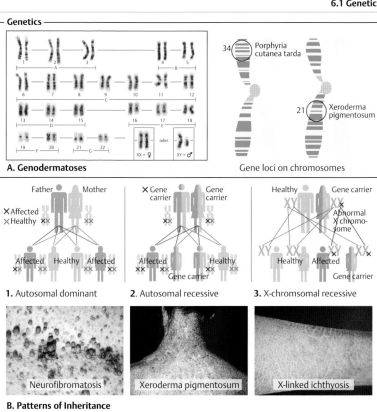

Genetics

A. Genodermatoses

Gene loci on chromosomes

Porphyria cutanea tarda 34

Xeroderma pigmentosum 21

1. Autosomal dominant

Father — Mother
× Affected
× Healthy ×× × ××
Affected Healthy Affected
×× × ×× × ××

2. Autosomal recessive

× Gene carrier — Gene carrier
×× ××
Affected Healthy
×× Gene carrier ××

3. X-chromsomal recessive

Healthy — Gene carrier
XY XX ×
Abnormal X chromosome
XY XX XY XX ×
Healthy Affected Healthy
Gene carrier

Neurofibromatosis

Xeroderma pigmentosum

X-linked ichthyosis

B. Patterns of Inheritance

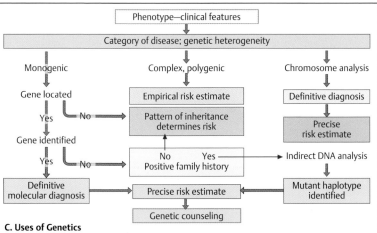

Phenotype—clinical features

Category of disease; genetic heterogeneity

Monogenic — Complex, polygenic — Chromosome analysis

Gene located — Empirical risk estimate — Definitive diagnosis

Yes — No — Pattern of inheritance determines risk — Precise risk estimate

Gene identified

Yes — No — No   Yes — Indirect DNA analysis
Positive family history

Definitive molecular diagnosis — Precise risk estimate — Mutant haplotype identified

Genetic counseling

C. Uses of Genetics

II Diagnosis of Dermatologic Diseases

A. Definition and Indications

In-vitro diagnosis of allergy involves the analysis of serum, blood, or other bodily fluids (such as nasal secretions), to identify the presence or concentration of immunoglobulins, mediators, or various reaction products. High levels of eosinophilic cationic protein likely reflect disease activity involving eosinophils. An elevated immunoglobulin E (IgE) level is one clue to a predisposition to allergic disorders, while the presence of specific IgE against certain pollen, coupled with an accurate history and in-vivo testing, help set the criteria for hyposensitization therapy.

On rare occasions, in-vitro procedures may even replace in-vivo studies. Examples include:

- patients with marked dermatographism in whom prick testing is unreliable
- patients with a history of severe skin reactions, in which re-exposure in vivo could re-induce a life-threatening toxic epidermal necrolysis
- patients who cannot stop taking antihistamines or corticosteroids to allow patch testing.

The disadvantage of in-vitro allergy testing is that is usually does not allow an assessment of the severity of the in-vivo situation. There is no clear correlation between antibody titer and the clinical severity of an allergic reaction.

B. Test Procedures

IgE. Allergen-specific immunoglobulins can be identified in a semiquantitative way by simple strip and ImmunoDOT (allergen as point on nitrocellulose) tests. Quantitative determination with a radio-allergosorbent test (RAST) or enzyme-linked immunosorbent assay (ELISA) is more complicated and expensive.

The principle of the test is identification of IgE that is directed against specific allergens. The allergens are attached to cellulose strips or disks, which are then incubated with patient serum. If IgE directed against a test allergen is present, it forms a complex. The strip or disk is then washed and the antigen–antibody complexes are either made visible with a chromogen or labeled with a radioactive substance and then measured with a scintillation spectrophotometer.

Total IgE. The total IgE is usually measured with ELISA and is only useful for orientation. The normal concentration is 17–450 ng/mL (2.4 ng/mL = 1 IU (international unit)/mL). Serum values over 240 ng/mL (100 IU/mL)

suggest atopy. Levels higher than 10 000 IU/mL are rarely reached. Markedly higher IgE levels are seen in pulmonary aspergillosis, parasitic infestations, some acquired immune defects, and with immunosuppression as in graft versus host disease (GVHD) and human immunodeficiency virus (HIV)/acquired immune deficiency syndrome (AIDS).

Multitests. In atopy screening, multitests are useful. A mixture of common allergens for type I allergy are bound to carrier or placed in solution. Test strips are less accurate. Positive results must be further investigated.

Specific IgE. Specific IgE is usually determined with RAST or enzyme marker systems. There are RASTs available for more than 500 allergens. Each test requires only 50 µL of serum or secretion. Standarized sera from allergic patients are used to check the accuracy of the determination and assess the strength of the reaction. While the IgE level is usually divided into 4–6 classes, these do not correlate well with the severity of allergic disease.

C. Cellular Allergen Stimulation Test

The cellular allergen stimulation test (CAST) measures the levels of leukotrienes D4, C4, and E4 after allergen stimulation. These are synthesized de novo in response to stimulation and are unlikely to reflect nonspecific processes. The CAST is sensitive and specific for type I reactions.

D. Eosinophilic Cationic Protein and Tryptase

Eosinophilic cationic protein (ECP) is released by activated eosinophils. The amount of ECP present is measured, after the blood has been allowed to clot causing eosinophil degranulation.

Tryptase is released during mast-cell degranulation and is useful for assessing both mast-cell activity in type I reactions and the number of mast cells in mastocytosis.

In-vitro Diagnosis of Allergy

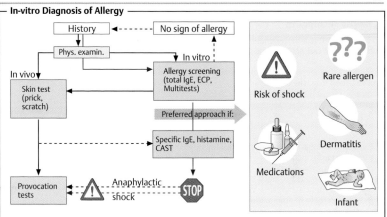

A. Definition and Indications

1. RAST, CAP

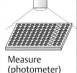 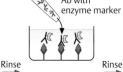 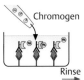

2. ELISA

B. Test Procedures

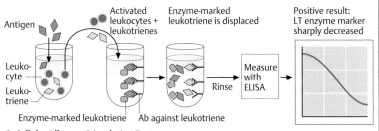

C. Cellular Allergen Stimulation Test

A. Biopsy Techniques

No specialty offers a better chance for correlation of clinical and pathological findings than dermatology.

The following steps will maximize information obtained from the biopsy:
- choose a fresh lesion that is not scratched or ulcerated
- depending on the lesion, punch, shave, or excisional biopsy may be appropriate. Shave biopsies are most appropriate for benign exophytic lesions; they should be avoided if melanoma is suspected
- do not grasp the specimen with forceps; crush artifact destroys much cellular detail. Shave and punch biopsies can be transferred directly to fixative without using forceps; a shave biopsy can be transferred on the scalpel blade, while a punch biopsy can usually be popped out and lifted up with scissors. Excisions should only be handled at the edge
- if excising tumor, label for orientation (Ch. 22.3). Follow local guidelines and confer with laboratory personnel on difficult cases. A marked photograph may be helpful for complex excisions where margin control is required
- rarely, adjacent or contralateral normal skin is needed for comparison, primarily when studying dermal thickness, or considering diagnoses like connective tissue nevus or morphea
- Provide the dermatopathologist with adequate clinical information. For example, not having the correct age of patient may severely hamper the diagnostic approach.

B. Staining Techniques

Routine. The standard stain for skin specimens is hematoxylin and eosin (H&E). The epidermis and adnexal structures are blue; the dermis, pink. When describing routine sections, eosinophilic means pink–red and basophilic means blue.

Special stains. Some structures can be better seen using other biochemical stains. Examples include:
- *Giemsa*—mast cells
- *periodic acid–Schiff* (PAS)—basal membrane, fungal elements
- *Masson–Fontana*—melanin
- *orcein*—elastic fibers
- *Van Gieson*—collagen, smooth muscle
- *Gram*—bacteria
- *Ziehl–Neelsen*—acid-fast bacteria
- *Congo red*—amyloid.

Immunostains. Immunostains use highly specific antibodies and marker system to identify individual cell markers. They are primarily used in tumor diagnosis, especially lymphomas, where most types of T and B cells are identified by combinations of antigens that are defined by the CD (cluster of differentiation). Other useful stains include:
- *Melan-A*—melanocytes
- *S 100*—melanocytes, nerves, Langerhans cells
- *HMB45*—melanocytes
- *smActin*—smooth muscles, pericytes
- *CD 1 a*—Langerhans cells
- *CD 3*—T cells
- *CD 4*—helper T cells
- *CD 8*—cytotoxic T cells
- *CD 20*—B cells
- *CD 30*—activated T cells (Ch. 23.1)
- *CD 34*—endothelial cells, dermatofibrosarcoma protuberans (Ch. 22.3)
- *CD 68*—macrophages
- *CD 117*—mast cells
- K_i-67—proliferation marker
- *Cytokeratin 20*—Merkel cells.

Immunofluorescence stains. Immunofluorescence stains are essential for diagnosing autoimmune bullous diseases (Ch. 7.3, 14.11, 15.1)

Note: A favorite old pathology saying is "Special stains only show one what one does not recognize in a different color." Virtually all diagnoses can be made on routine H&E sections. On the other hand, there are situations where an accurate diagnosis is not possible without special stains, such as when assessing a spindle-cell tumor (fibrous, smooth muscle, or neural origin) or evaluating a possible lymphoma. The clinician should suggest the likely clinical diagnosis and let the dermatopathologist decide which special stains are appropriate.

Histopathology

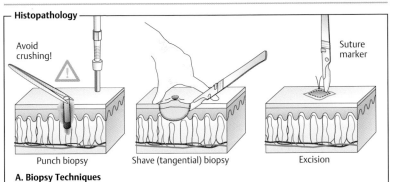

Avoid crushing!

Suture marker

Punch biopsy   Shave (tangential) biopsy   Excision

A. Biopsy Techniques

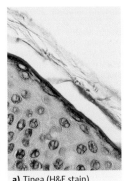

a) Tinea (H&E stain)

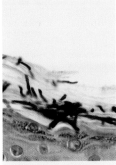

b) Tinea (PAS stain)

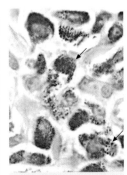

c) Mast cell with granules; arrows (Giemsa stain)

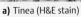

1. Special stains

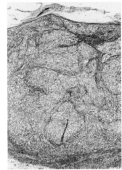

a) Melanoma (H&E stain)

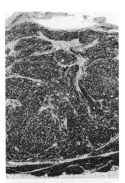

b) Melanoma (Melan-A stain)

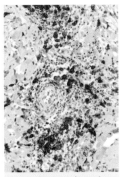

c) Lymphomatoid papulosis (CD30 stain)

2. Immunostains

B. Staining Techniques

C. Histological Features

Specific terms are applied to a variety of pathologic changes. Understanding them makes dermatology easier.

Epidermal changes

- *Hyperplasia*: thickened epidermis because of an increased number of cells
- *Acanthosis*: thickened stratum spinosum of the epidermis with enlarged cells
- *Hyperkeratosis*: thickened stratum corneum
- *Epidermal atrophy*: thinning of the entire epidermis, just 2–4 cell layers thick
- *Hypergranulosis*: the stratum granulosum is thickened (lichen planus)
- *Parakeratosis*: nuclei are retained in the stratum corneum
- *Dyskeratosis*: individual cell keratinization (Darier disease)
- *Apoptosis*: individual cell death, leaving eosinophilic cells (lichen planus, GVHD)
- *Papillomatosis*: church-spire pattern of epidermis (warts, seborrheic keratoses)
- *Acantholysis*: loss of connections between keratinocytes (pemphigus, Hailey–Hailey disease, herpes infections)
- *Hydropic or vacuolar change*: damage to the basal layer (lupus erythematosus)
- *Spongiosis*: epidermal edema with exocytosis of inflammatory cells.

Dermal changes

- *Incontinence of pigment*: melanin falls into the dermis following inflammation of the dermal–epidermal junction (DEJ)
- *Solar elastosis*: basophilic change in collagen after chronic sun exposure
- *Fibrosis*: thickening of the dermis through increased numbers of collagen fibers
- *Atrophy*: thinning of the dermis

D. Patterns of Inflammation

Ackerman's nine patterns of inflammation best cover the inflammatory changes of the skin and allow the easiest approach to diagnosis. They describe the pattern seen at scanning magnification and include:

- superficial perivascular dermatitis
- superficial and deep perivascular dermatitis
- vasculitis
- nodular or diffuse inflammation
- intraepidermal vesicular or pustular dermatitis
- subepidermal vesicular dermatitis
- follicular or perifollicular inflammation
- fibrotic dermatitis
- panniculitis—septal or lobular.

Each diagnostic category can be further subdivided. In the case of superficial perivascular dermatitis, it is important to identify the predominant inflammatory cell (neutrophil, lymphocyte, eosinophil). Similarly, one should look for changes in the basement membrane, or spongiosis.

E. Approach to Slides

- Extract the maximum clinical information.
- Look for tumor versus inflammation.

If tumor is present, determine the cell type, then whether it is benign or malignant.

- Benign tumors are symmetrical, and have a regular expanding border. Central necrosis or an inflammatory infiltrate are uncommon. Malignant tumors are asymmetrical with an irregular border. They may have central necrosis when they outgrow their blood supply and often have an inflammatory infiltrate as part of the immune response to tumor.

If inflammation is present, determine the pattern, and then look for associated clues to narrow the diagnosis.

- The inflammatory pattern can be determined at low–medium power. Never switch to high power before determining the basic pattern

> **Note:** The only two tumors that are likely to present with an inflammatory pattern are patch-stage mycosis fungoides and Langerhans cell disease.

Histopathology

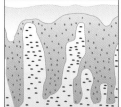

Papillomatosis

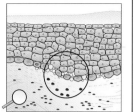

Hyperplasia

Vacuolar change

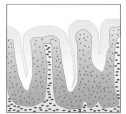

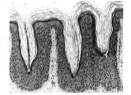

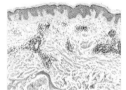

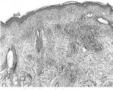

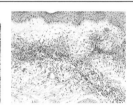

C. Histological Features

Superficial perivascular infiltrate

Superficial and deep perivascular infiltrate

Vasculitis

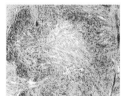

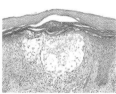

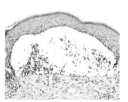

Nodular granulomatous infiltrate

Intraepidermal vesicular and pustular dermatitis

Subepidermal vesicular dermatitis

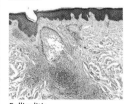

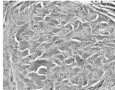

Folliculitis

Fibrosis

Septal panniculitis

D. Patterns of Inflammation

A. Types of Examination

There are two main types of immunofluorescence (IF) examination. In each case, fluorescent-labeled antibodies are used to identify immunoglobulins, complement, or fibrin.
Direct IF (DIF). Tissue specimen from the patient is stained with labeled antibody that specifically recognizes an antigen that characterizes either a cell or an intra- or extracellular glycoprotein. Examples include antibodies that recognize specific T-cell antigens (such as CD3), deposits of human immunoglobulin or complement.
.

Indirect IF (IIF). The patient serum is applied to control tissue (monkey esophagus, salt-split human skin), which is then counterstained with secondary antibody.

B. Technical Tips

- Perilesional skin is the preferred biopsy site, not blister.
- Biopsies must be frozen or fixed in Michel medium.
- Biopsies must be read promptly; prepared slides are only stable in the refrigerator for 2–3 days.

C. Examples of Uses

DIF revolutionized the diagnosis of autoimmune bullous diseases (Ch. 14.11, 15.1), starting by clearly showing the distinction between pemphigus vulgaris and bullous pemphigoid. The following features are seen on DIF and IIF:
- pemphigus vulgaris reveals IgG between keratinocytes in almost all cases. In pemphigus foliaceus, the binding is only in the upper layers of the epidermis. In paraneoplastic pemphigus, a variety of intercellular and basal layer antibodies are found
- bullous pemphigoid always displays complement with various Igs along the dermal-epidermal junction (DEJ)
- dermatitis herpetiformis shows granular deposits of IgA in the dermal papillae
- in systemic lupus erythematosus, a band of C3 and immunoglobulins is seen at the DEJ in nonlesional skin (lupus band test)
- in cutaneous lupus erythematosus, the same deposits are seen only in lesional skin.

IIF shows where antigens from a patient's serum attach to normal skin or other epithelial substrates.

- In pemphigus, they are intercellular, while in bullous pemphigoid they attach along the DEJ.
- In lupus erythematosus, antinuclear antibodies can be identified using cultured Hep-2 (laryngeal carcinoma) cells (Ch. 17.5).

D. Advanced Techniques

- Both ELISA and immunoblotting can replace IIF to identify serum antibodies. Commercially available ELISA tests for desmoglein 1 and 3, as well as the bullous pemphigoid antigens BP180 and BP230 have made diagnosis of pemphigus vulgaris and bullous pemphigoid more precise.
- Salt-split skin employs normal human skin incubated in 1 M (molar) NaCl; the split occurs at the level of the lamina lucida; bullous pemphigoid antibodies are found above the split, while epidermolysis bullosa acquisita and others are below it.
- *Antigen mapping* allows even more precise determination of the level of DEJ blister. A standard array of antibodies is used, staining from the uppermost lamina lucida on the basal cell membrane down to the anchoring fibrils in the upper papillary dermis.

E. Electron Microscopy

Ultrastructural examination played a key role in developing our understanding of the structure and function of the skin. In the past, electron microscopy was often used in diagnostic pathology, especially for tumor diagnosis and renal pathology. Today it has been generally replaced by immunohistochemistry which is simpler and cheaper.

Nonetheless, negative contrast electron microscopy is still the quickest way to identify viruses when an infection with herpes simplex or varicella-zoster virus is suspected. The large pox viruses, which cause orf and milker's nodule, can also be quickly identified. For years the identification of Birbeck granules—tennis-racket-shaped pinocytotic organelles in Langerhans cells—was required for the diagnosis of Langerhans cell histiocytosis. Today antibodies to langerin (CD207) stain the same structures.

Immunoelectromicroscopy is an even more complex procedure, combining electron microscopy and immune labeling to precisely identify the location of antigens within cells or tissues. It is primarily used for research, not for clinical diagnosis.

Immunofluorescence and Electron Microscopy

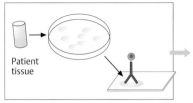

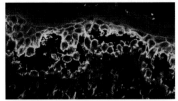

1. Direct immunofluorescence

Pemphigus vulgaris

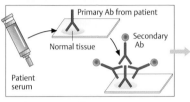

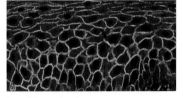

Primary Ab from patient

Secondary Ab

Normal tissue

Patient serum

2. Indirect immunofluorescence

Pemphigus vulgaris

A. Types of Examination

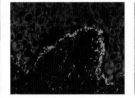

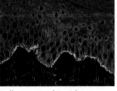

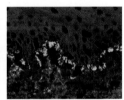

Dermatitis herpetiformis

Bullous pemphigoid

Lupus erythematosus (LE) with LE band

C. Examples of Uses

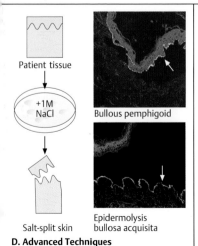

Patient tissue

+1M NaCl

Bullous pemphigoid

Herpes viruses with negative contrast

Salt-split skin

Epidermolysis bullosa acquisita

D. Advanced Techniques

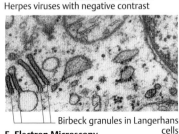

Birbeck granules in Langerhans cells

E. Electron Microscopy

7 Laboratory

A. Mycological Diagnosis

Diagnosis of dermatophyte infections. After disinfection, scales or pustules are scraped or opened with a sterile scalpel blade; on the nails, material can be filed or snipped off from dystrophic (discolored, crumbly) areas. The material is placed on a microscope slide with 10%–15% KOH solution and examined for the presence of fungal hyphae. No speciation is possible.

Histologic examination of a skin biopsy, or more commonly nail clippings, using PAS stain, is another way to demonstrate dermatophytes.

Material obtained in same way is cultured on Sabouraud glucose agar at 25 °C for up to 6 weeks. Macroscopic and microscopic observation of the culture makes speciation possible.

Wood light examination can help find *Trichophyton schoenleinii* and *Microsporum* spp., as infected hairs fluoresce green.

Diagnosis of yeast infections. *Candida* spp. can be cultured at 37 °C over 3 days. Speciation of the yeast colonies is made using a germ-tube test (immediate identification of *C. albicans*) or after subculture on rice agar. Other yeasts are identified on culture morphology and biochemical characteristics (assimilation, fermentation). *Malassezia* spp. are easily identified on KOH examination by the typical short hyphae and spherical yeast (spaghetti and meatballs). Culture on media containing olive oil is possible.

B. Bacteriologic Diagnosis

1. Direct identification. Bacteria can be directly identified in smears or biopsies. Smears are applied to a microscope slide, stained, and examined. The classic Gram stain employs a basic aniline dye such as gentian violet or crystal violet, which helps both identify and classify the bacteria. Gram-positive bacteria have a thicker peptidoglycan-rich cell wall than Gram-negative bacteria and thus resist decolorization. Ziehl–Neelsen and Fite stains are used to identify mycobacteria, while the Warthin–Starry and Dieterle stains are used for spirochetes.

New methods for direct identification of bacteria include direct immunofluorescence and fluorescent in situ hybridization.

The dark-field examination for diagnosing early syphilis uses an unstained blood-free tissue exudate, which is examined under a special microscope to visualize motile spirochetes.

2. Culture methods. Obtaining the material correctly is absolutely essential for successful and accurate culture of bacteria. Intact blisters or pustules are especially suitable. Cultures taken from erosions or ulcers are frequently contaminated with nonpathogenic organisms. Abscesses and inflamed nodules can be aspirated. When questions exist, the best way to obtain results, especially in immunocompromised patients with a broad potential pathogen spectrum, is to do a biopsy and culture the tissue.

3. Serological methods. Most bacteria induce an immune response and thus can be studied with serological methods. Serology often trails the clinical picture, so early false-negative results are common; similarly, an individual remains seropositive long after an infection has resolved, so late false-positive results occur. Sequential samples showing an increasing titer are reliable, but are more often used for epidemiologic than clinical studies.

4. Molecular-biological methods. In recent years, the use of molecular-biological tools such as polymerase chain reaction (PCR) has led to great advances in identifying microorganisms. Different subtypes of infectious organisms such as *Borrelia burgdorferi* can be separated using gel electrophoresis. Because the sensitivity has increased so much, particular attention must be paid to the clinical relevance of positive findings and to their therapeutic implications.

Mycology and Bacteriology

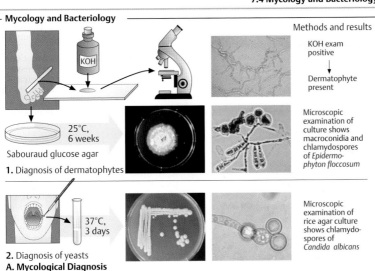

Methods and results

KOH exam positive
→
Dermatophyte present

Microscopic examination of culture shows macroconidia and chlamydospores of *Epidermophyton floccosum*

25°C, 6 weeks

Sabouraud glucose agar

1. Diagnosis of dermatophytes

37°C, 3 days

Microscopic examination of rice agar culture shows chlamydospores of *Candida albicans*

2. Diagnosis of yeasts

A. Mycological Diagnosis

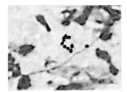

Gram stain of cocci

1. Direct identification

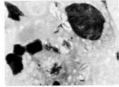

Ziehl–Neelsen stain of acid-fast rods

Darkfield image of *Borrelia burgdorferi* (from culture)

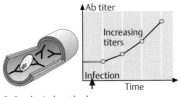

Smear   Biopsy   Culture

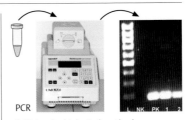

Colonies of *Staphylococcus aureus*

2. Culture methods

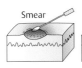

Ab titer

Increasing titers

Infection

Time

3. Serological methods

B. Bacteriologic Diagnosis

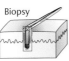

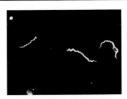

PCR

L NK PK 1 2

4. Molecular-biological methods

7 Laboratory

When an IgE-mediated allergic disease is suspected, there are several ways to try to determine the trigger or allergen. Skin tests, as well as in-vitro analysis of blood and other body fluids, can document a sensitization. The problem is deciding if the documented immunologic reaction is of clinical relevance and explains the patient's problem; whether a clinical hypersensitivity reaction truly correlates with an exposure to an expected allergen can only be determined by an exact history and perhaps provocation testing.

A. Requirements for Allergy Testing

Testability. The patient must be willing to be tested so that compliance can be expected. In addition, they should give signed permission once the risks and benefits have been explained.

Choice of test area. Skin tests cannot be performed in areas that are inflamed or have recently been inflamed. Patients with marked dermatographism (Ch. 17.1) or physical urticaria are difficult to test.

Contraindications
- Pregnancy, infancy
- Severe illnesses
- Use of immunosuppressive medications (corticosteroids)
- Use of medications that can cause erroneous test results (β-blockers, angiotensin-converting enzyme [ACE] inhibitors, antihistamines)
- Risk of severe life-threatening reaction to the test substance
- Current allergic problems that could make the test invalid
- Infection, especially in the organ to be tested

Intracutaneous tests are also contraindicated in those taking adrenergic antagonists.

Test substances (1). Test materials must contain a standardized allergen in a uniform concentration. When a test substance is made locally, it must be certain that:
- it is not irritating or toxic
- there is no risk of infection
- it has been tested on control individuals.

Test methods (1). The test methods must be completely standardized. For prick testing, this includes:
- testing on the inner aspect of the forearm
- keeping the test pricks 2 cm apart
- reading the test at 20 minutes
- standardized evaluation.

The results of the test are documented; for example, for prick tests, erythema and wheal formation are simply quantified.

Complications. Both skin and systemic provocation tests used to diagnose immediate hypersensitivity reactions can trigger severe systemic reactions, ranging from asthma to anaphylaxis. Severe reactions indicate that the patient has a marked and potentially dangerous sensitivity to the allergen.

Procedure. Skin and provocation tests should only be performed by trained personnel with resuscitation equipment available (2). If an anaphylactic reaction is possible, for example when Hymenoptera venom allergy is suspected, the following precautions are wise:
- a peripheral venous line should be placed
- increased observation period
- consider admitting the patient for testing.

Potential errors. Psychological factors can distort test results; this is a particular problem with food allergies where placebo-controlled, blinded testing is essential.

B. Exogenous Influences

Medications, especially corticosteroids, antihistamines, and psychopharmaceuticals, can reduce reactivity, while others such as β-blockers can increase it. If testing is started too soon after an allergic episode, the immune response still can be exhausted with false-negative results. Excessive type I reactions during testing can be seen with infections, immunizations, and excessive physical activity, as well in patients with mastocytosis and physical urticaria.

Overview of Allergy Testing

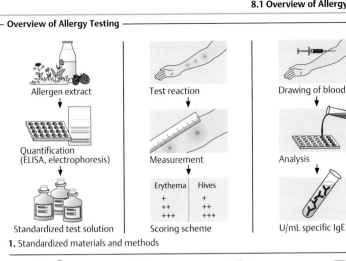

Allergen extract

↓

Quantification
(ELISA, electrophoresis)

↓

Standardized test solution

Test reaction

↓

Measurement

Erythema	Hives
+	+
++	++
+++	+++

Scoring scheme

Drawing of blood

↓

Analysis

↓

U/mL specific IgE

1. Standardized materials and methods

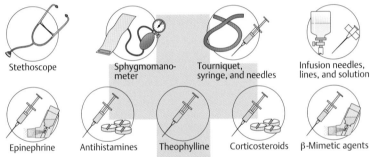

Stethoscope

Sphygmomano-
meter

Tourniquet,
syringe, and needles

Infusion needles,
lines, and solution

Epinephrine

Antihistamines

Theophylline

Corticosteroids

β-Mimetic agents

2. Emergency kit

A. Requirements for Allergy Testing

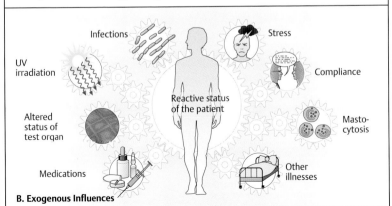

Infections

Stress

UV
irradiation

Compliance

Altered
status of
test organ

Reactive status
of the patient

Masto-
cytosis

Medications

Other
illnesses

B. Exogenous Influences

Blind screening is to be discouraged. It is wasteful and often leads to false-positive results that consume further time and energy. Instead, by considering the:

- general history
- allergy history
- clinical features of suspected allergic reaction,

the number of potential allergens can be sharply reduced. Then one can decide about:

- useful skin tests
- complementary in-vitro tests
- provocation tests to establish relevance.

A. Choice of Test Methods

Skin tests. For immediate allergic reaction, the rub, prick, scratch, and intracutaneous tests (Ch. 8.3) are all available. Dermatitic reactions are evaluated with patch testing to exclude or confirm allergic contact dermatitis (Ch. 8.4).

In-vitro tests. These are indicated:

- when in-vivo test results are unclear
- to support in-vivo test result
- when skin or provocation tests are not possible (pregnancy, infancy, medications, active disease).

Provocation tests. The clinical relevance of the history and allergen search can be explored with provocation tests. Under certain conditions, special test procedures should be considered, including:

- workplace-related *inhalation provocation tests* to simulate occupational exposure
- *oral provocation tests* combined with increased physical activity.

After hyposensitization with bee or wasp toxins, the success of therapy can be assessed by provoked sting testing.

In-patient testing is generally required to:

- evaluate severe reactions (asthma, anaphylaxis)
- increase observation times when a delayed reaction is suspected
- establish special test conditions, such as a strict additive-free diet.

B. Physical Urticaria

In approximately 10%–20% of patients with urticaria (Ch. 17.1), a physical or mechanical effect is the trigger.

1. Dermatographism. This common reaction pattern is tested on the upper aspect of the back by rubbing the skin with a tongue blade.

- An erythema known as *red dermatographism* normally develops within minutes.
- *Urticarial dermatographism* occurs when, in addition to or instead of erythema, urticaria develops. This is also called *factitial urticaria*.
- *White dermatographism* leads to a blanched area after stroking; it often reflects underlying atopic dermatitis (Ch. 14.4).

2. Pressure test. To diagnose *pressure* urticaria, some form of pressure test is used. A 10-cm-wide belt with 5 kg at each end is hung over the shoulder for 10–20 minutes. Alternatively, a standardized metal cylinder 5 cm in diameter is pressed against the thigh for 10–20 minutes. The pressure site is examined after 20 minutes and again after 2–4 hours, for signs of urticaria.

3. Warm/cold test. The skin is heated with an arm bath or a metal cylinder, both at 38–42 °C. The site is checked after 10–20 minutes and again after 2 hours. Cooling is achieved with a cold (5 °C) arm bath for 10 minutes or with a glass of iced water held against the skin for 3–10 minutes. In this test, urticaria after rewarming is the end point; rarely patients may develop angioedema (Ch. 17.1) in response to cold testing.

4. Sweat test. The diagnosis of cholinergic *urticaria* is confirmed with a sweat test. A hot bath (40–41 °C, 10 minutes) or physical activity in a sweat suit is used to induce tiny wheals, which are often not interpreted as urticaria.

Physical Testing

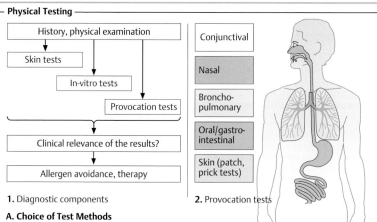

History, physical examination	Conjunctival
Skin tests	Nasal
In-vitro tests	Broncho-pulmonary
Provocation tests	Oral/gastro-intestinal
Clinical relevance of the results?	Skin (patch, prick tests)
Allergen avoidance, therapy	

1. Diagnostic components

2. Provocation tests

A. Choice of Test Methods

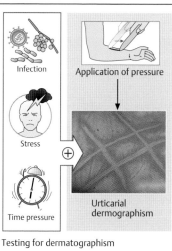

Infection

Stress

Time pressure

⊕

Application of pressure

Urticarial dermographism

Testing for dermatographism

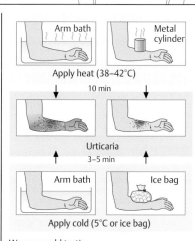

Arm bath

Metal cylinder

Apply heat (38–42°C)

10 min

Urticaria

3–5 min

Arm bath

Ice bag

Apply cold (5°C or ice bag)

Warm or cold testing

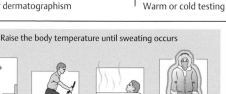

Raise the body temperature until sweating occurs

Stair climbing

Exercise bike

Hot bath 40–41°C

Warm clothes

Sweat Test

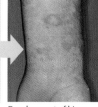

Development of hives

B. Physical Urticaria

A. Skin Tests

Immediate reactions can be assessed with rub, scratch, prick, and intracutaneous testing. The tuberculin test is a variant of the latter, used to assess delayed hypersensitivity.

1. The rub test. When contact urticaria or marked sensitization is suspected, the rub test is the least dangerous starting point. The allergen, such as animal hairs, plants, foodstuffs, medications, skin-care products, or latex products, is rubbed on the inner aspect of the forearm in a circular fashion. Development of hives is positive; a negative control and the use of at least 10 control individuals are required.

2. The scratch test. The skin of the inner aspect of the forearm is scratched to produce a 1 cm linear scratch without bleeding. The test substance is then rubbed on the site or crushed in 0.9 % NaCl solution and then a drop is applied. The negative control is 0.9 % NaCl solution, and the positive control is histamine solution. Control subjects should also be tested.

3. The prick test. The standard test for evaluating immediate hypersensitivity is the prick test. Drops of standardized allergen solutions are applied to the inner aspect of the forearm and then pricked with a lancet to make a 1 mm superficial defect without bleeding. Test series are available that cover most allergens associated with allergic rhinoconjunctivitis and asthma. Controls are 0.9 % NaCl solution and histamine solution. A positive reaction is a wheal at the site.

4. The intracutaneous test. This modification is used to increase the sensitivity when immediate hypersensitivity is suspected, to determine the reaction threshold (with Hymenoptera toxins) and to assess delayed hypersensitivity. Usually 0.02–0.05 mL of a sterile allergen solution is injected intracutaneously on the inner aspect of the forearm with a tuberculin syringe. A correct injection leads to a 2–3 mm "hive" caused by fluid expansion. Controls are 0.9 % NaCl solution and histamine solution.

In contrast to prick testing, more-dilute allergen solutions (1:100 to 1:10) are used; irritant reactions may still occur (for example to molds), making the interpretation of results difficult. Immediate reactions are assessed for erythema and wheal reaction after 20 minutes, 6 hours, and sometimes 24–48 hours. A positive reaction features a wheal with surrounding erythema and pseudopods. When delayed hypersensitivity is suspected, the reading is made after 2–4 days.

B. Tuberculin Test

The tuberculin test is the standard way to assess the presence of intact delayed hypersensitivity. Historically, delayed hypersensitivity was also called tuberculin-type hypersensitivity.

Indications. The test can only establish if a delayed hypersensitivity response to the test antigen has occurred via infection, exposure, or immunization. The time course of the sensitization is not clarified: a patient could have been recently sensitized or exposed as a child.

Procedure. The standard commercial antigen is purified protein derivative standard (PPD-S). Testing can be with a multiple tine needle (tine test) or as an intracutaneous test at varying dilutions. The tine test is pressed on the inner aspect of the forearm; it is not very precise and thus the Mantoux test with intracutaneous injection is preferred. The standard dosage is 10 IU (international units), but if an excessive reaction is expected, the reaction can be titrated starting with a 0.01 IU test dose.

Interpretation. In a positive test, a tiny papule develops 48–72 hours after injection. Using the standard 10 IU dosage, a 10-mm area of induration is positive.

In the past, almost every individual had been exposed to either tuberculosis or BCG (Bacillus Calmette–Guérin) vaccine, so a positive test was expected. Today in some western countries, that is no longer the case. A negative test occurs in all those who had neither tuberculosis nor BCG vaccine. In those previously exposed to tuberculin antigens, a negative test can reflect inborn or acquired immunodeficiency, sarcoidosis, or reduced cellular immunity because of corticosteroids, other medications, marked exposure to ultraviolet (UV) light, recent infections (measles, rubella), or immunizations.

Skin Tests I

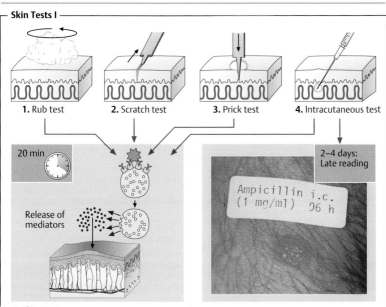

1. Rub test **2.** Scratch test **3.** Prick test **4.** Intracutaneous test

20 min

Release of
mediators

2–4 days:
Late reading

Ampicillin i.c.
(1 mg/ml) 96 h

A. Skin Tests

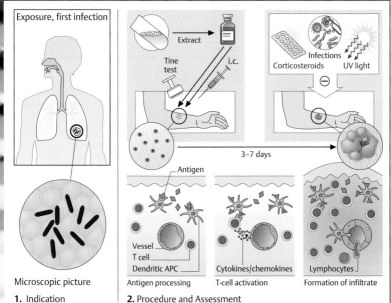

Exposure, first infection

Extract

Tine
test

i.c.

Infections
Corticosteroids   UV light

3–7 days

Antigen

Vessel
T cell
Dendritic APC

Cytokines/chemokines

Lymphocytes

Microscopic picture

1. Indication

Antigen processing

T-cell activation

Formation of infiltrate

2. Procedure and Assessment

B. Tuberculin Test

A. Patch Testing

Patch testing is used to identify allergens that could potentially be responsible for the allergic contact dermatitis variant of delayed hypersensitivity, a type IV reaction (Ch. 5.11). Usual test subjects are those with suspected contact allergies or unexplained dermatitis.

1. Procedure. Test substances are placed in small aluminum (Finn) chambers, taped to the back with hypoallergenic tape. Some allergens are available in impregnated test strips. The patches are left on the back for 48 hours, during which time the area must be kept dry. The sites are read 20 minutes after the patches have been removed (to allow reaction to the tape to resolve) and again after another 24–72 hours to capture late reactions. Reactions are graded as 0 to ++++ or as irritant (IR).

2. Problems. Causes of misleading results include:
- tests are applied to inflamed skin or during a flare of dermatitis
- tape irritation
- immunosuppression through medications or UV irradiation.

If multiple (≥5) positive reactions occur to unrelated substances, "angry back" syndrome should be suspected, with a state of excessive reactivity because of subclinical inflammation. In such a case, each individual allergen should be tested separately.

If patch tests are negative but clinical suspicion is high, then either repeated testing or a controlled-usage test is required. The latter involves applying the suspected substances twice daily to the inner forearm and then observing for a reaction after 5–7 days.

B. Test Substances

The suspected allergens are commercially available; most are in petrolatum but some come in aqueous solution. The standard patch-test series include the most common allergens; there are only minor differences between Europe and the USA. The following are included:
- metals like nickel, cobalt, chromium, and their salts
- chemicals used in rubber manufacture, such as thiuram and mercaptol mix
- para-phenylenediamine, a dye
- fragrances
- ingredients of topical medications such as wool wax alcohols, parabens, other preservatives, and active ingredients (neomycin, benzocaine).

In addition to the standard series, there are many specialized series, including preservatives, fragrances, rubber additives, plastic additives, and metals. In addition, special series are available for high-risk professions (dentist, hairdresser).

The choice of test substances may also be influenced by the distribution of the dermatitis. For example:
- periorbital—cosmetics, nail polish, hair products, eye medications
- hands—gloves, jewelry, hand-care products, occupational exposure.

Nonstandardized test substances must be applied in a nonirritative concentration and tested on controls. Their evaluation is very difficult, so they are best avoided.

C. Special Situations and Test Modifications

Immediate patch test. Triggers of contact urticaria can be patch tested for 30 minutes, read immediately and then after another 30 minutes. Included in this group are proteins from natural latex and many fruits and vegetables, as well as enzymes used in food preparation.

Atopy patch test (1). Immediate-type aeroallergens can also be tested in petrolatum or aqueous solutions. Patients with atopic dermatitis may react to house dust mites, pollen, or animal dander and hairs, identifying a potential worsening factor for their disease. If the patients are very sensitive, their atopic dermatitis may flare after exposure to the test allergen.

Photo patch test (2). If a light-induced contact allergy is suspected, the potential allergens are applied in duplicate to the back. One row is removed after 24 hours and the site irradiated with UVA (5 or 10 J/cm²). The two areas are then compared in the standard way.

Fixed drug eruption. Here the patch bearing the suspected trigger is applied to a site of previous involvement.

Skin Tests II

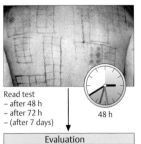

Read test
– after 48 h
– after 72 h
– (after 7 days)

48 h

Evaluation	
o	Negative
(+)	Erythema only
+	Erythema and infiltrate
++	Erythema and papules
+++	Erythema, papules, vesicles
++++	Erythema, vesicles, erosions
IR	Irritant reaction: sharp borders, decrescendo

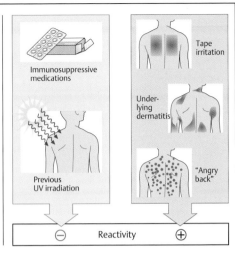

Immunosuppressive medications

Previous UV irradiation

Tape irritation

Under-lying dermatitis

"Angry back"

⊖ Reactivity ⊕

A. Patch Testing

Substance	Percent positive	Vehicle	Concen-tration
Nickelsulfate	12.9%	Petrolatum	5%
Fragrance mix	10.5%	Petrolatum	8%
Balsam of Peru	7.3%	Petrolatum	25%
p-Phenylene-diamine	4.5%	Petrolatum	1%

1. Contact allergen "hit list"

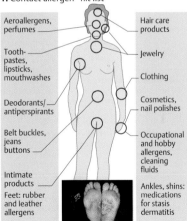

Aeroallergens, perfumes

Tooth-pastes, lipsticks, mouthwashes

Deodorants/antiperspirants

Belt buckles, jeans buttons

Intimate products

Feet: rubber and leather allergens

Hair care products

Jewelry

Clothing

Cosmetics, nail polishes

Occupational and hobby allergens, cleaning fluids

Ankles, shins: medications for stasis dermatitis

2. Typical allergens

B. Test Substances

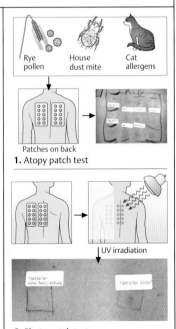

Rye pollen   House dust mite   Cat allergens

Patches on back

1. Atopy patch test

↓ UV irradiation

2. Photo patch test

C. Special Situations and Test Modifications

The two most important imaging procedures in dermatology are dermatoscopy and sonography. They both make it possible to conduct noninvasive studies in vivo without surgery, anesthesia, or ionizing radiation.

A. Dermatoscopy

Dermatoscopy (or dermoscopy) allows a more exact assessment of individual skin lesions; it has proven most useful in the assessment of pigmented lesions.

■ Technique

The dermatoscope consists of a magnifying lens, light source, and handle; the lens is applied directly to the skin. To minimize the alteration of light waves at the skin–air interface, either ultrasound gel, immersion oil or disinfectant spray is used as a coupling medium. The usual magnification is 10× with a mononuclear system, although higher magnifications and binocular systems are available. Systems are also available that are coupled to digital cameras and computers, as discussed below. The two-dimensional image of the epidermis and upper dermis is evaluated with regard to color, structural features, size, border, and symmetry.

Dermatoscopy is most often used to assess melanocytic lesions with the question—is it benign nevus, atypical nevus, or melanoma? In the hands of well-trained physicians, dermatoscopy has a sensitivity for melanoma of 90% and a specificity of 80%. Many other lesions, some of which clinically can be confused with melanocytic tumors, have typical dermatoscopic images; hemangioma, basal cell carcinoma, and seborrheic keratosis are included in this group.

■ Diagnostic Approach

When confronted with a pigmented lesion, the first question is—is it *melanocytic or nonmelanocytic?*

If any of the following are present (1):
- pigment network
- aggregated globules
- branched streaks

a melanocytic lesion is likely. Exceptions where none of these are found include amelanotic melanoma and blue nevus. If the lesion is melanocytic, then the ABCD rules of dermatoscopy are used to help determine whether it is benign or malignant (p. 69 A).

Nonmelanocytic lesions. If no network, globules, or stripes are seen, features of a nonmelanocytic lesion should be sought:
- a blue nevus (2) has a homogenous steel-gray color, which arises because the pigment is so deep that all other colors are absorbed, including the red component of the brown pigment, and only blue is reflected
- the typical changes of a seborrheic keratosis (3) are horn pseudocysts and pseudofollicular openings. In addition, structures resembling the gyri and sulci of the brain, or a fingerprint pattern may be seen. There is usually an irregular border with a moth-eaten appearance and a filmlike effect described as a "jelly sign"

> **Caution:** On the face, a flat seborrheic keratosis can be difficult to distinguish from a lentigo maligna, as the pigment may be concentrated in a perifollicular pattern mimicking a network.

- if red, blue-red, or red-black sharply defined lacunae are seen, the diagnosis is hemangioma (4) (often thrombosed) or another vascular tumor
- typical findings for a basal cell carcinoma (5) are maple-leaf–like structures as well as arborizing vessels. Other findings include a cartwheel pattern, ulceration, and a dirty-brown-gray color.

> **Caution:** If none of the structural features discussed above are identified after going through steps 1–5, then one must return to the starting point and consider the possibility of an unusual melanocytic lesion, most often an amelanotic melanoma.

Melanocytic lesions.
There are several methods of determining whether a pigmented lesion is malignant or not; the four most common are:
- ABCD rule of dermatoscopy (Stolz)
- modified pattern analysis (Soyer)
- Menzies' scoring methods
- seven-point checklist (Argenziano)

We have most experience with the ABCD rule and will describe it as an example. It is based on a semi-quantitative assessment of four features: asymmetry, border, color, and differential structures.
- *Asymmetry* is determined by placing two axes at 90° to one another over the lesion and trying to determine if there is mirror symmetry.

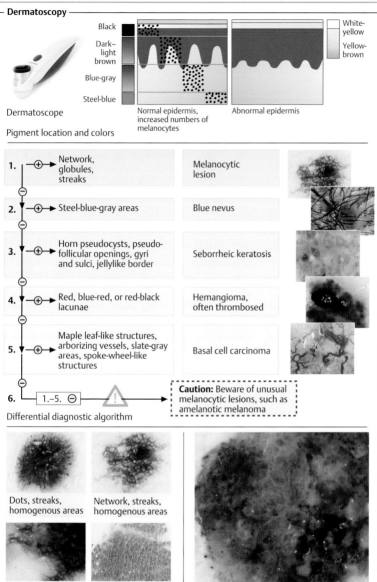

Dermatoscopy

Black
Dark–light brown
Blue-gray
Steel-blue

White-yellow
Yellow-brown

Dermatoscope

Pigment location and colors

Normal epidermis, increased numbers of melanocytes

Abnormal epidermis

1. ⊕→ Network, globules, streaks — Melanocytic lesion
⊖
2. ⊕→ Steel-blue-gray areas — Blue nevus
⊖
3. ⊕→ Horn pseudocysts, pseudo-follicular openings, gyri and sulci, jellylike border — Seborrheic keratosis
⊖
4. ⊕→ Red, blue-red, or red-black lacunae — Hemangioma, often thrombosed
⊖
5. ⊕→ Maple leaf-like structures, arborizing vessels, slate-gray areas, spoke-wheel-like structures — Basal cell carcinoma
⊖
6. 1.–5. ⊖ → **Caution:** Beware of unusual melanocytic lesions, such as amelanotic melanoma

Differential diagnostic algorithm

Dots, streaks, homogenous areas

Network, streaks, homogenous areas

Streaks, network, homogenous areas

Globules

Structural features

A. Dermatoscopy

Red, white, black, blue-gray, light brown, dark brown

Colors

- *Border* is assessed by dividing the lesion into eight segments, like cutting a cake, and each part is assessed for a sharp (suggesting melanoma) or more diffuse (suggesting nevus) border.

Caution: Clinically, a sharp border is more indicative of a benign lesion, as the clinical ABCD rule states (Ch. 24.2). Care must be taken not to let the paradox cause confusion.

- *Color* receives a value from 1 to 6, with the six possible colors of white (lighter than surrounding skin), red, tan, brown, blue-gray, and black. The color indicates where in the skin melanin (the main pigment) is found. The deeper light penetrates into the skin, the more red is absorbed. Thus, epidermal melanin is brown-black; upper dermis, brown to tan; and deeper dermis, blue-gray, as typified by blue nevus. White may be caused by a thickened stratum corneum or by areas of regression, while red reflects vascularization (p. 67, top).
- *Differential structures* include pigment network, structureless areas, branched streaks, globules, and dots, yielding a score of 1 to 5. The structural features give insight into the three-dimensional (3D) nature of the skin lesion. A regular network, typical for a benign nevus, results from the summation of the pigment over the rete ridges condensed into a 2D framework. Since melanin is present along the basement membrane zone, it is heavier, and thus darker, when looking down through the entire side of a rete ridge than when looking through just the tip. The globules and dots are nests of melanocytes; these are defined as <0.1 mm in diameter. Streaks reflect loss of the regular network at the periphery. If the ends of streaks are thickened, they are referred to as "pseudopods," which may be a clue to melanoma.
- *Total dermatoscopy score*—using a simple formula, the total dermatoscopy score (TDS) can then be calculated. If the TDS is 1–4.75, the lesion is clearly benign; if the value is >5.45, a melanoma is likely and histological evaluation mandatory. Lesions with values of 4.75–5.45 should be regarded as suspicious, and either excised or carefully monitored. They often correspond to what are clinically diagnosed as atypical or dysplastic nevi.

Caution: If the lesion is not a pigmented lesion, then the ABCD rule and TDS score are of no value.

Dermatoscopy is also very helpful in searching for the female mite in her tunnel in scabies (hang-glider sign at the end of the tunnel), as well as for identifying foreign bodies and tattoos (accidental and decorative).

B. Digital Dermatoscopy

Digital dermatoscopy brings many further advantages. Here a dermatoscope is combined with a digital camera so the images can be stored in a computer. This greatly facilities the time-consuming process of follow-up examinations looking for changing pigmented lesions, especially in patients with multiple atypical nevi. Such records are also of medicolegal value. The stored images can be used for continuous quality improvement, by comparing the clinical and dermatoscopic diagnosis to the final histologic diagnosis for those lesions that require excision. The digital dermatoscopy allows much greater magnification—up to 50× without a loss of quality. This is quite useful when analyzing nail pigment or searching for scabies mites.

In addition, there are a variety of elegant computer programs available that can apply the ABCD rule or any of the other approaches to automatically analyze a given image or compare two images of the same lesion taken at different times.

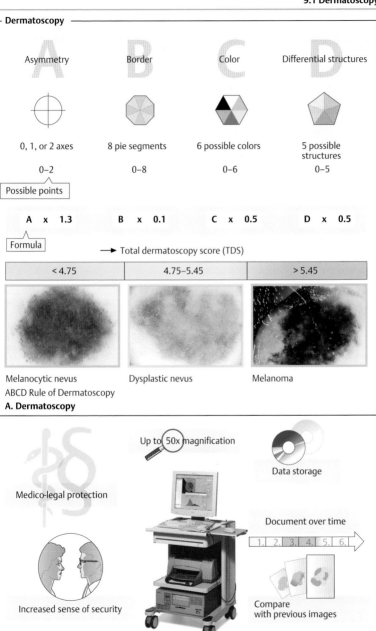

Dermatoscopy

Asymmetry | Border | Color | Differential structures

0, 1, or 2 axes | 8 pie segments | 6 possible colors | 5 possible structures

0–2 | 0–8 | 0–6 | 0–5

Possible points

A x 1.3 | B x 0.1 | C x 0.5 | D x 0.5

Formula

→ Total dermatoscopy score (TDS)

| < 4.75 | 4.75–5.45 | > 5.45 |

Melanocytic nevus | Dysplastic nevus | Melanoma

ABCD Rule of Dermatoscopy

A. Dermatoscopy

Up to 50x magnification

Data storage

Medico-legal protection

Document over time

1. 2. 3. 4. 5. 6.

Increased sense of security

Compare with previous images

B. Digital Dermatoscopy

A. Sonography

Sonography (also known as ultrasonography or ultrasound) is a noninvasive method of imaging structures by recording the reflections of ultrasonic waves directed into tissues. The higher the frequency of the waves, the better the resolution and the worse the penetration.

1. High-frequency sonography. The superficial structures of the skin can be imaged (skin sonography) using frequencies of 20–100 MHz. The maximum penetration with 20 MHz is 8 mm. This modality is primarily used to measure the tumor thickness of melanomas prior to surgery, but is also used for monitoring the therapeutic response of scleroderma.

2. 7.5-MHz sonography. This form is used primarily to evaluate subcutaneous lymph nodes and vessels. With frequencies of 7.5–3.5 MHz, depths up to 7 cm can be imaged.

A. Lymph node sonography. When staging melanoma, and then during tumor follow-up, the primary tumor site, lymphatic drainage path, regional lymph nodes, and superficial cervical, axillary, and inguinal lymph nodes are evaluated. Cutaneous and subcutaneous metastases can be identified, and normal lymph nodes separated from enlarged inflamed lymph nodes and those bearing metastases. Sonography makes earlier diagnosis of lymph node involvement possible, and thus contributes to an improved prognosis.

Typical features of postinflammatory *lymph nodes* are:
- long-oval form
- nonsharp border
- echo-poor uniform peripheral rim
- homogenous echo-rich center
- hilus visualized.

Lymph nodes metastases, in contrast, show:
- rounded form
- sharp border
- missing or irregular peripheral rim
- nonhomogenous echo-poor center
- absent hilus.

Melanoma metastases can be identified in lymph nodes with a sensitivity of 90%, as compared with around 50% with palpation. The specificity is around 98% with sonography, which is superior in all aspects to computed tomography for studying lymph nodes.

B. Differential diagnosis of subcutaneous masses. Sonography often makes it possible to distinguish between a seroma, hematoma, or recurrence following lymph node excision. Other subcutaneous structures such as lipomas (round to oval masses with reduced internal echogenicity combined with echo-rich fibrous septa producing cloudy appearance) and cysts (round, sharply bordered, increased dorsal image with lateral shadowing "comet tail") also have typical sonographic patterns.

Areas of calcification almost completely reflect the waves and are thus echo rich. In addition, foreign bodies such as glass, metal, or wood splinters can be identified, as well as iatrogenic foreign bodies such as stents, catheters, filler materials, or even sutures. Depending on the material, they may be echo rich or echo poor, but often have bizarre shapes or surface features.

■ Angiologic Sonography

Sonography using the Doppler or duplex techniques is an essential part of the evaluation of the vascular system. Chronic venous insufficiency, peripheral arterial occlusion, thrombophlebitis, or a deep vein thrombosis can all be diagnosed (Ch. 25.2).

B. Other Imaging Procedures

When staging melanomas or cutaneous lymphomas, routine x-rays, computed tomography, and magnetic resonance imaging are all employed, especially when dealing with thicker tumors. Positron emission tomography (PET) combined with computed tomography seems to have greater sensitivity in identifying melanoma. Because of their increased glucose metabolism, it can identify metastases using radioactive markers.

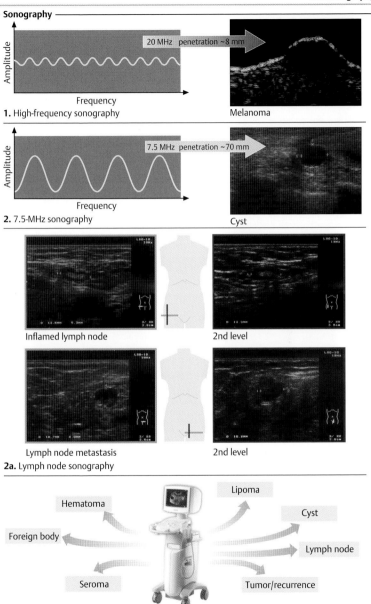

Sonography

1. High-frequency sonography

20 MHz penetration ~8 mm

Amplitude — Frequency

Melanoma

2. 7.5-MHz sonography

7.5 MHz penetration ~70 mm

Amplitude — Frequency

Cyst

Inflamed lymph node

2nd level

Lymph node metastasis

2nd level

2a. Lymph node sonography

Hematoma

Lipoma

Foreign body

Cyst

Lymph node

Seroma

Tumor/recurrence

2b. Differential diagnosis of subcutaneous masses

A. Sonography

9 Imaging Procedures

III Treatment of Dermatologic Diseases

The factors to consider when using topical therapy are the active ingredients, vehicle, correct method of application, and condition of the skin to be treated. Topical therapy should be preferred over systemic therapy because it has far fewer side effects, but it must always be borne in mind that it is much more difficult and time-consuming for patients, especially those with chronic diseases.

A. Interactions between Medications and Skin

The goal of most topical medications is penetration through the stratum corneum and passage into the epidermis and upper dermis, with direct action on skin. Uptake into the dermal vessels and lymphatics, with subsequent systemic action, are usually undesirable. Patches (estrogens or pain medications, for example) and topical nitroglycerin ointment are common exceptions.

There are several steps between application of a topical agent and its local or systemic action. At each step of the process, the active ingredient (AI) must be more soluble or driven by a concentration gradient so that it further penetrates the skin.

- *Liberation*—release of the AI from the vehicle
- *Adsorption*—binding of the AI to skin structures, such as the stratum corneum
- *Absorption*—uptake of the AI from the vehicle; for example, into the lipid film because of increased lipid solubility
- *Penetration*—usually reserved for passage through the stratum corneum, the major barrier
- *Permeation*—passage through other barriers, such as the rest of the epidermis, the basement membrane zone, dermis, and vessel endothelium
- *Resorption*—uptake into the vessel, and thus systemic effects

Clinical correlate: Some medicines (many corticosteroids) are stored in the stratum corneum, which serves as reservoir. Others are released to the skin via eccrine sweat, with a "sprinkler effect."

B. Vehicles

The choice of the vehicle is one of the critical tasks in topical prescribing.

Types of vehicles

- *Cream*—two forms: oil in water and water in oil; cosmetically most acceptable; non-occlusive
- *Lotion*—thin cream, easier to apply
- *Solution*—alcoholic vehicle
- *Ointment*—greasy or occlusive
- *Gel*—semi-solid; converts to liquid when rubbed into the skin
- *Paste*—ointment plus powder; protective, as for diaper rash
- *Shake lotion*—water and powder; cooling
- *Lacquer*—special type of solution which leaves behind a film when dry, as in medicated nail polish

Clinical correlate: Proper choice of the vehicle can be more important than the choice of medication. Ointments for dry skin; creams for general use; gels and lotions for easy application; solutions for the scalp; shake lotions for drying.

C. Compounding

Standard commercial products have the advantages of having tested combinations of active ingredient and vehicle to ensure both delivery of the drug and stability of the product. Some dermatologists compound prescriptions. The advantages are cost savings and an ability to minutely adjust dosages, as in anthralin therapy. Disadvantages are difficulty finding a willing pharmacist, decreased shelf life, and risk of incompatibility. Only approved or registered formulations should be compounded.

D. Tricks for Topical Prescribing

1. *Provide enough medication*—30–60 mg of cream is required to cover the entire body; make the calculations and you will see that most often far too little medicine is prescribed.
2. *Keep it simple*—complex instructions, applying different medicines at different times to different areas, are futile and cause confusion; this is not an improvement.
3. *Be aware of costs*—there are tremendous variations in the costs of medications. For example, topical calcineurin inhibitors cost considerably more than roughly equivalent topical corticosteroids.

Principles of Topical Therapy

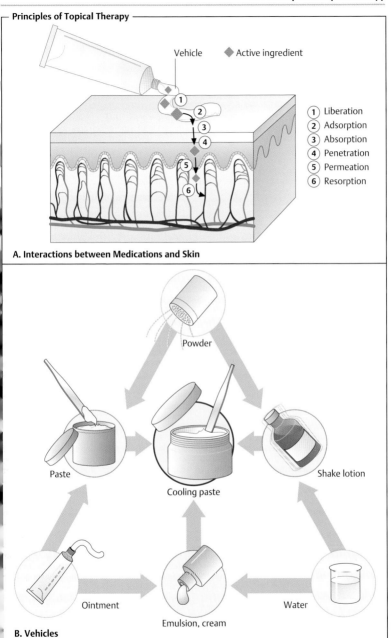

Vehicle ◆ Active ingredient

1. Liberation
2. Adsorption
3. Absorption
4. Penetration
5. Permeation
6. Resorption

A. Interactions between Medications and Skin

Powder

Paste

Cooling paste

Shake lotion

Ointment

Emulsion, cream

Water

B. Vehicles

Corticosteroids. Modern dermatologic therapy without corticosteroids is unthinkable. The introduction of the first synthesized corticosteroids dramatically expanded the arsenal of anti-inflammatory drugs. The initial euphoria was replaced by a somber realization of the multitude of side effects. Today the pendulum has swung in the other direction, and many patients are afraid of using even modest amounts of low-potency corticosteroids topically, a fear that is not justified.

Immunomodulators. Immunomodulators is a sweeping term referring to all medications that are designed to influence the immune system. They may suppress overexuberant or incorrect immune responses, such as when treating autoimmune diseases, or, less commonly, enhance the immune response, as with imiquimod in treating warts.

A. Structure and Potency

Corticosteroids are members of the steroid family and are synthesized in the adrenal cortex. Their basic framework is the cyclopentanoperhydrophenanthrene ring, which can then be modified:

- halogenation with fluoride or chloride atoms leads to increased potency (clobetasol propionate with three halogen molecules is a potent example)
- esterification (introduction of acids as side chains) leads to increased penetration (betamethasone-17-valerate)
- double esterification instead of halogenation leads to fewer side effects (hydrocortisone butyrate and prednicarbate).

Topical corticosteroids are divided into four classes in Germany, ranging from I = weak to IV = very strong. There is considerable variation within the four classes. In the USA, the classes range from 1 to 7, with 1 being very strong.

For topical use, corticosteroids are available as creams, emollient creams, ointments, gels, lotions, solutions, and impregnated tape. Crystallized suspensions are available for intralesional use, for example in treating keloids. In addition, nasal sprays and turbo-inhalers are widely used for allergic rhinitis and asthma, delivering the medication directly to the affected mucosa.

Systemic corticosteroids are usually given orally, since they are absorbed rapidly and completely, with a maximum plasma level reached after 1–2 hours. They are subdivided based on their potency and duration of action:

- *short* (hydrocortisone, prednisolone)
- *medium* (triamcinolone, fluocortolone)
- *long* (dexamethasone, betamethasone).

Most systemic therapy can be accomplished with prednisolone; it is simplest to learn just one corticosteroid and learn it well. With 20 mg or more of prednisolone daily, the adrenal axis is completely suppressed. Side effects are rare with 5 mg or less daily. If a single daily dose is used, it should be given in the morning to mimic the body's circadian rhythm of cortisone secretion.

Intravenous (IV) corticosteroids are the mainstay of emergency treatment of anaphylaxis or severe drug reactions (Ch. 17.1).

Intramuscular and subcutaneous routes of administration are rarely needed, and should be avoided.

B. Mechanisms of Action

Corticosteroids are anti-inflammatory, antiproliferative, immunosuppressive, and vasoconstrictive. They have both genomic and nongenomic mechanisms of action. In lower doses, corticosteroids work via two cytosolic receptors, glucocorticoid receptor (GR)-α and GR-β. They migrate as a dimer to the nucleus, attach to the genomic deoxyribonucleic acid (DNA), and then modify or regulate its transcription. The formation of inflammatory mediators (IL-1, TNF-α, prostaglandins, and leukotrienes) is downregulated. With doses of 200–300 mg of prednisolone or equivalent, the receptors are overloaded and nongenomic mechanisms take over. Via nonspecific interactions with the cell membrane or binding to membrane-bound corticosteroid receptors, membrane stability is increased. Of particular importance is stabilization of the lysosomal membranes, which reduces the release of inflammatory mediators, providing a significant anti-inflammatory effect.

Inflammatory edema is reduced as the increased capillary permeability is reduced. This change also decreases the migration of white blood cells and mast cells into the tissue. In addition, corticosteroids lead to an increase in the circulating neutrophils, while, in contrast, the number of lymphocytes drops (via redistribution in the spleen, lymph nodes, and bone marrow), as do the levels of monocytes, eosinophils, and basophils. The cytotoxicity of T cells is reduced and the migration of macrophages is inhibited by upregulation of the migration inhibitory factor (MIF).

The antiproliferative effect occurs because of inhibition of DNA synthesis and interference with mitosis in the G1 and G2 cell-cycle phases. The synthesis of collagen and other matrix components by fibroblasts is also suppressed, helping to explain the frequent cutaneous atrophy.

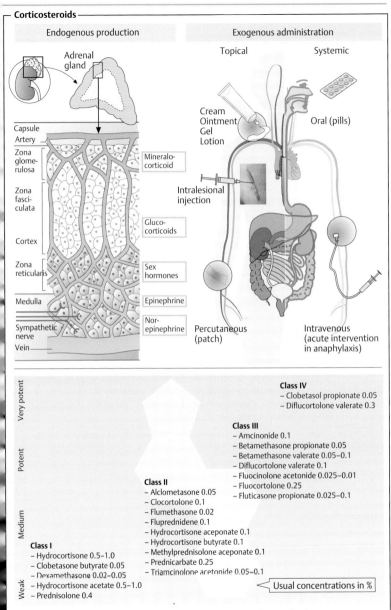

Corticosteroids

Endogenous production

Exogenous administration

Topical

Systemic

Adrenal gland

Cream
Ointment
Gel
Lotion

Oral (pills)

Capsule
Artery
Zona glomerulosa

Mineralo-corticoid

Zona fasciculata

Intralesional injection

Gluco-corticoids

Cortex

Zona reticularis

Sex hormones

Medulla

Epinephrine

Sympathetic nerve

Nor-epinephrine

Vein

Percutaneous (patch)

Intravenous (acute intervention in anaphylaxis)

Very potent

Class IV
– Clobetasol propionate 0.05
– Diflucortolone valerate 0.3

Potent

Class III
– Amcinonide 0.1
– Betamethasone propionate 0.05
– Betamethasone valerate 0.05–0.1
– Diflucortolone valerate 0.1
– Fluocinolone acetonide 0.025–0.01
– Fluocortolone 0.25
– Fluticasone propionate 0.025–0.1

Class II
– Alclometasone 0.05
– Clocortolone 0.1
– Flumethasone 0.02
– Fluprednidene 0.1
– Hydrocortisone aceponate 0.1
– Hydrocortisone butyrate 0.1
– Methylprednisolone aceponate 0.1
– Prednicarbate 0.25
– Triamcinolone acetonide 0.05–0.1

Medium

Class I
– Hydrocortisone 0.5–1.0
– Clobetasone butyrate 0.05
– Dexamethasone 0.02–0.05
– Hydrocortisone acetate 0.5–1.0
– Prednisolone 0.4

Weak

Usual concentrations in %

Classification of topical corticosteroids (German classification after Niedner)

A. Structure and Potency

10 Medical Therapy

C. Indications and Side Effects

■ Topical Therapy

Indications. Topical therapy is indicated for most forms of dermatitis (atopic, nummular, allergic contact, irritant contact), granulomatous disorders, and autoimmune disease (for example, lichen planus or cutaneous manifestations of lupus erythematosus). It is also useful to reduce the need for systemic steroids in disorders like bullous pemphigoid. Topical corticosteroids are contraindicated for the dermatitis resulting from fungal infections.

Side effects. The topical side effects of corticosteroids are dependent on the strength of the agent, and the site and duration of application. The periorbital region and genitalia are particularly susceptible, while the scalp, palms of the hands, and soles of the feet are almost impervious. Findings include persistent erythema (rubeosis), telangiectases, dermal atrophy, and an increased tendency to bruise. Hirsutism and an acneiform eruption may also occur. A common problem is the rebound effect; when topical corticosteroids are stopped, the underlying condition often rebounds with a vengeance. This is particularly common in psoriasis.

Important contraindications are acne, rosacea and perioral dermatitis. A frequent scenario is that a patient, often one who is treating perioral dermatitis, gets initial improvement with corticosteroids, but then develops therapy-related side effects like steroid acne, which are mistaken for a recurrence of the disease, leading to further use of higher-potency agents and inducing a vicious cycle of corticosteroid abuse.

> **Caution:** When using very potent agents, treating wide areas, or managing young patients, there may be sufficient absorption of topical agents to induce systemic side effects.

■ Systemic Therapy

Indications. Allergic reactions with systemic involvement, refractory inflammatory dermatoses, autoimmune diseases, and granulomatous disorders are the most common indications.

Administration. Patients usually start with prednisolone 0.5–2 mg/kg daily; the goal is to get below 6 mg of prednisolone after 3–6 weeks, as this is the Cushing threshold. In chronic disease, the prednisolone should always be combined with steroid-sparing immunosuppressive agents. Do not forget calcium and vitamin D for osteoporosis prophylaxis. If long-term therapy is anticipated, get an ophthalmologic examination (to check for pre-existing cataracts or glaucoma) and determine tuberculosis status. Gastric ulcers should be prevented with H_2-receptor antagonists.

Side effects. The side effects are summarized as iatrogenic Cushing syndrome; they include diabetes mellitus, hypertension, increased susceptibility to infections, reactivation of tuberculosis, osteoporosis, aseptic bone necrosis (usually of the femoral head), gastrointestinal ulcers, insomnia, increased appetite, mood changes, seizures, and eye problems (both cataracts and glaucoma). In addition, all the cutaneous features may develop. The rebound effect is even more prominent than with topical agents, and an Addisonian crisis may occur if the corticosteroids are stopped while the adrenal axis is suppressed or if adrenal atrophy has occurred so the organ is unable to respond.

Corticosteroids

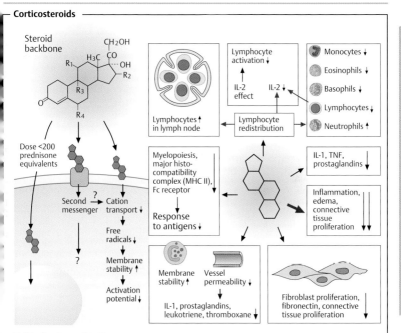

B. Mechanisms of Action

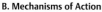

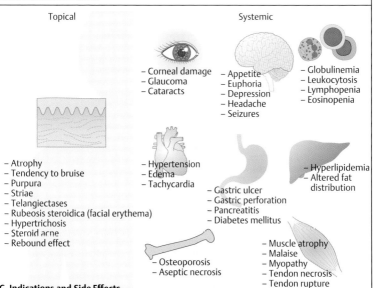

Topical

Systemic

– Corneal damage
– Glaucoma
– Cataracts

– Appetite
– Euphoria
– Depression
– Headache
– Seizures

– Globulinemia
– Leukocytosis
– Lymphopenia
– Eosinopenia

– Atrophy
– Tendency to bruise
– Purpura
– Striae
– Telangiectases
– Rubeosis steroidica (facial erythema)
– Hypertrichosis
– Steroid acne
– Rebound effect

– Hypertension
– Edema
– Tachycardia

– Gastric ulcer
– Gastric perforation
– Pancreatitis
– Diabetes mellitus

– Hyperlipidemia
– Altered fat distribution

– Osteoporosis
– Aseptic necrosis

– Muscle atrophy
– Malaise
– Myopathy
– Tendon necrosis
– Tendon rupture

C. Indications and Side Effects

A. Calcineurin Inhibitors

The calcineurin inhibitors are macrolide lactones, which have similar immunosuppressive effects to corticosteroids. The best-known member of the group is ciclosporin A (CyA), which has been a mainstay of antirejection therapy in transplantation medicine for many years. CyA is too large a molecule for topical use. The macrolides tacrolimus (FK506) and pimecrolimus are smaller molecules, and can penetrate the skin in optimized vehicles. Tacrolimus is available as a 0.03% and 0.1% ointment, while pimecrolimus comes as a 1.0% cream. Related substances such as rapamycin (sirolimus) are undergoing clinical testing.

Mechanisms of action. The macrolides form intracellular complexes—CyA with cyclophilin, tacrolimus and pimecrolimus with macrophilin 12 (FK506-binding protein)—which then inhibit calcineurin. This in turn blocks the dephosphorylation of NFAT (nuclear factor of activated T cells), which inhibits the synthesis of IL-2 and other cytokines. Proliferation and activation of T cells is blocked, leading to immunosuppression. Calcineurin inhibitors also act on transcription repressors. They indirectly attenuate the key cell cycle regulator p53; this may be relevant for the increase in UV- or virally-induced cancers during treatment with these agents. There is little systemic absorption of either agent.

Topical use. Tacrolimus and pimecrolimus are only approved for atopic dermatitis. Case reports and randomized studies suggest they may be useful for a variety of other inflammatory dermatoses, including lichen planus (especially mucosal disease), lupus erythematosus, and pyoderma gangrenosum.

Immediately after application, there may be a burning sensation; this unpleasant effect disappears shortly and most patients develop a tolerance so that they have less burning. There is no cutaneous atrophy, in contrast to corticosteroids. Although topical immunosuppressive agents are generally not associated with increased carcinogenesis, the patient should use light-protection or light-avoidance measures.

Systemic use. CyA is approved for treating severe psoriasis and refractory atopic dermatitis systemically. Other indications include pyoderma gangrenosum, Behçet disease, severe lupus erythematosus, and refractory lichen planus.

The most common side effects are impaired renal function and hypertension, both of which often require discontinuation of therapy. Hypertrichosis and gingival hyperplasia are also common

Caution: Systemic calcineurin inhibitors increase the risk of UV-induced cutaneous squamous cell carcinomas in all patients. In solid organ transplant patients the risk increases up to 100-fold. Metastasis is also more common. Thus the patients must practice light protection or avoidance and should not receive phototherapy after long-term therapy with calcineurin inhibitors.

B. Azathioprine

Azathioprine (AZT) inhibits inosine monophosphate dehydrogenase, which interrupts DNA synthesis, and blocks the proliferation of T and B cells.

Indications. Indication are bullous autoimmune diseases, dermatomyositis, lupus erythematosus, and pyoderma gangrenosum, as well as severe atopic dermatitis and lichen planus. Therapy usually starts with 100–150 mg AZT with 0.5–1.0 mg/kg prednisolone daily. After clinical improvement, the AZT dose should be continued and prednisolone tapered to 5 mg daily. AZT takes 4–6 weeks to show any clinical effects.

Side effects. These include macrocytic anemia, gastrointestinal problems, central nervous system (CNS) disorders, flu-like symptoms, and hair loss, as well as leukopenia and hepatotoxicity, especially with reduced activity of thiopurine-S-methyltransferase (TPMT). Therefore TPMT should be checked prior to use. Complete blood count (CBC) and liver values should be monitored closely. Patients should not take allopurinol together with AZT.

C. Mycophenolate Mofetil

Mycophenolate mofetil (MMF) works in a similar way and is approved for use in solid organ transplants. It does not interact with allopurinol, does not depend on TPMP, and is less hepatotoxic than AZT, but more myelosuppressive.

Calcineurin Inhibitors, Azathioprine, and Mycophenolate Mofetil

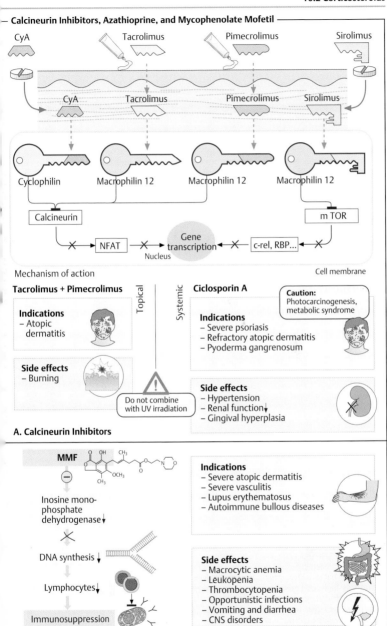

Mechanism of action

Nucleus

Cell membrane

Tacrolimus + Pimecrolimus

Topical | Systemic

Indications
– Atopic dermatitis

Side effects
– Burning

Do not combine with UV irradiation

Ciclosporin A

Caution:
Photocarcinogenesis, metabolic syndrome

Indications
– Severe psoriasis
– Refractory atopic dermatitis
– Pyoderma gangrenosum

Side effects
– Hypertension
– Renal function↓
– Gingival hyperplasia

A. Calcineurin Inhibitors

MMF

Inosine mono-phosphate dehydrogenase↓

DNA synthesis ↓

Lymphocytes↓

Immunosuppression

Indications
– Severe atopic dermatitis
– Severe vasculitis
– Lupus erythematosus
– Autoimmune bullous diseases

Side effects
– Macrocytic anemia
– Leukopenia
– Thrombocytopenia
– Opportunistic infections
– Vomiting and diarrhea
– CNS disorders

C. Mycophenolate Mofetil

10 Medical Therapy

A. Definition

Biologicals are medications based on natural molecules. Today the term is applied to agents that mimic or inhibit mediators, especially in the inflammatory process. Common targets include cytokines such as TNF, adhesion molecules, and molecules involved in the activation or silencing of immune responses.

B. Anti-TNF Therapy

TNF is a cytokine that regulates multiple functions including embryonal development, metabolism, angiogenesis, and immune response. It transmits its signal primarily via TNF receptors.

■ Functions of TNF

In high concentrations, TNF can destroy tumor cells, but in lower concentrations it stimulates tumor growth, vessel formation, and inflammation. In bacterial infections and septic shock, TNF is responsible for the fever and circulatory collapse, but also for control of the pathogenic bacteria. TNF is critical for the recruitment of neutrophils into tissues. For this reason, TNF antagonists increase the risk of more severe infections with bacteria, mycobacteria, and yeasts. They also suppress fever, chills, and pain, masking the early signs of infection. TNF antagonists make sense in diseases dominated by neutrophils, such as psoriasis, psoriatic arthritis, rheumatoid arthritis, and inflammatory bowel disease.

■ Therapy with TNF Antagonists

Indications. These agents are widely used for rheumatoid arthritis and inflammatory bowel disease. The classic dermatologic indication is severe psoriasis of the skin, nails, or joints that has not responded to fumaric acid, photochemotherapy, or methotrexate. When used early, they help protect against chronic damage of arthritis and nail disease. Excellent patient compliance is also required. TNF antagonists have a good safety profile, and only their high price prevents them being used even more widely. With TNF blockade, the risk of mycobacterial and bacterial infections, even with saprophytic bacteria like *Staphylococcus epidermidis*, is high. Latent tuberculosis, marked cardiac insufficiency, and demyelinating diseases must be ruled out. On the other hand, sarcoidosis seems to respond favorably to TNF-antagonists.

Etanercept. This TNF-receptor fusion protein binds in serum to free TNF and lymphotoxin-β. The usual dose is 25–50 mg subcutaneously twice weekly. An effect is first seen after 8 weeks; in 3 months the Psoriasis Area and Severity Index (PASI) has improved by 75% in one-third of patients.

Infliximab. A chimeric monoclonal immunoglobulin (Ig)G1 anti-TNF antibody, infliximab is given i. v., and shows the most rapid effects. With a dose of 3–5 mg/kg at 0, 2, and 8 weeks, the PASI improves by 75% in 80% of patients during the first 10 weeks.

Adalimumab and Golimumab. These two recombinant fully humanized monoclonal anti-TNF antibodies are administered subcutaneously. For psoriatic arthritis, 40 mg of adalimumab or 50 mg of golimumab are given every 2 weeks. After 24 weeks, two-thirds of patients show a PASI improvement of 75%.

C. Anti-IL-12/IL-23p40 Therapy

Inflammation in diseases like psoriasis and rheumatoid arthritis is initiated by antigen-presenting cells (APCs), CD4+, and helper T cells, T_{H1} and T_{H17}. Large amounts of IL-17 and IL-23 are found in the skin of patients with acute psoriasis. Accordingly, psoriasis improves when T cells are depleted or when T_{H1} cells and T_{H17} are deviated to T_{H2} cells through IL-4 therapy. Another approach to treating psoriasis is administration of antibodies that neutralize IL-12/IL-23p40, the common chain for IL-12 and IL-23 and thus block the T_{H1}/T_{H17} response.

Ustekinumab. This monoclonal antibody binds to the entire IL-12/IL-23p40 complex. Since the specific IL-12p35 and IL-23p19 monomers alone are not biologically active, the effects of IL-12 and IL-23 are effectively limited. In clinical studies, the injection of 90 mg ustekinumab every 3 months produced a 75% PASI improvement in 60% of patients.

Briakinumab. Another anti IL-12/IL-23 monoclonal antibody, briakinumab failed to receive approval in 2011 because of an increased risk of major cardiac events, early appearance of squamous cell carcinomas and increased numbers of increased infections. This rejection has cast a cloud over the use of the almost identical ustekinumab.

D. New Compounds

New small molecules that interfere with cytokine signaling through Janus kinases are under clinical evaluation.

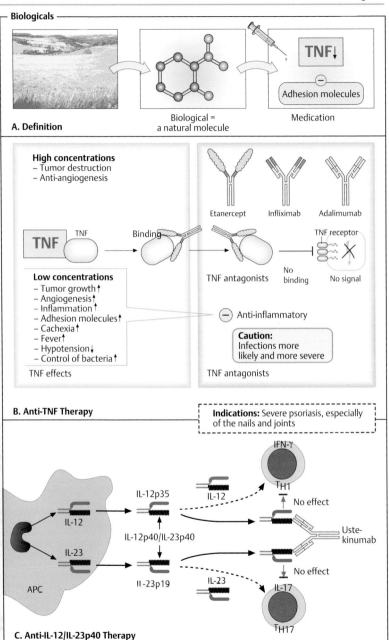

Biologicals

A. Definition

Biological = a natural molecule

Medication

TNF↓

— Adhesion molecules

B. Anti-TNF Therapy

High concentrations
– Tumor destruction
– Anti-angiogenesis

Etanercept   Infliximab   Adalimumab

TNF

Binding

TNF receptor

TNF antagonists

No binding

No signal

Low concentrations
– Tumor growth↑
– Angiogenesis↑
– Inflammation↑
– Adhesion molecules↑
– Cachexia↑
– Fever↑
– Hypotension↓
– Control of bacteria↑

TNF effects

— Anti-inflammatory

Caution:
Infections more likely and more severe

TNF antagonists

Indications: Severe psoriasis, especially of the nails and joints

C. Anti-IL-12/IL-23p40 Therapy

IL-12

IL-23

APC

IL-12p35

IL-12p40/IL-23p40

IL-23p19

IL-12

IL-23

IFN-γ

TH1

No effect

Uste-kinumab

No effect

IL-17

TH17

10 Medical Therapy

83

A. Immunostimulators

Currently, four groups of medications are used for stimulating or enhancing the immune response in dermatologic patients:
- interleukin 2 (IL-2)
- interferon (IFN)
- toll-like receptor agonists
- T-cell activating antibodies

There are also many other agents such as β-blockers, which are also immunomodulatory. In addition, the immunostimulatory role often depends on the nature of usage; in certain situations, the same drugs may be immunosuppressive. Another problem is that cytokines work in vivo only over short distances in high concentrations. Thus, when they are given i.v., they easily reach toxic concentrations and are effective for too short a period of time. To address this problem, they are ideally combined with stabilizers.

B. Interleukin 2

The first cytokine to be used in tumor therapy was IL-2. When used in high toxic concentrations, IL-2 can induce a remission in about 10% of patients with metastatic melanoma. It is approved for this usage in the USA. There are two different methods of administration.
- With systemic use, there are very severe side effects including edema, capillary leakage syndrome, and marked cardiovascular overload, so that patients often require intensive care.
- In contrast, intratumoral IL-2 is less toxic with fewer and milder systemic effects, but also with only local antitumor activity.

The total dosage of 6×10^6 IU (international units) for each day of injection is so small that only malaise and, occasionally, fever develop. There are studies suggesting that 50% of the treated metastases regress. Only lesions that are less than 0.5 cm seem to respond; larger ones are not influenced. Intratumoral IL-2 injections are symptomatic, not curative, but may be of great benefit in special situations.

C. Interleukin 12

IL-12 is probably the most promising molecule in antitumor therapy. There are many reasons for this. IL-12 probably does not distinguish itself via effector functions, but instead by profoundly influencing the differentiation of activated T cells, inducing proinflammatory, antitumoral T cells. In addition, it has a strong anti-angiogenesis action.

D. Interferons

Among the interferons (IFNs), IFN-α and IFN-β are best established therapeutically. *IFN-β* is used as an anti-inflammatory cytokine in patients with multiple sclerosis. In contrast, *IFN-α* helps to induce proinflammatory antitumoral T_{H1} cells. Its anti-angiogenesis action is less marked than that of IL-12. The usual dose is 3–6 million IU three times weekly.

It is most widely used in chronic hepatitis C infection (usually in pegylated form). It is also effective against Kaposi sarcoma and hairy cell leukemia. In dermatology, it is used as adjuvant therapy for cutaneous lymphomas, especially mycosis fungoides, and melanoma. It is approved for prophylactic treatment of high-risk melanoma patients following excision of the tumor, and is also incorporated into many protocols for metastatic disease, both as a single agent and an adjuvant. Side effects of IFN-α include flu-like signs and symptoms, as well as bone marrow suppression.

E. Toll-like Receptor Agonists

A recent development in immunostimulation is the discovery of agents which directly influence the innate immune response via activation of toll-like receptors (TLRs). TLRs are highly conserved structures on macrophages/monocytes and some epithelial cells, which are pattern-recognition receptors recognizing archaic bacterial and viral structures or nucleic acid sequences and alerting the immune system. Imiquimod is a topical agent that stimulates TLR7 and activates an innate local response. It is approved for treating genital human papillomavirus (HPV) infections, but also seems effective for superficial cutaneous tumors such as superficial basal cell carcinoma, actinic keratosis, and even lentigo maligna. Other TLR agonists are incorporated into vaccines as adjuvants; they have been developed for indications as diverse as ragweed desensitization and breast cancer therapy.

F. CTLA-4 Antagonists

New data show that ipilimumab and tremelimumab, monoclonal antibodies directed against CTLA-4 (Ch. 5.4), can induce long-term remission in about 10% of patients with metastatic melanoma; at the same time, they carry the risk of triggering autoimmune diseases. Anti-CTLA-4 antibodies impair T-cell silencing through the CTLA-4 receptor molecule and thus induce broad, poorly controlled activation of pre-activated memory T cells.

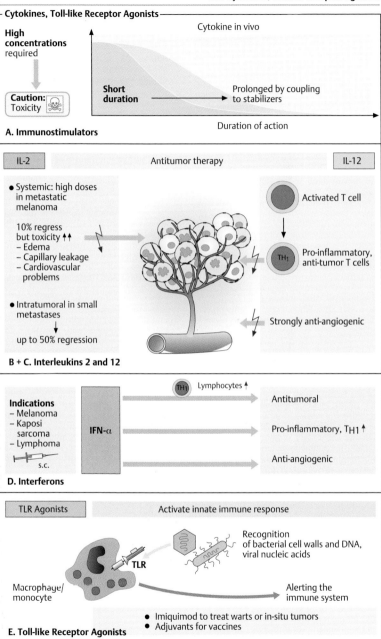

Cytokines, Toll-like Receptor Agonists

Cytokine in vivo

High concentrations required

Caution: Toxicity

Short duration

Prolonged by coupling to stabilizers

Duration of action

A. Immunostimulators

IL-2 · Antitumor therapy · IL-12

Activated T cell

- Systemic: high doses in metastatic melanoma

  10% regress but toxicity ↑↑
  – Edema
  – Capillary leakage
  – Cardiovascular problems

- Intratumoral in small metastases

  up to 50% regression

TH₁ · Pro-inflammatory, anti-tumor T cells

Strongly anti-angiogenic

B + C. Interleukins 2 and 12

Indications
– Melanoma
– Kaposi sarcoma
– Lymphoma

s.c.

IFN-α

TH₁ Lymphocytes ↑

Antitumoral

Pro-inflammatory, TH1 ↑

Anti-angiogenic

D. Interferons

TLR Agonists · Activate innate immune response

Recognition of bacterial cell walls and DNA, viral nucleic acids

TLR

Macrophage/ monocyte

Alerting the immune system

- Imiquimod to treat warts or in-situ tumors
- Adjuvants for vaccines

E. Toll-like Receptor Agonists

10 Medical Therapy

85

III Treatment of Dermatologic Diseases

A. Thalidomide

Thalidomide was introduced in the 1960s, primarily in Germany, as a safe, nonaddictive sedative recommended especially for controlling morning sickness during pregnancy. Tragically, it was a potent teratogen, impairing limb development in particular; more than 5000 affected children were born in Germany before the drug was removed from the market. Not surprisingly, it is difficult to obtain today and not available in every market. Thalidomide has a variety of anti-inflammatory and immunomodulatory effects which were later discovered. It blocks the release of cytokines like TNF and impairs both phagocytosis and chemotaxis in neutrophils.

Indications. Thalidomide (or its more effective analog lenalidomide) is part of most protocols for multiple myeloma. In addition, it is the most effective treatment for type II leprosy reactions. It is also used in discoid lupus erythematosus, Behçet disease, pyoderma gangrenosum, Langerhans cell disease, severe aphthae, and refractory prurigo nodularis.

Side effects. The teratogenicity makes its use in women of child-bearing potential almost impossible. In addition, many patients experience neurotoxicity with a peripheral polyneuropathy.

B. Chloroquine

Chloroquine and its derivative hydroxychloroquine were developed to replace quinine in malaria therapy. They have an anti-inflammatory action, blocking lysosomal activity and impairing the release of proinflammatory cytokines. The usual dose is 200–400 mg daily, with the lower dose required for long-term therapy. In porphyria cutanea tarda (PCT), chloroquine forms porphyrin complexes, which are more easily excreted by the kidney.

> **Caution:** In PCT, a much lower dose is used—50–100 mg twice weekly. The usual dosage causes PCT to flare.

Indications. Indications are lupus erythematous, including reticular erythematosus mucinosis (REM) syndrome, Behçet disease, granuloma faciale, and, at low doses, porphyria cutanea tarda. It is also used extensively in rheumatoid arthritis.

Side effects. The main problem is retinal toxicity; a baseline ophthalmologic examination and then regular re-examinations are wise. At doses of 200 mg daily or lower, ocular problems are rare.

> **Caution:** Prior to starting therapy, glucose-6-phosphate dehydrogenase (G6PD) deficiency and pregnancy should be excluded.

C. Fumaric Acid Esters

Fumaric acid esters are the most widely used systemic agent for psoriasis in Germany, but scarcely available in the rest of the world. Although they have been used for many years, a standardized product first became available in 1995. Fumaderm® contains dimethyl fumarate and ethyl hydrogen calcium fumarate. The single agent dimethyl fumarate has been shown to be effective in early trials in multiple sclerosis.

The combination is given orally, starting with a very low dose and increasingly gradually following published protocols. The final effective level varies tremendously; there may be an 18-fold range. This is probably the safest long-term systemic therapy for psoriasis.

Mechanisms of action. Dimethyl fumarate functions by interacting with the thiol system. As reduced glutathione levels increase, redox-sensitive kinases are blocked. They, in turn, hamper the transfer of the transcription factor (nuclear factor) NF-κB from the cytosol to the nucleus. This has a strong anti-inflammatory effect, as NF-κB facilitates the transcription of genes that code for inflammatory mediators (TNF or IL-8) and adhesion molecules.

Indications. Dimethyl fumarate is approved for moderate to severe psoriasis. With long-term use, it also produces improvement in psoriatic arthritis. Small series suggest it is effective in cutaneous sarcoidosis and granuloma annulare.

Side effects. At the start of therapy, at least 60% of patients have gastrointestinal problems, with nausea, vomiting, and diarrhea, as well as flushing. This is mainly because of overdosage. It is usually not necessary to interrupt therapy. Instead, the dose should be increased very slowly, keeping in mind the tremendous individual variations in effective and tolerated levels. Aspirin can help ameliorate these symptoms. In addition, neutropenia, lymphopenia, and eosinophilia may develop. Rarely, there may be impaired hepatic or renal function.

— Thalidomide, Chloroquine, and Fumaric Acid Esters —

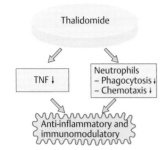

Thalidomide

TNF ↓

Neutrophils
– Phagocytosis ↓
– Chemotaxis ↓

Anti-inflammatory and
immunomodulatory

**Many restrictions on use
but helpful in:**
– Leprosy
– Lupus erythematosus
– Behçet disease
– Pyoderma gangrenosum

Side effects
– Teratogenicity
– Polyneuropathy

Caution: Cannot
use in women of
child-bearing age

A. Thalidomide

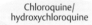

Chloroquine/
hydroxychloroquine

Malaria

Stabilization
of lysosomal
membranes

Porphyrin

Chloroquine

Release of pro-
inflammatory cytokines
and enzymes

Anti-inflammatory

Indications
– Lupus erythematosus,
including REM syndrome
– Behçet disease
– Porphyria cutanea tarda (much lower
dose)

Side effects
– Retinopathy

Caution: Exclude G6PD deficiency
before starting

B. Chloroquine

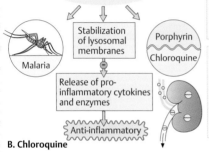

Fumarate/dimethyl
fumarate

Thiol system

Reduced glutathione ↑

Redox-sensitive transcription factors ↓

NF-κB   Nucleus

Cell

TNF, IL-6, IL-12, IL-23 ↓
Adhesion molecules ↓

Anti-inflammatory

Indications
– Psoriasis (marked to severe)

Sarcoidosis
Granuloma annulare

Occasionally
helpful;
not approved

Side effects
– Nausea, vomiting
– Seizures
– Flushing
– Neutropenia and lymphopenia
– Eosinophilia
– Impaired hepatic and renal function

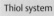

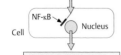

C. Fumaric Acid Esters

10 Medical Therapy

87

A. Nonsteroidal Anti-inflammatory Agents

Nonsteroidal anti-inflammatory agents (NSAIDs) are among the most widely employed medications worldwide. They are analgesic, anti-inflammatory, and antipyretic, with a host of other effects.

Mechanism of action. Just like the prototype agent aspirin or acetylsalicylic acid, many of the NSAIDs are acidic (diclofenac, ibuprofen, indometacin, piroxicam, azapropazone). They all block prostaglandin synthesis by inhibiting cyclo-oxygenase (COX). Newer substances more selectively block COX1 or COX2. In the latter case, there are fewer gastrointestinal effects but an increased cardiovascular risk. Others block leukotriene release by inhibiting lipoxygenase, or are direct leukotriene receptor antagonists (montelukast, zafirlukast). Many of the NSAIDs influence both COX and lipoxygenase to varying degrees and may also modify leukocyte function.

Indications: topical. Bufexamac is similar to diclofenac and was widely used topically in Germany as a replacement for low-potency steroids because of the fear of these agents among the general population, especially in parents and pediatricians. It is either ineffective or certainly not as effective as 1 % hydrocortisone, and also such a potent contact allergen that it was removed from the market in 2010.

Diclofenac combined with hyaluronic acid is approved for treating actinic keratoses. It is not as effective or quick-acting as topical 5-fluorouracil but causes less inflammation, apparently because it interferes with carcinogenesis rather than destroying tissue. The COX inhibition seems to block a key inflammatory step in tumor development. The long-term use of low dose aspirin may reduce the risk of carcinoma of the colon by as much as 50 %.

Indications: systemic. NSAIDs are used for all conditions with musculoskeletal or articular pain, such as rheumatoid arthritis, gout, and polychondritis. They are also effective for superficial thrombophlebitis. In dermatology, they are also often prescribed for patients with erythema nodosum, zoster, erysipelas, or pressure urticaria. In addition, both systemic and topical NSAIDs can help suppress a sunburn reaction if given soon enough after exposure; unfortunately, this is usually impossible because patients present with the burn, not the history of recent exposure.

NSAIDs also have a tumor-protective function in patients with multiple colonic polyps (Gardner syndrome, Ch. 30.3), slowing the progression of polyps into carcinomas, but this benefit must be weighed against other long-term side effects, especially gastrointestinal disease.

The leukotriene inhibitors are approved for asthma, but are also used with varying degrees of success for atopic dermatitis, urticaria, and other allergic reactions.

Side effects. The main problem is gastrointestinal signs and symptoms, especially gastric and duodenal ulcers. In addition, asthma attacks and reduced renal function occur in individuals at risk. Some NSAIDs also cause agranulocytosis. While there are considerable differences between classes, NSAIDs are responsible for a variety of cutaneous drug reaction, including severe skin reactions.

B. Dapsone

Dapsone has been used for over 50 years as a mainstay of leprosy therapy. It is both antibacterial and anti-inflammatory.

Mechanisms of action. As the scientific name diamino-diphenyl sulfone (DADPS) suggests, dapsone is an aniline derivative in which two aniline groups are bound by a sulfone group. Dapsone interferes with COX and lipoxygenase metabolism and impairs phagocytosis, chemotaxis, and lymphocyte function, especially blocking IL-6-dependent inflammation. Just like sulfonamides, it blocks dihydrofolic acid synthesis and is bactericidal against *Mycobacterium leprae*, so that it is a mainstay of all leprosy protocols. Dapsone is administered orally; the usual dose is 50–150 mg daily.

> **Caution:** Prior to therapy, G6PD deficiency and pregnancy must be excluded. Monitor for hematologic problems, especially methemoglobinemia.

Indications. Indications are leprosy, dermatitis herpetiformis, subcorneal pustulosis, bullous pemphigoid, other autoimmune (mainly IgA-associated) bullous diseases, erythema elevatum et diutinum, and other neutrophilic disorders.

Side effects. Possible side effects are methemoglobulinemia, hemolytic anemia, agranulocytosis (rare), and hepatic toxicity.

Nonsteroidal Anti-inflammatory Agents and Dapsone

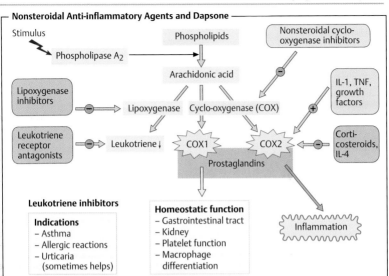

Leukotriene inhibitors

Indications
– Asthma
– Allergic reactions
– Urticaria
  (sometimes helps)

Homeostatic function
– Gastrointestinal tract
– Kidney
– Platelet function
– Macrophage
  differentiation

Inflammation

Nonsteroidal cyclo-oxygenase inhibitors

Indications
– Thrombophlebitis
– Erythema nodosum
– Arthritis (many types)
– Adjunct for zoster, erysipelas,
  sunburn, pressure urticaria

Side effects
– Gastrointestinal ulcers
– Asthma
– Impaired renal function
– Drug exanthems, phototoxicity
– Agranulocytosis (agent specific)

A. Nonsteroidal Anti-inflammatory Agents

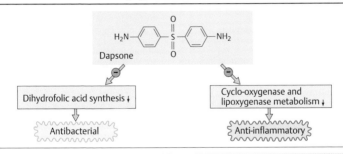

Dapsone

Dihydrofolic acid synthesis ↓

Antibacterial

Cyclo-oxygenase and
lipoxygenase metabolism ↓

Anti-inflammatory

Indications
– Leprosy
– Dermatitis herpetiformis
– Bullous pemphigoid
– Linear IgA dermatosis
– Erythema elevatum et diutinum

Side effects
– Methemoglobulinemia
  ► Hemolytic anemia
– Hepatic toxicity
– Agranulocytosis

B. Dapsone

Cytostatic agents are used in dermatology to treat metastatic melanoma, squamous cell carcinoma, Merkel cell carcinoma, and some lymphomas, as well as in severe autoimmune disorders where they function as immunosuppressive agents by reducing lymphocyte functions. There are several types of agents that act at different points in the cell cycle or cell metabolism. All somewhat selectively kill or damage more rapidly dividing cells, which in most instances includes tumor cells. Those normal tissues that also divide rapidly are especially likely to be damaged during therapy. Problems may include:

- anagen effluvium by damaging the hair bulb
- diarrhea and intestinal erosions or ulcers because of reduced epithelial turnover
- bone marrow suppression
- immunodeficiency because of reduced levels of lymphocytes
- fertility problems because of germ cell damage
- DNA damage, which can be teratogenic damaging offspring, as well as carcinogenic in the patient themselves
- increased risk of secondary malignancies, such as leukemia.

To maximize the cytotoxic effects on the tumor cells, and minimize the side effects, cytostatic agents are usually administered in combination, in complex chemotherapy protocols.

The most common side effect is nausea, but serotonin antagonists given prior to chemotherapy help to control this problem.

Mechanisms of action. There are several major categories of agents with different mechanisms of action. They include:

- indirect DNA interaction through:
  - inhibitors of mitosis (vincristine, vinblastine, paclitaxel)
  - antimetabolites (folic acid antagonists, purine and pyrimidine analogs)
- direct DNA interaction through:
  - alkylating agents (cyclophosphamide, dacarbazine, temozolomide, carboplatin)
  - tumoricidal antibiotics (etoposide, doxorubicin, epirubicin)
- molecular therapy (imatinib, bexarotene, tretinoin).

A. Indirect Inhibition of DNA Function

■ Antimitotic Agents

Vincristine and vinblastine are known as vinca alkaloids, because they are derived from the Madagascar periwinkle *Catharanthus roseus*, which was also known as *Vinca rosea*. They stop mitosis in metaphase by inhibiting the contractile protein tubulin, which is a main component of the spindle. Vincristine is neurotoxic, while vinblastine is myelosuppressive and may also cause paralytic ileus.

Indications. Indications are Kaposi sarcoma, lymphoma, and Langerhans cell disease, in combinations for melanoma.

The *taxanes* paclitaxel and docetaxel block spindle formation by inhibiting depolarization of the microtubules. They are widely used in oncology, in dermatology for Kaposi sarcoma, and as second-line therapy for melanoma.

> **Caution:** Side effects include polyneuropathy and hypersensitivity syndrome.

Colchicine is a toxic alkaloid, derived from *Colchicum autumnale*, the autumn crocus, which also inhibits the spindle. The classic indication for colchicine is to treat gout. It is used in dermatology for Behçet disease, leukocytoclastic vasculitis, and other conditions involving neutrophils. Gastrointestinal toxicity is usually the dose-limiting factor.

■ Antimetabolites

1. Folic acid antagonists

Folic acid analogs serve as a false substrate for dihydrofolate reductase, which converts dihydrofolic acid to tetrahydrofolic acid. This in turn interferes with the synthesis of thymidine and purines, which blocks DNA synthesis, and, in higher doses, protein synthesis. This block can be bypassed by the administration of tetrahydrofolic acid (leucovorin).

The most important member of the group is methotrexate (MTX), which is both cytotoxic and immunomodulatory. It is generally given once weekly, either orally or parenterally, in doses of 15–25 mg. In psoriasis, the Weinstein regimen is sometimes used—3 doses of 5–7.5 mg, every 12 hours, once weekly.

Indications. Indications are moderate to severe psoriasis, psoriatic arthritis, pityriasis rubra pilaris, autoimmune dermatoses (bullous diseases, lupus erythematosus, dermatomyositis), and sarcoidosis. Because of the extensive experience with MTX, it is often used as a steroid-sparing agent in these and other settings. It is also used for advanced mycosis fungoides.

> **Note:** MTX can be effectively and safely combined with phototherapy, anti-TNF or anti-IL-12/IL-23 therapy.

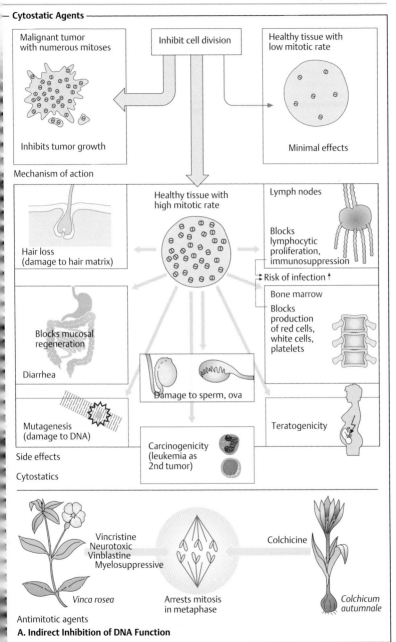

Cytostatic Agents

Malignant tumor with numerous mitoses

Inhibit cell division

Healthy tissue with low mitotic rate

Inhibits tumor growth

Minimal effects

Mechanism of action

Healthy tissue with high mitotic rate

Lymph nodes

Blocks lymphocytic proliferation, immunosuppression

Risk of infection ↑

Hair loss (damage to hair matrix)

Bone marrow

Blocks production of red cells, white cells, platelets

Blocks mucosal regeneration

Diarrhea

Damage to sperm, ova

Mutagenesis (damage to DNA)

Teratogenicity

Carcinogenicity (leukemia as 2nd tumor)

Side effects

Cytostatics

Vincristine Neurotoxic Vinblastine Myelosuppressive

Colchicine

Vinca rosea

Arrests mitosis in metaphase

Colchicum autumnale

Antimitotic agents

A. Indirect Inhibition of DNA Function

10 Medical Therapy

91

Side effects. Contraception is essential for both women and men. A side effect is liver fibrosis or cirrhosis, especially if combined with alcohol. Some groups recommend liver biopsy after a total dose of 1.5 g. Newer results from patients with rheumatoid arthritis show that the risk of liver damage was overestimated. Rare but severe reactions include alveolitis, bone marrow depression, and renal damage.

2. Nucleic acid analogs

Purine and pyrimidine analogs are false bases (6-mercaptopurine, 5-fluouracil) or nucleosides with the wrong sugar moiety (cytarabine). They block DNA/RNA (ribonucleic acid) synthesis, or lead to the formation of incorrect DNA sequences. 6-Mercaptopurine is formed in vivo from its inactive precursor azathioprine, which is frequently used as an immunosuppressive agent (Ch. 10.3). In combination with corticosteroids, it serves as a steroid-sparing drug.

> **Caution:** Thiopurine-S-methyltransferase (TPMT) deactivates 6-mercaptopurine; determine levels of this enzyme prior to therapy. Metabolism of 6-mercaptopurine is blocked by allopurinol, so the two cannot be combined.

Indications. Indications are bullous autoimmune diseases, lupus erythematosus, dermatomyositis, and vasculitis.
Side effects. Side effects are bone marrow depression and abnormal liver function tests; contraception is not mandatory.

B. Direct DNA Interactions

These substances bind directly, or after being metabolized in a covalent fashion to DNA bases, leading to cross-links or breaks, as well as inducing apoptosis signals.

■ Alkylating Agents

Cross-linking of DNA interferes with uncoiling and splitting. Long-term low-dose therapy predisposes to the development of rapidly dividing secondary malignancies. The active metabolite of cyclophosphamide causes hemorrhagic cystitis. Dacarbazine is metabolized in the liver and temozolomide in the tumor cells, to the active methyl diazonium form. The latter two are front-line therapy for melanoma. Alkylating agents cause severe nausea at the start of therapy and modest myelosuppression after 21 days.

The platins (cisplatin, carboplatin, oxiplatin) are especially effective at forming cross-links. They cause marked nausea, myelosuppression, peripheral neuropathy, and nephrotoxicity. They are used in combination with taxanes in melanoma, as back-up therapy. Fotemustine is a nitrosourea alkylating agent used in melanoma.

■ Cytostatic Antibiotics / Topoisomerase Inhibitors

These cause breaks in DNA strands as they fit into the double helix and produce free oxygen radicals. Doxorubicin (**caution:** cardiac toxicity) and daunorubicin are used for vascular tumors. They are usually administered in liposomal preparations, which reduce their toxicity and increase delivery to vascular cells.

Epirubicin and etoposide are used in protocols for metastatic Merkel cell and squamous cell carcinomas.

C. Molecular Therapy

This refers to a heterogenous group of small molecules and antibodies that have been developed to inhibit specific molecules. Retinoids also fall into this group.

Imatinib is a tyrosine kinase inhibitor, which inhibits the signals of platelet-derived growth factor and related tyrosine kinases. It is effective for disorders that feature an abnormality of the c-Kit receptor in its intracellular component.
Indications. Dermatofibrosarcoma protuberans, and, less often, mastocytosis and acral melanoma if c-kit mutation is in right location.

Epidermal growth factor receptor (EGFR) inhibitors often cause a rosacea-like eruption, whose severity correlates with a better response. They may be effective in combination for metastatic squamous cell carcinoma. Angiogenesis inhibitors are just starting to be employed.

A new approach to melanoma therapy is the targeted inhibition of the MAPK signaling pathway. Vemurafenib interferes with the mutated BRAFV600 and improves survival rates of patients with metastatic melanoma but may also cause other cancers.

D. Topical Use

Both 5-fluorouracil and podophyllotoxin are used topically. They induce a severe toxic dermatitis which is effective against actinic keratoses, warts, condyloma, and Bowen disease.

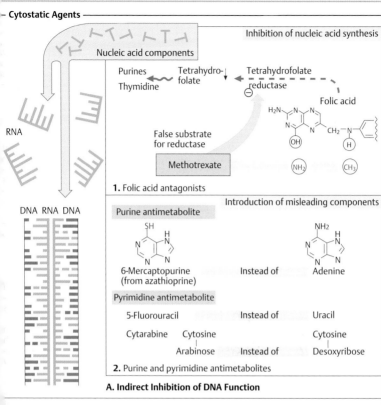

Cytostatic Agents

Inhibition of nucleic acid synthesis

Nucleic acid components

Purines
Thymidine ← Tetrahydro-folate ← Tetrahydrofolate reductase ⊖ ← Folic acid

H₂N

False substrate for reductase

Methotrexate

1. Folic acid antagonists

Introduction of misleading components

Purine antimetabolite

SH

6-Mercaptopurine (from azathioprine)   Instead of   Adenine   NH₂

Pyrimidine antimetabolite

5-Fluorouracil   Instead of   Uracil

Cytarabine   Cytosine   Cytosine
                    Arabinose   Instead of   Desoxyribose

2. Purine and pyrimidine antimetabolites

RNA

DNA RNA DNA

A. Indirect Inhibition of DNA Function

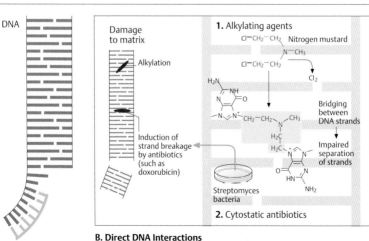

DNA

Damage to matrix

Alkylation

Induction of strand breakage by antibiotics (such as doxorubicin)

Streptomyces bacteria

1. Alkylating agents

Cl—CH₂—CH₂   Nitrogen mustard
        N—CH₃
Cl—CH₂—CH₂   Cl₂

H₂N
        NH
        O
        N⁺—CH₂—CH₂—N   CH₃
        H₂C
        H₂C—N⁺
        O
        HN
            NH₂

Bridging between DNA strands

Impaired separation of strands

2. Cytostatic antibiotics

B. Direct DNA Interactions

A. Patient–Bacteria Interactions

When bacteria inhabit the skin or epithelial surface, the term *colonization* is used. Colonization requires not only the presence of the appropriate physiologic bacteria but also proper keratinocyte function and normal intercellular space composition. If pathogenic bacteria cross the epithelial barrier and enter the tissue, then an *infection* is present, but the innate immune system usually controls the invaders without producing clinical signs and symptoms. If these first defense mechanisms are unsuccessful, then an infectious disease develops, often with fever, malaise, and other more specific clinical features.

B. Site of Action

The ideal antibiotic kills or inhibits bacteria while causing little or no damage to the host cells. Attractive sites of action are bacterial cell walls, which are not present in humans.

C. Mechanisms of Action and Resistance

Bacteria may be killed (*bactericidal effect*) or they may remain alive but be unable to duplicate (*bacteriostatic effect*).

If an agent is only effective against a limited number of bacteria, it has a narrow spectrum (such as penicillin G which only works against streptococci or *Treponema pallidum*). Broad-spectrum antibiotics attack many different microbes.

If bacteria are not affected by an antibiotic because of their natural metabolism, there is *natural resistance*. If resistance develops in an initially sensitive strain, as a result of a mutation or transfer of genetic material, then this is referred to as *acquired resistance.*

In many settings, resistance is transferred when a bacterium acquires a resistance plasmid from another strain. The more often an antibiotic is employed, the more likely it is that resistant strains will develop. As resistant strains are exposed to other antibiotics, then multiresistant strains develop such as methicillin-resistant *Staphylococcus aureus* (MRSA) and multidrug-resistant *Mycobacterium tuberculosis.*

Note: When giving antibiotics:
- have a definite indication! Many skin diseases can be treated with topical disinfectants, which can be just as effective without any risk of developing resistance
- try to choose an agent with a narrow spectrum aimed against the organism most likely to be present. Do not routinely use broad-spectrum antibiotics. If the clinical situation warrants initial use of a broad-spectrum agent, perform bacterial culture and sensitivity studies and switch to a more specific agent as soon as feasible
- reserve antibiotics such as vancomycin for problem situations like MRSA infection in an ill patient
- do not use antibiotics in topical form that the patient may later need systemically. The risk of sensitization is high.

D. Classes of Antibiotics

■ 1. Inhibitors of Cell-wall Synthesis

Bacteria are surrounded by a stable cell wall which protects the cell membrane from breaking under high osmotic pressure. The cell wall consists of a network or frame of linked peptidoglycans. The building blocks, two acetylated amino sugars with a peptide chain, are synthesized in the bacteria, pass through the cell membrane, and then link into the meshwork by transpeptidases. Gram-positive bacteria have a much thicker cell wall.

Inhibitors of cell-wall synthesis are bactericidal, because the cells burst when they lack a stable wall. Agents in this group include β-lactam antibiotics (penicillins and cephalosporins), as well as glycopeptide antibiotics such as vancomycin, which competitively block the addition of glycosylated peptides.

Penicillins. Penicillins are bactericidal, inhibiting transpeptidase. The basic substance is penicillin G (benzylpenicillin), which was isolated from the mold *Penicillium notatum*. The backbone of the molecule is *6-aminopenicillanic acid* (which is not antibacterial) with a four-member β-lactam ring which blocks the transpeptidase.

Penicillin is eliminated rapidly by the kidneys; the half-life is around 30 minutes. The duration of action can be enhanced by:
- using a high dose, to ensure the minimum inhibitory concentration of the antibiotic in the serum is exceeded for a longer time

Antibacterial Agents

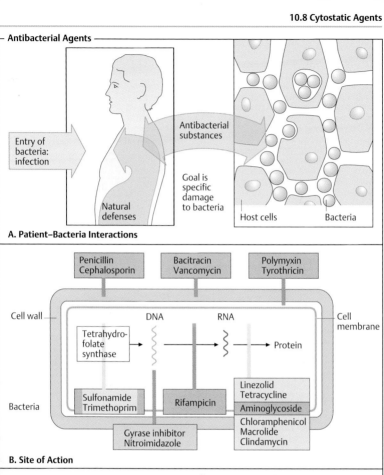

Antibacterial substances

Entry of bacteria: infection

Goal is specific damage to bacteria

Natural defenses

Host cells   Bacteria

A. Patient–Bacteria Interactions

Penicillin
Cephalosporin

Bacitracin
Vancomycin

Polymyxin
Tyrothricin

Cell wall

DNA   RNA

Cell membrane

Tetrahydro-folate synthase → DNA → RNA → Protein

Bacteria

Sulfonamide
Trimethoprim

Rifampicin

Linezolid
Tetracycline
Aminoglycoside
Chloramphenicol
Macrolide
Clindamycin

Gyrase inhibitor
Nitroimidazole

B. Site of Action

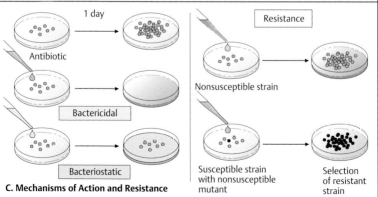

1 day

Resistance

Antibiotic

Bactericidal

Nonsusceptible strain

Bacteriostatic

Susceptible strain with nonsusceptible mutant

Selection of resistant strain

C. Mechanisms of Action and Resistance

- administering probenecid, which competitively inhibits renal acid secretion and thus delays the excretion of penicillin G
- using intramuscular depot products, where penicillin G is combined with substances with positive amino groups (procaine, benzathine) forming poorly soluble salts which then, over time, release the antibiotic.

Depot preparations are routinely used in treating syphilis and for prophylaxis in patients with recurrent erysipelas.

Penicillin G is well tolerated, but can lead to allergic reactions in up to 5% of users—typically a macular exanthem but in some instances anaphylactic shock (<0.05%). One must always enquire about penicillin allergy, as it is so common. Some 5%–10% of those with penicillin allergy will also react to cephalosporins because they share the β-lactam ring. In very high doses, or when administered intrathecally, penicillin G can causes seizures.

Disadvantages of penicillin G include:

- narrow spectrum
- it is only used parenterally, as stomach acids split the lactam ring, inactivating the drug
- bacterial β-lactamases, such as penicillinase in staphylococci, inactivate penicillin G making the organisms resistant.

The properties of the penicillin can be changed by substituting the β-lactam ring, making the agents:

- acid stable and suited for oral use (penicillin V, oxacillin, amoxicillin)
- resistant to penicillinase—isoxazolyl-l-penicillins (oxacillin, dicloxacillin, flucloxacillin) are effective against staphylococci
- have a wider spectrum—the aminopenicillin amoxicillin is also effective against Gram-negative bacteria (*E. coli, Salmonella*). The carboxypenicillins (ticarcillin) and acyl aminopenicillins (mezlocillin, piperacillin) are even effective against some pseudomonas species. These agents can be combined with penicillinase inhibitors (clavulanic acid, sulbactam) further increasing the spectrum.

Indications: penicillinase-resistant agents are needed for staphylococcal infections such as impetigo, furuncles and carbuncles, severe paronychia, and secondary infections in atopic dermatitis. Broad-spectrum derivatives are used for borreliosis (children and pregnant women) and listeriosis.

Cephalosporins. This group also works by blocking transpeptidases and is thus bactericidal. They are acid resistant but poorly absorbed, so most are given parentally, although some (cephalexin) are used orally. They are penicillinase resistant and have a broad spectrum.

Indications: recurrent erysipelas, neuroborreliosis, severe Gram-negative infections.

Side effects: well tolerated, these drugs may interact with anti-penicillin antibodies, and there is occasional nephrotoxicity, bleeding (vitamin K antagonist), and alcohol intolerance.

Other inhibitors of cell-wall synthesis. Glycopeptide antibiotics such as vancomycin inhibit the transfer of glycosylated amino peptides through the cell membrane. They are effective against Gram-positive bacteria.

Indications: these are a last-resort choice for severe MRSA infection, as well as being one option for pseudomembranous colitis (proliferation of *Clostridium difficile* in the gut as a complication of antibiotic therapy).

■ 2. Inhibitors of Tetrahydrofolic Acid Synthesis

Tetrahydrofolic acid (THF) is a coenzyme for the synthesis of purines and amino acids. THF is formed from dihydrofolic acid (DHF) through DHF-reductase.

Sulfonamides. This large group of antibiotics resembles para-aminobenzoic acid and serves as a false substrate for synthesis of DHF, with a bacteriostatic action.

Trimethoprim. Trimethoprim blocks bacterial DHF-reductase, which is more sensitive than the human enzyme; it rarely causes bone marrow depression.

Co-trimoxazole. This is a combination of trimethoprim and the sulfonamide sulfamethoxazole. Through the combined mode of action, the antibacterial action is more effective, while the risk of resistance is reduced.

Indications: Gram-negative infections, especially Gram-negative toe web infections but also other cutaneous lesions. Co-trimoxazole is also used for toxoplasmosis prophylaxis and both prophylaxis and therapy of *Pneumocystis jirovecii* pneumonia in HIV/AIDS patients.

Side effects: hemolytic anemia in patients lacking G6PD; neurotoxicity and hepatotoxicity, and a common cause of severe skin reactions, including toxic epidermal necrolysis.

> **Caution:** Do not use in late pregnancy or in newborns because of the risk of kernicterus.

Antibacterial Agents

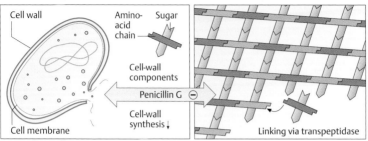

Action of penicillin G

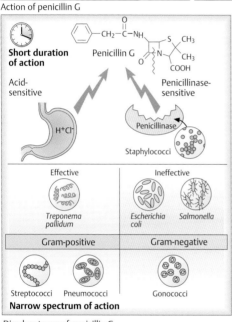

Short duration of action

Acid-sensitive

Penicillin G

Penicillinase-sensitive

Penicillinase

Staphylococci

Effective	Ineffective
Treponema pallidum	Escherichia coli Salmonella
Gram-positive	Gram-negative
Streptococci Pneumococci	Gonococci

Narrow spectrum of action

Disadvantages of penicillin G

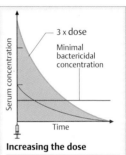

Increasing the dose

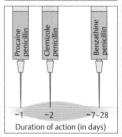

Procaine penicillin   Clemizole penicillin   Benzathine penicillin

~1   ~2   ~7–28

Duration of action (in days)

Depot forms

Alternatives

	Acid	Penicillinase	Spectrum
Penicillin V	Resistant	Sensitive	Narrow
Oxacillin	Resistant	Resistant	Narrow
Amoxicillin	Resistant	Sensitive	Broad

Derivatives of penicillin G

Cephalexin	Resistant	Resistant, but sensitive to cephalosporinase	Broad

Cephalosporin

1. Inhibitors of cell-wall synthesis

D. Classes of Antibiotics

■ 3. Inhibitors of DNA Function

The enzyme gyrase alters the spatial orientation of the DNA molecule by opening and closing strands.
Gyrase inhibitors (quinolones). Gyrase inhibitors block the closing of opened strands and thus have a bactericidal effect. The old substance nalidixic acid is only effective against Gram-negative bacteria; the newer substances such as ofloxacin, ciprofloxacin, and norfloxacin have a broader spectrum and achieve high systemic concentrations.
Indications: skin and soft-tissue infections, pelvic inflammatory disease, prostatitis, gonorrhea.
Side effects: neurotoxicity (confusion, seizures), gastrointestinal disturbances, macular exanthem, cartilage damage.

Caution: Do not use during pregnancy or in nursing mothers or in children.

Metronidazole (nitroimidazole). This damages DNA in obligate anaerobic bacteria, and is thus bactericidal.
Indications: orally for anaerobic and protozoan infections; agent of choice for *C. difficile*. Used topically in rosacea and perioral dermatitis for anti-inflammatory effects.
Rifampicin. Rifampicin blocks transcription of RNA polymerase and is bactericidal and effective against a broad spectrum of Gram-positive and Gram-negative bacteria, especially mycobacteria.
Indications: leprosy and tuberculosis; sometimes for chronic staphylococcal infections.

■ 4. Inhibitors of Protein Synthesis

A variety of antibiotics hamper protein synthesis, usually by interfering with ribosomal function. Since there are some similarities between mitochondrial and bacterial ribosomes, there is a risk of toxicity.
Tetracyclines. Tetracycline, or more often its derivatives doxycycline and minocycline, consist of four aromatic rings and irreversibly bind to 30S ribosomes and thus inhibit binding of aminoacyl-tRNA to the DNA on the 70S ribosome. They have a broad spectrum of action against intracellular bacteria but are bacteriostatic. They also have an anti-inflammatory effects at low doses. Resistance is common.
Indications: infections with mycoplasma, chlamydia, borrelia and atypical mycobacteria; widely used in acne and rosacea for anti-inflammatory effects, also topically.

Side effects: gastrointestinal disturbances—tetracycline is inactivated via complex formation with milk or antacids (thus it should be taken 2 hours before or after meals); this is less of a problem with derivatives.

Caution: Do not use in combination with isotretinoin or acitretin because of the risk of pseudotumor cerebri.

Aminoglycosides. This group irreversibly binds to the 30S ribosome stopping initiation of synthesis, as well as leading to misreading errors. These drugs are bactericidal and useful primarily against Gram-negative bacteria. They are not effective against anaerobic bacteria as oxygen is required for their uptake, and they work poorly against intracellular bacteria. They work in synergy with β-lactams, which damage the cell wall and enhance their entry. Resistance is common.
Representative members include gentamicin, tobramycin, amikacin, streptomycin, and neomycin. Spectinomycin is similar and also blocks 30S ribosomes but does not cause misreading errors.
Indications: infections with Gram-negative anaerobic bacteria. Spectinomycin is used against gonorrhea. Neomycin is widely used topically.

Note: While other aminoglycosides (especially gentamicin) are available for topical use, they should be avoided, as the risk of sensitization is high and then the patient may be deprived of a life-saving systemic drug because of cross-reactions.

Side effects: ototoxicity and nephrotoxicity.
Macrolides. Erythromycin and its less acid-labile derivatives azithromycin, clarithromycin, and roxithromycin block the movement of the ribosome complex along the mRNA (messenger RNA), and are primarily bacteriostatic for Gram-positive bacteria. They are often used in patients with penicillin allergy or when organisms are resistant.
Indications: infections with streptococci and staphylococci (widespread resistance in many communities), mycoplasma, chlamydia, and borrelia.
Lincosamides. Clindamycin is a synthetic chlorinated analog of lincomycin. It is bacteriostatic against Gram-positive and Gram-negative bacteria. In the skin, it should be reserved for resistant staphylococcal infections and for streptococcal infections in patients with peni-

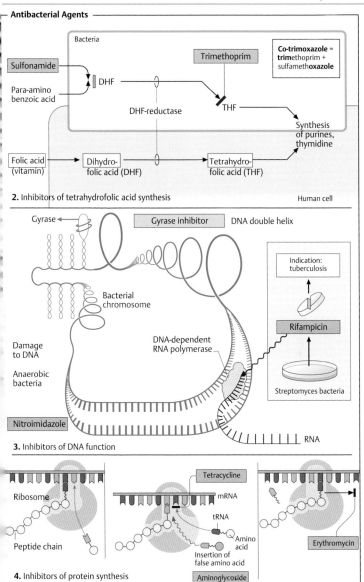

Antibacterial Agents

Bacteria

Co-trimoxazole = **trim**ethoprim + sulfameth**oxazole**

Sulfonamide

Para-amino benzoic acid

DHF

Trimethoprim

DHF-reductase

THF

Synthesis of purines, thymidine

Folic acid (vitamin)

Dihydro-folic acid (DHF)

Tetrahydro-folic acid (THF)

2. Inhibitors of tetrahydrofolic acid synthesis

Human cell

Gyrase

Gyrase inhibitor

DNA double helix

Bacterial chromosome

Damage to DNA

Anaerobic bacteria

DNA-dependent RNA polymerase

Indication: tuberculosis

Rifampicin

Streptomyces bacteria

Nitroimidazole

RNA

3. Inhibitors of DNA function

Ribosome

Peptide chain

Tetracycline

mRNA

tRNA

Amino acid

Insertion of false amino acid

Aminoglycoside

Erythromycin

4. Inhibitors of protein synthesis

D. Classes of Antibiotics

cillin allergy. It should be avoided for minor infections or acne. It is widely used topically for acne.

> **Caution:** There is a risk of pseudomembranous colitis caused by *Clostridium difficile.*

E. Topical Antibiotics

Topical antibiotics should be used reluctantly because of two risks. They may increase the level of resistant microorganisms in a community, not just in a patient. This has been demonstrated for the use of topical erythromycin in acne and the development of resistant staphylococci in family members. The second problem is the development of allergic contact dermatitis to the topical antibiotics; for many years, neomycin was the leading topical sensitizer. Once a patient is sensitive to a topical antibiotic, they generally cannot use the systemic agent or any related drugs because of the risk of a hematogenous allergic contact dermatitis or baboon syndrome (Ch. 29.1).

Topical antibiotics are used primarily for bacterial skin infections, especially simple impetigo, wound infections, and acne (erythromycin and clindamycin). Their use should be carefully considered.

Effective agents that are not used systemically and that rarely cause allergic contact dermatitis are listed next.

Fusidic acid. This is widely used in Europe for impetigo and erythrasma; it inhibits elongation factor in Gram-positive bacteria. There is a very low risk of sensitization or resistance.

Mupirocin. This is used primarily for impetigo and other superficial skin infections, as well for prophylaxis in patients with nasal colonization with staphylococci. It is even effective against MRSA.

Retamulpin. This is one of the pleuromutilins, antibiotics widely employed systemically in animal medicine; it was recently released for topical use against staphylococci and streptococci.

F. Disinfectants

> **Note:** Whenever possible, disinfectants should be used instead of topical antibiotics. The risk of developing resistant strains is almost zero.

There are many categories of disinfectants including oxidizing agents, alcohols, aldehydes, halogens, phenols, tensides, and organic acids. They function by denaturing proteins, reacting with nucleic acids, or damaging enzymes. Disinfectants are most effective against bacteria (Gram-positive > Gram-negative > mycobacteria). They generally do not destroy spores and only a few are virucidal (formaldehyde).

The most commonly used *wound disinfectants* are povidone-iodine, octenidine, and triclosan. Older favorites such as hydrogen peroxide, potassium permanganate, and the whole spectrum of dyestuffs (gentian violet, brilliant green, and many more) are best avoided, as they are clearly less effective.

Hand disinfection prior to surgery is best accomplished with iodine tinctures, chlorhexidine solution, and alcoholic mixes.

Hand disinfection between patients is accomplished with alcohols, aldehydes, phenols, or tensides. Agents that are applied, rubbed, and wiped are more effective than washing hands between patients.

Surfaces and instruments can be cleaned with tensides, aldehydes, halogens, and phenols. Here the agents can be more toxic because skin compatibility is not an issue.

Antibacterial Agents

Cave

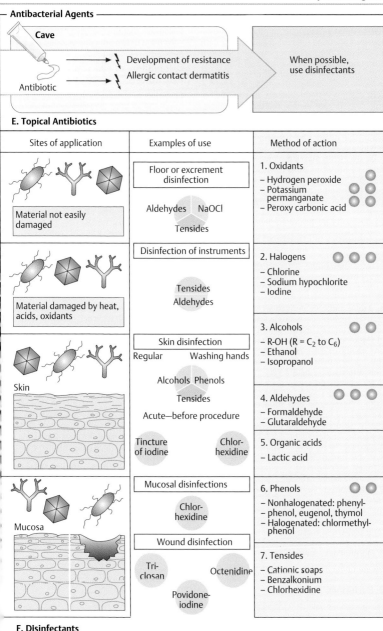

Antibiotic → Development of resistance

→ Allergic contact dermatitis

When possible, use disinfectants

E. Topical Antibiotics

Sites of application	Examples of use	Method of action
Material not easily damaged	Floor or excrement disinfection — Aldehydes / NaOCl / Tensides	1. Oxidants – Hydrogen peroxide – Potassium permanganate – Peroxy carbonic acid
Material damaged by heat, acids, oxidants	Disinfection of instruments — Tensides / Aldehydes	2. Halogens – Chlorine – Sodium hypochlorite – Iodine
Skin	Skin disinfection — Regular / Washing hands — Alcohols / Phenols / Tensides — Acute—before procedure — Tincture of iodine / Chlorhexidine	3. Alcohols – R-OH (R = C_2 to C_6) – Ethanol – Isopropanol
		4. Aldehydes – Formaldehyde – Glutaraldehyde
		5. Organic acids – Lactic acid
Mucosa	Mucosal disinfections — Chlorhexidine — Wound disinfection — Triclosan / Octenidine / Povidone-iodine	6. Phenols – Nonhalogenated: phenyl-phenol, eugenol, thymol – Halogenated: chlormethyl-phenol
		7. Tensides – Cationic soaps – Benzalkonium – Chlorhexidine

F. Disinfectants

10 Medical Therapy

Most fungal infections are localized, and limited to the skin, hair, nails, or mucosa. Systemic mycoses affecting internal organs vary greatly in different geographie regions and are more common in immunocompromised individuals (HIV/AIDS, leukemia, chemotherapy). There is a broad array of topical antifungal agents as well as some systemic choices. As with the terminology for antibiotics, the terms *fungicidal* (killing the fungi) and *fungistatic* (inhibiting growth) antimycotics are used. Another parallel is the distinction between narrow- and broad-spectrum antimycotic agents.

To selectively attack the fungi and spare the human cells, many modern antimycotic agents interfere with the formation of the fungal cell wall, for example by inhibiting ergosterol synthesis or by forming damaging pores in the wall.

A. Inhibitors of Ergosterol Synthesis

Ergosterol is a crucial component of the cytoplasmic membrane of fungal cells and is not found in human cells. The following agents interfere with various steps in ergosterol synthesis:

1. Azole/imidazole derivatives. Azoles are effective against dermatophytes, yeasts, and molds, primarily in a fungistatic fashion. Most of the older azoles (clotrimazole, miconazole, and many others) are poorly absorbed and thus used primarily topically. Ketoconazole is best absorbed at acid levels, is highly lipophilic, and is currently primarily used topically, although it was introduced as a systemic agent. Fluconazole and itraconazole are the two systemic azoles available, and are used for severe skin infections, onychomycosis, and systemic involvement. Voriconazole and posaconazole are new substances designed for systemic fungal infections, especially in immunosuppressed hosts.

Side effects: hepatotoxic, teratogenic.

2. Allylamines (squalene epoxidase inhibitors). This group is very effective against dermatophytes, but less useful for yeasts and molds. Terbinafine is used systemically and topically, while naftifine is only available for topical use.

3. Morpholines. Amorolfine is used as a cream or nail lacquer.

B. Pyridones

The pyridones have as wide a spectrum as the azoles. They are chelators and form reactive oxygen free radicals, with a fungicidal action.

Ciclopirox olamine is used topically for involvement of the skin, mucosa, and nails.

C. Inhibitors of Cell Wall or DNA Synthesis

Griseofulvin. Griseofulvin is derived from a mold and is only effective against dermatophytes. It is only effective systemically and is deposited in newly formed keratin of the skin, hair, and nails. It functions by inhibiting the cell spindle and interfering with the production of chitin, a key component of the cell wall. In the skin, one sometimes speaks of a "sprinkler effect," as griseofulvin is secreted in the eccrine sweat. It must be given until the keratinized structures have been completely renewed, which means 12–24 months for nails, limiting its utility.

Flucytosine. Flucytosine is converted into 5-fluorouracil by a cytosine deaminase found in fungi and yeasts but not in humans. It then functions as a false metabolite interfering with DNA/RNA synthesis, with a fungicidal effect. Although it was introduced for candidiasis, it is also effective against dermatophytes. It is rapidly absorbed, well tolerated, and can be combined with amphotericin B to reduce toxicity.

D. Polyene Antibiotics

These pore-forming agents such as amphotericin B and nystatin are produced by *Streptomyces* species. They complex with sterols in the cell membranes of fungi to form pores. The increased permeability has a fungicidal effect. Amphotericin B is poorly absorbed and must be given i. v. Nowadays, it is generally administered in its liposomal form, and used for systemic fungal infections and leishmaniasis. Oral nystatin is only effective in the gastrointestinal tract. Topical nystatin is only effective against yeasts; topical amphotericin B also works against dermatophytes but is very expensive and rarely used.

Antimycotic Agents

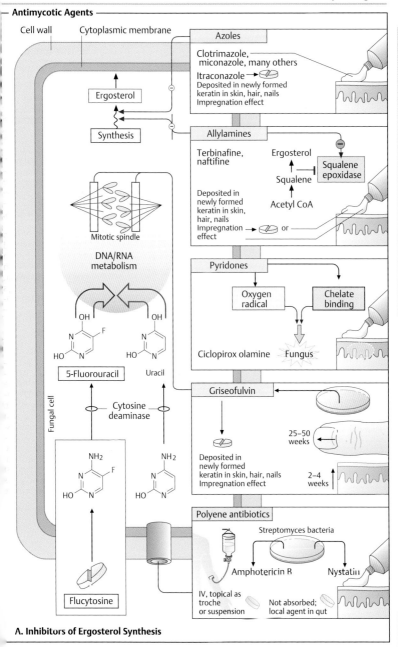

A. Inhibitors of Ergosterol Synthesis

A. Mechanisms of Action

Most virustatic agents generally interfere with DNA synthesis by providing false DNA building blocks (purines, pyrimidines, pyrophosphates), which block DNA polymerase. The points of attack against retroviruses like HIV are reverse transcriptase or proteases. Other agents inhibit uncoating or removal of the lipid shell, which is an important step in binding to the cell membrane needed for the introduction of nucleic acids into the host cell. Others inhibit the manufacture of a new viral capsule; protease inhibitors work in this way.

Since all these agents are virustatic, inhibiting viral growth but not killing viruses, it is important that they are started as soon as possible in the course of the infection. For example, in recurrent herpes simplex, they should be given at the first warning sign.

■ Systemic Agents

Aciclovir. Aciclovir is the most widely used antiviral agent. It is usually given orally but should be administered systemically in severe infections or immunocompromised hosts.

Aciclovir is a guanine analog. After phosphorylation and then activation by thymidine kinase, aciclovir functions as a false building block, interrupting viral DNA polymerase. Since viral thymidine kinases are 300× more effective than human thymidine kinase in activating aciclovir, the effects are almost entirely limited to the virally infected cells.

Indications: herpes simplex, zoster.
Side effects: renal and CNS toxicity.

Caution: Aciclovir is eliminated by the kidneys. When given i.v., it can cause acute renal failure. Thus, with preexisting impairment of renal function, creatinine levels must be monitored and the dose reduced.

Valaciclovir. Valaciclovir is a prodrug that is converted to aciclovir in the body. It thus has increased bioavailability but is otherwise similar and given orally.

Famciclovir/penciclovir. Famciclovir is the prodrug for penciclovir and offers better bioavailability. These newer nucleosides work in the same way as aciclovir to inhibit DNA polymerase. They have a longer intracellular half-life so that lower doses are effective.

Indications: herpes genitalis, zoster.
Side effects: nausea, CNS toxicity.

Brivudin. This agent is another inhibitor of DNA polymerase but in vitro is 100-fold more effective than aciclovir. It can be used orally in a single daily dose. It is effective against varicella zoster virus (VZV) and herpes simplex virus (HSV)1 but not against HSV2.

Indication: zoster in immunocompetent adults.
Side effects: nausea.

Caution: Brivudin cannot be given with 5-fluorouracil and other 5-fluoropyrimidines. There must be a 4-week interval. A metabolite of brivudin irreversibly inhibits dihydropyrimidine dehydrogenase, which is required for the metabolism of pyrimidines, leading to increased levels and potentially fatal toxic side effects from 5-fluorouracil.

Foscarnet. Foscarnet is a pyrophosphate analog which blocks the binding site for pyrophosphates on viral DNA polymerase.

Indications: infections with aciclovir-resistant herpes viruses and severe cytomegalovirus infections in HIV/AIDS.
Side effects: cardiac, renal, and hematopoietic toxicity.

■ Topical Agents

The effectiveness of topical virostatic agents is minimal. Aciclovir cream is approved for recurrent herpes labialis, but we only employ aciclovir systemically. Foscarnet 2% cream can be used to treat herpes simplex infections. Idoxuridine, another nucleoside analog, is effective for herpes keratitis.

Antiviral Agents

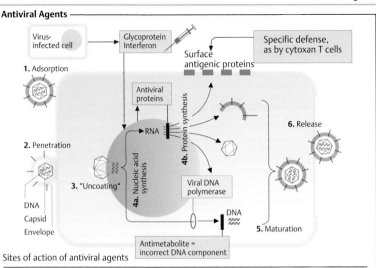

Sites of action of antiviral agents

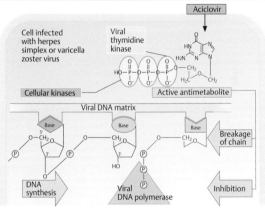

Mechanism of action of aciclovir

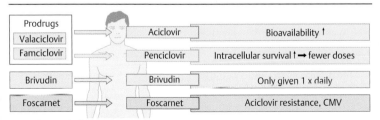

Metabolism and advantages of various agents

A. Mechanisms of Action

B. Antiviral Agents in HIV/AIDS

HIV infections are always treated with a combination of 3–4 different agents—just as with tuberculosis—to ensure increased effectiveness with fewer side effects and a reduced risk of inducing resistant strains. The latter is particularly important, as HIV is a rapidly mutating virus so that new resistant strains are rapidly selected for. The term used is HAART (highly active antiretroviral therapy), or, more neutrally, cART (combined antiretroviral therapy). This approach cannot eradicate HIV and thus produces no cures, but accomplishes the following, as it:

- dramatically reduces the viral load
- improves the immune status
- reduces the number of opportunistic infections and AIDS-defining illnesses
- prevents or improves AIDS-related wasting
- greatly increases life expectancy.

Available anti-HIV agents include:

- nucleoside analogs = nucleoside reverse transcriptase inhibitors (NRTIs)
- nonnucleoside reverse transcriptase inhibitors (NNRTIs)
- protease inhibitors (PIs)
- fusion inhibitors
- entry inhibitors (chemokine receptor antagonists).

Nucleoside reverse transcriptase inhibitors. After HIV enters a host cell, it uses reverse transcriptase to convert the viral RNA into double-stranded DNA, which is then incorporated into the host genome by another viral enzyme, integrase. NRTIs serve as false substrates; when they are built into the DNA chain by reverse transcriptase, they cannot be linked, leading to disruptions. They are excreted renally and thus have few interactions with the many medications metabolized by the liver.

Side effects: most side effects are mediated via mitochondria, as they also metabolize nucleosides. They include gastrointestinal disturbances (nausea, vomiting, diarrhea), headache, lactic acidosis, peripheral neuropathy, and lipodystrophy.

Non-nucleoside reverse transcriptase inhibitors. NNRTIs bind directly to reverse transcriptase and near the site where substrates are bound and inhibit its function. They are well tolerated and have a conveniently long half-life, so the patient must take fewer pills, but resistance develops readily. A single point mutation can lead to resistance, with cross-resistance to other NNRTIs. They are metabolized in the liver by the cytochrome P450 system.

Side effects: these vary greatly depending on the agent; nevirapine is associated with hepatotoxicity and allergic reactions (skin reactions in 20%), and efavirenz with CNS toxicity.

Protease inhibitors. PIs bind to the active center of the viral protease enzyme and block splitting of the viral gag-pol polyproteins, so that noninfectious viral particles are produced. They have been a valuable addition to therapeutic regimens, but have to be taken quite often due to a short half-life and must be taken up many times daily. They are also metabolized in the liver by the cytochrome P450 system, so many drug interactions are possible.

Side effects: lipodystrophy and dyslipidemia, presumably through mitochondrial damage; hepatotoxicity.

Fusion inhibitors. The prototype of this new substance class is enfuvirtide (formerly T-20), which inhibits gp41 which is essential for fusion of the viral and host-cell membranes. Thus, it blocks the transfer of viral RNA into host cells.

Entry inhibitors. Maraviroc, another new agent, blocks the chemokine receptor CCR5 which HIV gp120 uses as a coreceptor after binding to CD4 on helper T cells. Some HIVs also use CXCR4; a tropism assay must be performed to see if the drug is likely to help a given patient.

■ Combined Antiretroviral Therapy

cART or HAART typically involves 2 NRTI + 1 PI or 1 NNRTI or 1 additional NRTI. Many combination products are available to make compliance easier. The starting point for therapy is controversial; at the latest it should be started if there are 5×10^4 HIV copies/mL or <300 CD4+ T cells/µL (Chapter 37.1). The decision to start cART is based on:

- viral load
- immune status
- HIV type
- the resistance pattern of the virgin virus
- anticipated compliance (some regimens have many more pills than others)
- comedications
- comorbidities

The patient should be counseled at length about the choice of regimen, side effects, and effects on daily life. Once cART has been started, it is a lifelong therapy that should not be interrupted, because of the greatly increased risk of selecting out resistant strains.

Antiviral Agents

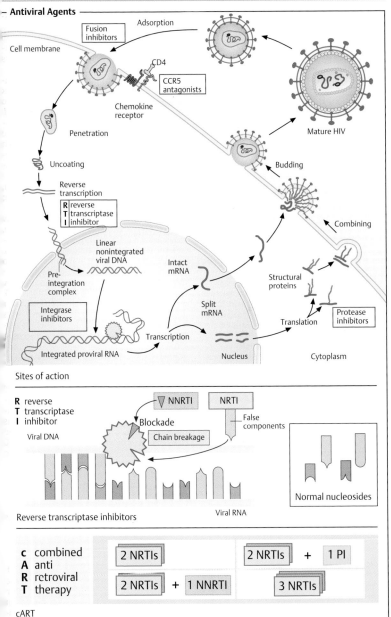

Sites of action

Reverse transcriptase inhibitors

cART

B. Antiviral Agents in HIV/AIDS

Antiparasitic agents are used against *ectoparasites* such as mites, lice, and fleas, as well as against *endoparasites* like gastrointestinal worms. For dermatology, the most important agents are those used against ectoparasites:

- acaricides—against mites
- insecticides—against insects, primarily lice
- repellents.

A. Acaricides/Insecticides

Permethrin. This is a partially synthetic *pyrethroid*, synthesized from extracts from chrysanthemums. Like its natural precursors, it has neurotoxic effects on parasites, which develop because it blocks the closure of sodium channels. The excess intracellular sodium leads to nerve paralysis.

Permethrin 5% is effective against both scabies and lice; it is available as a cream or solution for application to hairy areas. It is well tolerated and clearly the safest agent of this class in pregnancy, nursing, or infancy. Resistance is not much of a problem with scabies, but is seen increasingly with lice.

Side effects: irritation, pruritus, burning.

Hexachlorocyclohexane (lindane). Another neurotoxic agent, lindane was the mainstay of scabies and lice therapy for a long time, but was removed from most markets in 2008 because of neurotoxicity in infants. It remains a safe agent in older children and adults.

Side effects: neurotoxicity (seizures, permanent damage) after marked absorption in infants, especially those with damaged skin or who are treated too often.

Benzoyl benzoate. A safe antiscabies agent that is, unfortunately, only moderately effective. It is officially approved for pregnancy, nursing, and infancy, but should be viewed as a second-line choice.

Other options. *Goldgeist forte* is a natural pyrethrum extract (25% in alcohol) from flowers of *Chrysanthemum cinerariaefolium*. It is used in Germany against lice and their nits. Allethrin is another pyrethroid but not as effective as permethrin. *Crotamiton* has intrinsic antipruritic properties and is toxic to scabies mites by an unknown mechanism, but is only marginally effective.

Note: A key aspect of treating scabies or pediculosis is the careful examination and simultaneous treatment of all contact individuals; otherwise a ping-pong effect develops. Small epidemics are not uncommon in kindergartens, schools, and nursing homes.

Ivermectin. This old veterinary product is the only systemic agent approved for treating human ectoparasites. It can be given in a single dose of 200 µg/kg, perhaps repeated in one week, to treat scabies. It is especially effective is trying to deal with epidemics in nursing homes, but is also often used for crusted scabies, recurrent (proven) scabies, and in immunosuppressed patients. It can also be used to treat lice, but its main indications are to treat helminthic infestations.

B. Repellents

Repellents are used to keep biting insects away from the skin. They are most often used against mosquitoes, especially to reduce the risk of malaria transmission, but also help against horse flies and other flies. They have some effectiveness against ticks. All repellants should be combined with mechanical protection (long-sleeved clothing, mosquito nets). Agents include DEET (diethyl toluamide), picaridin, and a variety of natural repellants including sesquiterpenes (especially isolongifolenone from turpentine), garlic, eucalyptus oil, and citronella.

C. Antihelmintic Agents

The most common agents are albendazole (10–15 mg/kg daily) or mebendazole (100–200 mg daily). Treatment varies from 3 to 14 days, depending on the parasite, and is often repeated once. *Echinococcus multilocularis* requires longer courses.

Other choices include praziquantel, niclosamide, pyrvinium pamoate, and pyrantel pamoate (for enterobiasis) and diethylcarbamazine or ivermectin for filariasis or onchocerciasis. Ivermectin has such an excellent safety profile that it is being used in a worldwide effort to eradicate onchocerciasis (river blindness) and is also helping to reduce the prevalence of lymphatic filariasis.

Antiparasitic Agents

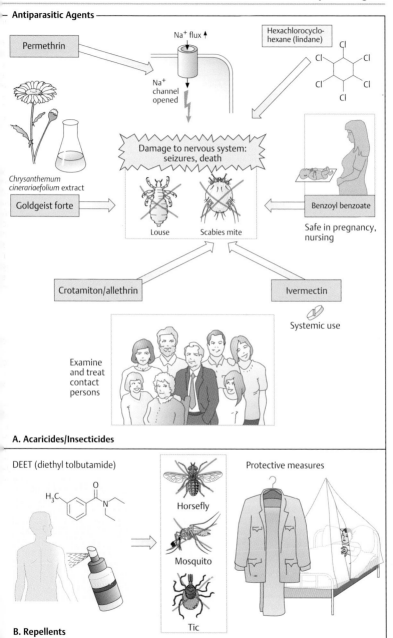

Na⁺ flux ↑

Permethrin

Na⁺ channel opened

Hexachlorocyclo-hexane (lindane)

Damage to nervous system: seizures, death

Chrysanthemum cinerariaefolium extract

Goldgeist forte

Louse   Scabies mite

Benzoyl benzoate

Safe in pregnancy, nursing

Crotamiton/allethrin

Ivermectin

Systemic use

Examine and treat contact persons

A. Acaricides/Insecticides

DEET (diethyl tolbutamide)

H₃C

O

Horsefly

Mosquito

Tic

Protective measures

B. Repellents

The retinoids include derivatives of vitamin A acid (retinol) and substances with different chemical structures but related biological activity. Three generations of retinoids are available:

- *nonaromatic retinoids*: tretinoin (all-trans retinoic acid = ATRA), isotretinoin (13-cis-retinoic acid), and alitretinoin (9-cis-retinoic acid)
- *monoaromatic retinoids*: acitretin, etretinate, and motretinide
- *polyaromatic retinoids*: adapalene, tazarotene and bexarotene.

Mechanisms of action. The retinoids belong to the steroid superfamily and bind to either specific nuclear receptors (RAR and RXR) or cytoplasmic retinoid-binding proteins (CRBPs). They enhance epidermal differentiation while inhibiting sebum production and neutrophil chemotaxis.

■ Systemic Retinoids

Isotretinoin. This drug revolutionized the treatment of severe acne as it is sebum suppressive, anticomedogenic, and anti-inflammatory. It is used orally, and absorption is enhanced by fatty meals. All retinoids are stored in body fat, but isotretinoin is excreted over a matter of weeks. Isotretinoin is also used for severe rosacea, Gram-negative folliculitis, and pustular psoriasis. Combined with psoralen plus UVA (PUVA) (Re-PUVA), it is used for psoriasis, lichen planus, and mycosis fungoides. Finally, it provides skin tumor prophylaxis in patients with nevoid basal cell carcinoma syndrome, xeroderma pigmentosum, and following organ transplantation.

> **Note:** The usual dose is 10–20 mg daily; it is just as effective as, and better tolerated than, the higher doses that were formerly used.

Acitretin. This is the active metabolite of etretinate, which is no longer used. It has an extremely long half-life, with traces found in the body years after concluding therapy. It may be combined with topical measures and/or phototherapy. The main indications are severe psoriasis (including nail involvement, pustular psoriasis, and psoriatic erythroderma (as Re-PUVA), as well as Darier disease, Hailey–Hailey disease, ichthyosis, palmoplantar keratoderma, pityriasis rubra pilaris, and severe lichen planus. The efficacy is similar to isotretinoin.

Bexarotene. This selectively binds to the RXR. It is used for cutaneous T-cell lymphoma, where it can be combined with methotrexate, interferon-α, or extracorporeal photophoresis.

Alitretinoin. This is a new agent that binds to both RXR and RAR. It is approved for severe chronic hand dermatitis; 10–30 mg daily or every other day for 3 months often brings good improvement.

Side effects. The main problem for all retinoids is teratogenicity. All are contraindicated during pregnancy and nursing.

> **Caution:** Women capable of becoming pregnant need to use contraception for 1 month before and 2 months after taking isotretinoin. With acitretin, contraception for 2 years from the conclusion of treatment is wise. Blood donations are not allowed.

All the other side effects are strictly dose related. They include elevated triglycerides (worse with bexarotene), dry skin and mucosa (especially ocular), paronychia, staphylococcal pyodermas, alopecia (acitretin), musculoskeletal problems (isotretinoin), and hypothyroidism (bexarotene). Abnormal laboratory findings include altered liver and kidney function, anemia, and thrombocytemia,

There has been much discussion of an increased risk of depression and suicide in teenagers taking isotretinoin, but this has not been confirmed with controlled studies.

■ Topical Retinoids

Isotretinoin, tretinoin and adapalene. All are approved for acne; since they attack the primary microcomedo, they can be used in almost every patient. They are also used to treat actinically damaged skin and improve wrinkling.

Tazarotene. This is approved for psoriasis, but it is not dramatically effective and expensive.

Bexarotene. This is approved for topical treatment of cutaneous T-cell lymphoma.

Alitretinoin. A topical formulation is available for Kaposi sarcoma, but is of limited effectiveness.

Side effects. All topical retinoids cause erythema, burning, and dryness.

> **Caution:** Topical retinoids should also be avoided during pregnancy. While the risk of fetal damage is immeasurably small, the medicolegal situation dictates this caution.

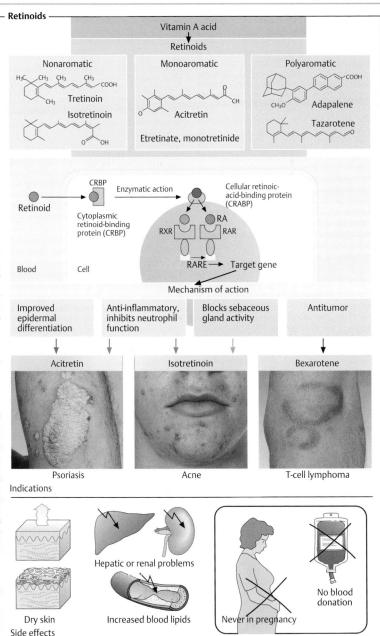

Retinoids

Vitamin A acid
↓
Retinoids

Nonaromatic

Tretinoin

Isotretinoin

Monoaromatic

Acitretin

Etretinate, monotretinide

Polyaromatic

Adapalene

Tazarotene

Retinoid → CRBP — Enzymatic action → Cellular retinoic-acid-binding protein (CRABP)

Cytoplasmic retinoid-binding protein (CRBP)

RXR   RA   RAR

RARE → Target gene

Blood   Cell

Mechanism of action

Improved epidermal differentiation

Anti-inflammatory, inhibits neutrophil function

Blocks sebaceous gland activity

Antitumor

Acitretin

Isotretinoin

Bexarotene

Psoriasis

Acne

T-cell lymphoma

Indications

Dry skin

Hepatic or renal problems

Increased blood lipids

Never in pregnancy

No blood donation

Side effects

10 Medical Therapy

A. Antihistamines

Histamine is a natural biogenic amine which is stored in mast cells, basophils, and platelets. It is the most important mediator of type I (immediate hypersensitivity) allergic reactions and pseudoallergic urticaria. Histamine influences cells via four different cell membrane receptors, all coupled to G protein:

- H_1 receptor: allergic and pseudoallergic reactions
- H_2 receptor: stimulation of gastric secretion, vasodilation, cardiac stimulation
- H_3 receptor: neurotransmitter release in the CNS
- H_4 receptor: chemotaxis of immune and inflammatory cells.

Mechanisms of action. Antihistamines are competitive antagonists acting on the histamine receptors. The older products were nonspecific and had numerous side effects; the newer agents are receptor specific, with H_1 blockers used for allergic disease and H_2 blockers for gastric protection. Agents are available to block H_3 and H_4 receptors but they are not yet of clinical relevance.

First-generation H_1 blockers (chlorpheniramine, clemastine, diphenhydramine) are lipophilic, cross the blood–brain barrier, and are sedative. This side effect is often used therapeutically, as sedation may be desirable in those with severe pruritus. Other side effects include paradoxical excitement in children, cardiac rhythm disturbances and weight gain. *Second-generation* H_1 blockers (cetirizine, loratadine) do not cross the blood–brain barrier, and are much more suitable for daytime use, as they do not interfere with driving or work. *Third-generation* agents are enantiomers (levocetirizine) or metabolites (desloratadine, fexofenadine) of the second generation. Cyproheptadine is a H_1 blocker that also blocks serotonin receptors.

Indications. *Systemic—oral:*
- allergic rhinitis
- allergic conjunctivitis
- urticaria.

Antihistamines should be taken regularly throughout the entire pollination season. Nasal or ocular hypersecretion is reduced and pruritus diminished.

Note: Mild to moderate allergic rhinitis and conjunctivitis tend to respond better to antihistamines than does chronic urticaria.

Systemic i.v.: antihistamines are a mainstay of the initial treatment of anaphylaxis; the i.v. route ensures more rapid action.

Caution: Always enquire about comedications. Patients with liver disease or taking other medications that are metabolized by the hepatic cytochrome P450 system are at risk for developing toxic levels of antihistamines, leading to disturbances of cardiac rhythm. Terfenadine was removed from the market because this risk was so high. Other common dermatologic drugs metabolized by this system include ciclosporin, erythromycin, oral contraceptives, and many systemic antifungal agents. Grapefruit also hampers the metabolic process.

Topical: H_1 blockers are available as eye or nose drops to reduce systemic effects. They are not dramatically effective via this route.

B. Antipruritic Agents

Selective serotonin reuptake inhibitors (SSRIs). These agents are usually employed as antidepressive agents and anti-emetics. They selectively block serotonin transport, so that serotonin can have a longer action at the nerve synapse, sometimes with antipruritic effects. They are not approved for this indication.

Tricyclic antidepressants. Older tricyclic antidepressants have antihistaminic, antiserotonin and sedative actions. Doxepin blocks both H_1 and H_2 effects and is sedating; it is frequently used for chronic refractory urticaria, but in much lower dosages than for psychiatric uses.

Opiate antagonists. Naloxone and other opiate antagonists may be used for severe pruritus, especially that associated with cholestasis.

Topical. The most important approach is regular lubrication, perhaps employing an agent containing urea. Topical polidocanol is a local anesthetic that is relatively effective on the skin. The caine family of local anesthetics (benzocaine) is frequently included in over-the-counter remedies for sunburn and insect bites, but these should be avoided as they often cause allergic contact dermatitis. Topical antihistamines are also potent sensitizers and also should be avoided. Topical corticosteroids are not especially effective at treating itch that is due to dermatitis.

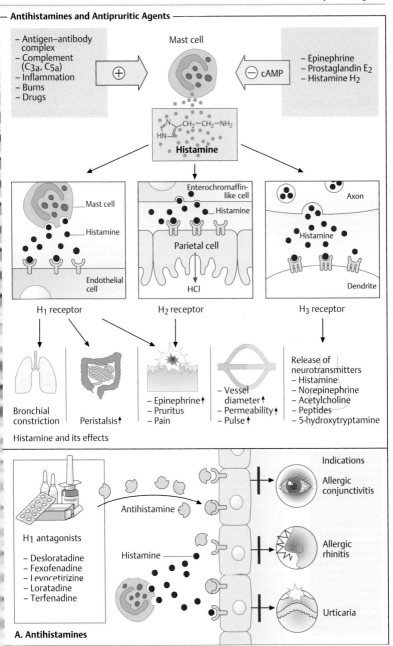

A. Antihistamines

A. Keratolytics

Keratolytics are used to remove keratin from the stratum corneum. They have been used in disorders of keratinization, acne, and cosmetic dermatology. Examples include:

- salicylic acid
- urea
- azelaic acid
- benzoyl peroxide
- α-hydroxy acids (fruit acids).

Salicylic acid. The original source was willow trees (*Salix* spp.). Salicylic acid is a cyclic β-hydroxy acid that is keratolytic as well and fungicidal and bactericidal. It is added to dithranol at 1% for oxidative protection. It can be incorporated into creams or ointments, but also comes as an impregnated plaster for localized use. The antiseptic effects are achieved with 1% concentration; the keratolytic effects increase with increasing levels. Usual levels are 0.5%–2.0% for widespread use and 10%–40% for small areas.

Indications: warts, calluses, corns (10% salicylic acid ointments under occlusion; 40% salicylic acid plasters), psoriasis (to remove heavy scales and let other medications work better); ichthyosis, palmoplantar keratoderma; acne (mild peeling). It is often helpful for superinfected crusted lesions. Crusted scalp lesions may respond to 2.5% salicylic acid in olive oil.

Side effects: salicylic acid is always irritating and drying; when used on larger areas, there is a risk of absorption and salicylism (tinnitus, nausea, vomiting).

> **Caution:** Never use in infants or small children or in the last trimester. The risk of fatal salicylism is considerable because of increased absorption and sensitivity.

Urea. Both keratolytic and humectant, urea binds water in the skin. It increases the penetration of corticosteroids, allowing less-potent products to be used. It is a mainstay of dry-skin-care products, and is also used in ichthyosis. In a special 40% formulation, it is used to soften nails for removal or can be combined with antifungal agents. It burns on initial application, making its use in children difficult.

Azelaic acid. This is a natural dicarboxylic acid synthesized by *Malassezia* spp., it has antimicrobial and keratolytic effects. It is used in acne and rosacea as a 20% cream or 15% gel. Side effects include burning and irritation.

Benzoyl peroxide. This strong oxidative agent is keratolytic and antibacterial. It is used in many forms in acne, and in higher concentrations for chronic wounds. It, too, is irritating and drying. It may stain or bleach clothing or hair.

α-Hydroxy acids. Also known as fruit acids, these agents are widely used for skin peeling and rejuvenation. Lactic acid in an optimized vehicle is useful for dry skin and ichthyosis.

B. Antiproliferative Agents

Vitamin D analogs. Modified forms of vitamin D_3 (calcipotriol, calcitriol, and tacalcitol) influence keratinocyte differentiation by binding to specific receptors. They are used in mild to moderate psoriasis, where they are about as effective as medium-strength corticosteroids, with far fewer side effects. Combination products are available where they are mixed with corticosteroids.

Side effects: irritation; hypercalcemia when applied to wide areas (>30% of body surface) or damaged skin.

Dithranol. Dithranol (cignolin or anthralin) is the oldest topical psoriatic medication and has been proven safe even for long-term use. Its mechanism of action is poorly understood. It is used for chronic stable psoriasis. It is used in increasing concentrations (1/32 to 2%), applied once daily in hospital, and often combined with methotrexate or phototherapy. It is messy and expensive and is now more often used in higher concentrations (3%–4%) in an easily-removed cream base for short periods (minute therapy or short contact therapy) for localized disease.

Side effects: irritation and burning; discoloration. Sometimes an irritant dermatitis may develop many hours after application. A bit of irritation is needed; *psoriasis disappears in the fires of dithranol.* It can cause hyperpigmentation of the periphery, so treated areas appear pale (psoriatic pseudoleukoderma). Severe reactions may be pustular.

Other agents. Coal tars and slate tars were previously used extensively for psoriasis and other inflammatory skin diseases but they have been replaced by more effective, less messy approaches. In addition, there are theoretical concerns about their carcinogenicity.

— Keratolytics and Antiproliferative Agents —

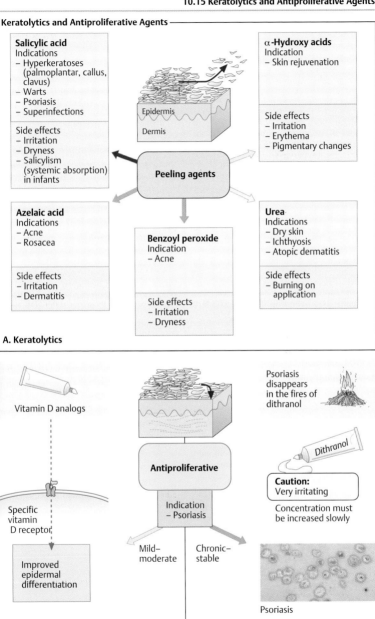

Salicylic acid
Indications
– Hyperkeratoses (palmoplantar, callus, clavus)
– Warts
– Psoriasis
– Superinfections

Side effects
– Irritation
– Dryness
– Salicylism (systemic absorption) in infants

α-Hydroxy acids
Indication
– Skin rejuvenation

Side effects
– Irritation
– Erythema
– Pigmentary changes

Epidermis
Dermis

Peeling agents

Azelaic acid
Indications
– Acne
– Rosacea

Side effects
– Irritation
– Dermatitis

Benzoyl peroxide
Indication
– Acne

Side effects
– Irritation
– Dryness

Urea
Indications
– Dry skin
– Ichthyosis
– Atopic dermatitis

Side effects
– Burning on application

A. Keratolytics

Vitamin D analogs

Psoriasis disappears in the fires of dithranol

Antiproliferative

Dithranol

Caution:
Very irritating

Concentration must be increased slowly

Specific vitamin D receptor

Indication
– Psoriasis

Improved epidermal differentiation

Mild–moderate

Chronic–stable

Psoriasis

1. Vitamin D analogs

2. Dithranol (anthralin, cignolin)

B. Antiproliferative Agents

A. Antiperspirants

Aluminum salts, tap water iontophoresis and botulinum toxin are the main choices in treating hyperhidrosis.

Aluminum salts. Aluminum chloride and aluminum chloride hexahydrate cause the sweatduct pores to close, reducing the flow of sweat. They are used in low concentrations in antiperspirant sticks, sprays and roll-ons. They are available in concentrations up to 20% in solutions or roll-ons for control of hyperhidrosis under medical supervision.

Indication: axillary hyperhidrosis.

Side effect: irritation.

Botulinum toxin A. This agent inhibits sweating by blocking the release of acetylcholine following stimulation of sympathetic nerves. It is injected intradermally at the site of excessive sweating; the dose depends on the agent used and the site. The effect lasts for 4–8 months; then it must be repeated.

Indications: axillary hyperhidrosis is the usual indication. When the hands or feet are treated, regional anesthesia is helpful to reduce the pain of injection.

Tap water iontophoresis. This approach is most useful for palmoplantar hyperhidrosis (Ch. 26.3).

B. Medications for Disturbances of Pigmentation

Depigmenting agents. The most important agents are hydroquinone and its derivatives. They are tyrosine analogs that block melanin synthesis. The main indication is melasma. The usual concentration is 2%–4%; they can be combined with tretinoin and low-potency corticosteroids (Kligman formula).

Side effects: irritation, hypopigmentation, milia, ochronosis (higher concentrations).

Repigmenting agents. The most common clinical situation is vitiligo. A rule of thumb is, the fresher the lesions and the darker the background skin, the more likely it is that repigmentation will be successful. Options include:

- photo- or photochemotherapy with narrow-band UVB or PUVA. Problems include burning pale skin and hyperpigmentation of peripheral normal skin
- topical corticosteroids (**caution:** skin atrophy with long-term use) or topical calcineurin inhibitors (**caution:** do not combine with phototherapy) may help in early lesions

- expert use of camouflage makeup is often the most satisfactory if least glamorous approach. It can be combined with sun protection
- melanocyte transplantation is often a last resort. It is only recommended for small areas of stable vitiligo and best reserved for specialty centers. The results appear patchy and may not please the patient. Subsequent phototherapy is mandatory.

C. Skin Cleansers and Protective Agents

There are few, if any, skin conditions that require special cleansing. Daily washing with soap or synthetic detergents and water is almost always all that is required to remove accumulated dirt and oils. Soaps are sodium or potassium salts of free fatty acids and thus alkaline, damaging the acid mantle of the skin and often irritating. Pure soaps are not necessarily mild soaps. Soaps may not be tolerated by patients with dry or damaged skin,

Synthetic detergents (syndets) can be adjusted to any pH; the most commonly used ones are set at around 5.5 and do not damage the acid mantle. They are better tolerated by patients with atopic dermatitis and other forms of irritated skin.

Protective agents are designed primarily for an occupational setting, but they can also be useful for homemakers with hand dermatitis. Some agents more effectively protect against either water or oils. Most provide skin maintenance care as well, containing emollients. The problem is always to provide protection without interfering with function. Patients should be carefully counseled; some protectants contain fluorescent dyes so it is easier to check for adequate coverage.

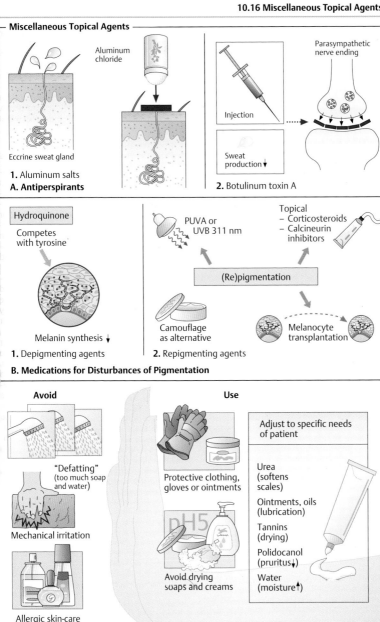

Miscellaneous Topical Agents

Aluminum chloride

Eccrine sweat gland

1. Aluminum salts
A. Antiperspirants

Injection

Parasympathetic nerve ending

Sweat production ↓

2. Botulinum toxin A

Hydroquinone

Competes with tyrosine

PUVA or UVB 311 nm

Topical
– Corticosteroids
– Calcineurin inhibitors

(Re)pigmentation

Melanin synthesis ↓

Camouflage as alternative

Melanocyte transplantation

1. Depigmenting agents
2. Repigmenting agents

B. Medications for Disturbances of Pigmentation

Avoid

Use

"Defatting" (too much soap and water)

Mechanical irritation

Allergic skin-care products

Protective clothing, gloves or ointments

Avoid drying soaps and creams

Adjust to specific needs of patient

Urea (softens scales)

Ointments, oils (lubrication)

Tannins (drying)

Polidocanol (pruritus↓)

Water (moisture↑)

C. Skin Cleansers and Protective Agents

A. Ultraviolet Radiation

Visible light covers the spectrum with wavelengths from 400 to 800 nm, with the familiar rainbow ranging from violet-blue at 400 nm through green, yellow, orange, and finally red at 800 nm. Visible light plays a role in only a few rare diseases, but is incorporated into laser intense pulsed light (IPL) and photodynamic therapy (PDT). Infrared light warms tissues primarily by heating water; it too plays little role in disease.

In contrast, ultraviolet (UV) light plays a significant role in skin aging and many diseases, is widely used in therapy, and has been the subject of extensive research because of its interactions with the immune system and other biological effects. The two main types of UV radiation are UVB (280–320 nm) and UVA (320–400 nm). UVC (200–280 nm) and x-rays do not reach the earth's surface. UVB is responsible for most DNA damage, while UVA only causes damage indirectly by generating reactive oxygen species (ROS), mainly in the dermis, at very high energy levels. On the other hand, almost all phototoxic and photoallergic reactions are caused by UVA.

B. Principles of Phototherapy

Phototherapy usually involves UVA or UVB; exceptions are some lasers and photodynamic therapy. Inflammatory skin diseases such as psoriasis or atopic dermatitis are most often treated, but tumors (early-stage mycosis fungoides) or pruritus are other important indications. Phototherapy is immunomodulatory and also causes structural alterations in the epidermis so that the UV sensitivity decreases due to epidermal thickening (in German, *Lichtschwiele* or "light callus").

Both fluorescent and high-pressure lamps are available to deliver UVB and UVA. The therapeutic spectrum can be modulated by the type of tube, the inert gas chosen, treating the inside of the light source, and employing filters. Typical sources include broad-spectrum UVB (280–320 nm) tubes, UVB 311 nm tubes, UVA (320–400 nm) tubes and UVA₁ (340–400 nm) high-pressure lamps. The dose must always be measured as the amount of energy applied to a surface area (mJ/cm² or J/m²) and never in time units, as each machine requires different times to deliver a given energy level, and the output generally decreases as a tube or lamp ages.

Caution: If a phototherapy unit is not correctly calibrated and exact dosage plans followed, there is a risk of potentially fatal burns.

PDT, IPL and some lasers also use visible light. Here, the idea is to concentrate energy in such as way as to use radiation to produce localized changes in individual tissues, such as vessels or even tumor cells.

C. UVB Phototherapy

UVB causes sunburn. The minimal dose that causes visible slight erythema is designated as the minimal erythema dose (MED). This value increases in darker skin, ranging from 20 to 40 mJ/cm² for type I skin to around 120 mJ/cm² for type III. Both MED and sunburn itself typically appear after 12–24 hours.

When UVB phototherapy is performed, the patient starts with 50% of the MED and is treated up to five times weekly. The patient must be checked for erythema before each treatment. The goal of treatment is to increase the dose to a point where it almost causes erythema, adjusting the dose daily or every second day. Typically, the dose is increased by 20% each time, until an individualized maximum dose is reached.

Today, narrow-band UVB (311 nm) is widely used. It delivers roughly one-tenth as much energy as broad-spectrum UVB but is more effective for many disorders including psoriasis, atopic dermatitis, and mycosis fungoides. UVB 311 nm is also effective in vitiligo and produces a more attractive copper-brown color than regular UVB. For uremic pruritus, broad-spectrum UVB is effective, but 311 nm is no helpful. Since UVB 311 nm is delivered at a 10 fold dose, extreme care must be taken when switching from this to broad-spectrum UVB, to avoid severe burns.

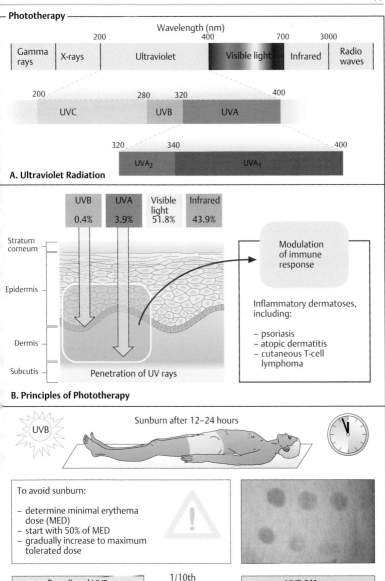

— Phototherapy —

A. Ultraviolet Radiation

B. Principles of Phototherapy

C. UVB Phototherapy

To avoid sunburn:

– determine minimal erythema dose (MED)
– start with 50% of MED
– gradually increase to maximum tolerated dose

Sunburn after 12–24 hours

1/10th as strong

Broadband UVB — Uremic pruritus

UVB 311nm — Psoriasis, atopic dermatitis, lymphoma, vitiligo

Wavelength (nm)

Gamma rays | X-rays | Ultraviolet | Visible light | Infrared | Radio waves

UVC | UVB | UVA

UVA₂ | UVA₁

UVB 0.4% | UVA 3.9% | Visible light 51.8% | Infrared 43.9%

Stratum corneum
Epidermis
Dermis
Subcutis

Penetration of UV rays

Modulation of immune response

Inflammatory dermatoses, including:

– psoriasis
– atopic dermatitis
– cutaneous T-cell lymphoma

11 Physical Modes of Therapy

D. UVA and UVA₁ Phototherapy

UVA irradiation alone causes almost no erythema and after long exposure produces a brown to gray-brown pigmentation. UVA causes two pigmentation reactions. Immediate pigment darkening (IPD) occurs after 30 minutes when existing melanin is oxidized or otherwise altered, while delayed tanning (DT) appears after 24 hours and involves synthesis of new melanin.

In nature, UVA has no measurable acute effects, because the UVB-induced sunburn drives the patient out of the light before enough UVA can be received to cause changes. UVA penetrates more deeply into the skin. UVA is not very effective therapeutically; it is sometimes combined with UVB to treat atopic dermatitis, as the combination provides more relief from pruritus.

UVA_1, which has no erythematous effects, is given in very high doses. Low-dose UVA_1 with $20-30 \, J/cm^2$ has 1000 times more energy than typical UVB therapy. Mid-range ($30-50 \, J/cm^2$) and high-dose ($50-60 \, J/cm^2$) UVA_1 has anti-inflammatory and antisclerotic effects through the induction of matrix metalloproteinases. This makes it suitable for treating morphea and systemic sclerosis. UVA_1 is also effective for atopic dermatitis and some forms of graft versus host disease (GVHD).

E. Photochemotherapy

UVA is responsible for a variety of phototoxic and photoallergic reactions by activating chemical ring structures. One of these structures is 8-methoxypsoralen (8-MOP). After the topical and systemic use of 8-MOP, very tiny doses of UVA can cause phototoxic reactions. This combination of psoralen (8-MOP) plus UVA is known as PUVA and is widely used therapeutically. About 2 hours after ingestion or 10–20 minutes after topical application of 8-MOP, the skin becomes very sensitive to UVA light. The minimal phototoxic dose (MPD) is $0.5-3 \, J/cm^2$, depending on skin type. This same dose is received with 4–20 minutes' exposure to sunlight. UVA passes through window glass, so this offers no protection.

PUVA therapy was initially introduced for psoriasis, where for several decades it was the mainstay of outpatient treatment of severe disease, along with methotrexate. Today there are many more options for psoriasis, and PUVA is used for a far wider spectrum of diseases.

With PUVA therapy, an attempt is made once again to administer an almost erythemal dose. The MPD is determined and the dose increased regularly. PUVA erythema is delayed for 2–3 days, so PUVA is generally given for 2 days, followed by a day's pause, and then evaluation for erythema and adjustment of dose. Typical schedules are then 2 days' PUVA–1 day pause–2 days' PUVA, or treatment every other day.

The most important indications are psoriasis, early mycosis fungoides, atopic dermatitis, vitiligo, lichen planus, scleroderma, GVHD, and even polymorphic light eruption (hardening the patient so they later tolerate sunlight). All diseases are best treated 3–4 times weekly, but there are differences. Psoriasis and vitiligo should be treated close to the erythema level, while with mycosis fungoides and GVHD much lower levels should be used, adjusted to the severity of the skin disease.

PUVA can be given orally with irradiation 2 hours after ingestion of 0.6 mg/kg 8-MOP. The genitalia and noninvolved areas should be covered during therapy. Following treatment the skin and eyes must be protected from sunlight for 8 hours, requiring UVA-protective glasses, and either avoidance, protective clothing, or sunscreens.

To reduce the systemic exposure to 8-MOP and the need for post-treatment eye protection, bath PUVA was developed. Here, patients bathe in water containing 0.5–1.0 mg/L 8-MOP at 20–25 °C and then immediately afterward are irradiated with, initially, 30%–50% of the oral PUVA dose. While bath PUVA is technically challenging, it is effective, safer, and makes the rest of the patient's life easier.

Topical PUVA therapy following application of an 8-MOP cream is another option for localized disease; unfortunately 8-MOP creams are difficult to prepare and the indicated 8-MOP concentrations unreliable

> **Caution:** Concentrated 8-MOP solutions are extremely toxic and must always be accurately diluted.

The main problem of PUVA is the increased risk of squamous cell carcinoma in patients who have received more than 300–500 treatments, which is a number easily achieved in severe psoriasis that requires lifelong therapy. When the patient also receives ciclosporin or calcineurin inhibitors, this risk is dangerously elevated. In contrast, combined use with methotrexate does not increase the risk.

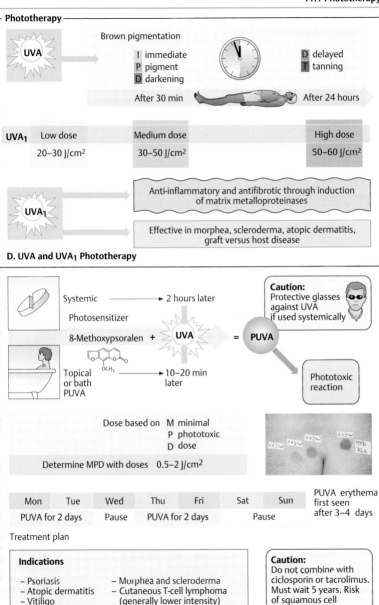

Photography

Brown pigmentation

I immediate
P pigment
D darkening

D delayed
T tanning

After 30 min   After 24 hours

UVA₁	Low dose	Medium dose	High dose
	20–30 J/cm²	30–50 J/cm²	50–60 J/cm²

Anti-inflammatory and antifibrotic through induction of matrix metalloproteinases

Effective in morphea, scleroderma, atopic dermatitis, graft versus host disease

D. UVA and UVA₁ Phototherapy

Systemic ⟶ 2 hours later

Photosensitizer

8-Methoxypsoralen + UVA = PUVA

Caution:
Protective glasses against UVA if used systemically

Topical or bath PUVA ⟶ 10–20 min later

Phototoxic reaction

Dose based on M minimal
                P phototoxic
                D dose

Determine MPD with doses 0.5–2 J/cm²

Mon	Tue	Wed	Thu	Fri	Sat	Sun
PUVA for 2 days		Pause	PUVA for 2 days		Pause	

PUVA erythema first seen after 3–4 days

Treatment plan

Indications

– Psoriasis
– Atopic dermatitis
– Vitiligo
– Morphea and scleroderma
– Cutaneous T-cell lymphoma (generally lower intensity)

Caution:
Do not combine with ciclosporin or tacrolimus. Must wait 5 years. Risk of squamous cell carcinoma↑

E. Photochemotherapy

A. Photodynamic Therapy

Cells that are actively metabolizing selectively take up porphyrins, making them more sensitive to phototoxic reactions. Such reactions damage cells through the formation of highly toxic singlet oxygen (O^-). This property can be used therapeutically by exposing carcinomas in situ to a topical porphyrin 5-aminolevulinic acid (5-ALA), which penetrates well into these cells. Inside the cells, 5-ALA is metabolized to protoporphyrin IX, which then interacts with light to produce singlet oxygen.

After the topical porphyrins have been applied for 2 hours in absolute darkness (the treated area is covered with aluminum foil), the skin is irradiated with polychromatic (incoherent) light. Since 5-ALA is selectively taken up by abnormal cells, these suffer far greater damage and preferential tumor destruction, with relative sparing of normal adjacent tissues.

The maximum depth of action is 2–3 mm, so that when basal cell carcinomas or squamous cell carcinomas are treated, there is significant risk of leaving an untreated deep component. Such residual tumors may be difficult to detect and cause considerable problems. Thus we limit the use of photodynamic therapy (PDT) to carcinomas in situ, such as actinic keratoses and Bowen disease.

B. Radiation Therapy

Ionizing radiation (or x-rays) has been widely replaced in dermatology because of improvements in both topical and surgical therapy. In the past, radiation therapy was used to treat inflammatory cutaneous disorders such as psoriasis or acne; today its use is limited to oncologic therapy.

Nonetheless, a basic understanding is essential, as cutaneous damage from radiation therapy still occurs, especially from iatrogenic exposure or even accidents like Chernobyl. Important terms include the tissue dose, measured in gray (Gy), and the tissue half-value depth (HVD). Roughly speaking, inflammatory disease responds to 2–3 Gy (although this is no longer used), lymphomas and Kaposi sarcoma to 20–30 Gy, and solid carcinomas (basal cell carcinoma, squamous cell carcinoma) to 50–60 Gy. Half of the dose should be administered to the bottom of the tumor—this is the significance of HVD.

The goal of radiation therapy is to maximize exposure in the tumor tissue and to minimize it in normal tissue. The eyes, cartilage, and bone are especially sensitive and must be protected or avoided. The mucosa is especially sensitive, and mucositis is almost impossible to avoid when the oral cavity is exposed. Adjusting the dosage parameters, especially the distance of the source from the skin, and altering the quality of the emitted x-rays allows the depth of damage to be precisely controlled. Rapid electron beam therapy probably offers the most exact method of treating skin tumors.

The total dose is only a rough guideline: the individual dose and the frequency with which it is given ultimately determine the effectiveness. Thus, the tendency today is toward many small doses (2–5 Gy) delivered frequently. In the past, a basal cell carcinoma might have been treated with seven doses of 8 Gy; today 15 doses of 4 Gy are more usual. This results in much less damage to adjacent skin.

The total safe dose for skin is around 60 Gy. When this is exceeded, nonhealing ulcers may develop. Thus, any one area can usually only be treated once or twice with x-rays. Ten years after skin is exposed to ≥10 Gy, it has an increased risk for the development of secondary tumors. This is a problem following treatment of breast carcinomas (with postirradiation angiosarcomas), lymphomas, and testicular tumors, even though sophisticated radiation therapy for internal tumors offers many ways of minimizing skin exposure.

Cutaneous lymphomas and limited Kaposi sarcoma are currently the most frequent indications for therapy with ionizing radiation.

C. Cryotherapy

In cryotherapy, the skin is frozen with liquid nitrogen ($-100°C$), which is usually administered with a spray device. The freeze–thaw cycles lead to cell damage and blister formation, both of which contribute to the therapeutic effect. Cryotherapy is most widely used for actinic keratoses and warts. The latter must be frozen more aggressively and often require multiple treatments. Deep cryotherapy for treatment of solid tumors is possible, but requires more complex equipment and cryoprobes to ensure that a killing dose is administered to the depth of the tumor. The main disadvantages of deep cryotherapy are pain and lack of histological control.

Photodynamic Therapy, Radiation Therapy, and Cryotherapy

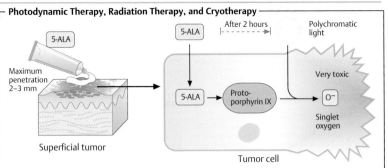

A. Photodynamic Therapy

Indications	Total dose	
Lymphoma, Kaposi sarcoma	~20–30 Gy	**Caution:** The following are easily damaged:
Basal cell carcinoma	~50–60 Gy	– eyes
Squamous cell carcinoma	~50–60 Gy	– cartilage
		– bone

If total skin dose >10 Gy, → then risk for skin cancer↑ after 10 years

Lifetime tissue dose 60 Gy

B. Radiation Therapy

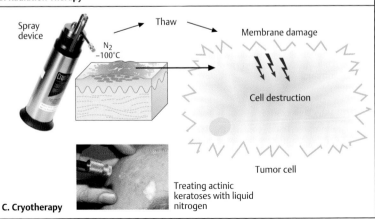

Spray device

N₂ –100°C

Thaw

Membrane damage

Cell destruction

Tumor cell

Treating actinic keratoses with liquid nitrogen

C. Cryotherapy

LASER is an acronym for *l*ight *a*mplification by *s*timulated *e*mission of *r*adiation. Laser light is generated by sending radiation through a crystal, gas, or liquid, thus bundling the rays. Laser emissions are always monochromatic and coherent, with a small diameter.

A. Principles of Laser Therapy

Laser therapy always involves destruction of tissue. In the skin, it is possible to destroy deeper structures in a highly localized and selective way. The target is a chromophore (hemoglobin, melanin, tattoo pigment), which determines the appropriate wavelength, duration of pulse, and beam size.

The thermal relaxation time (TRT) is the length of time it takes for uptake of energy and transfer to adjacent tissues. If the exposure time is less than the TRT, the target tissue will be damaged without affecting the surrounding tissue. The classic example is hemoglobin in a blood vessel. Lasers can release energy in several ways.

A continuous-wave (cw) laser releases a constant beam of light, where the duration of exposure determines the energy transmitted to tissue. Pulsed lasers can be long-pulsed, such as the pulsed dye laser working in the millisecond range, or very short-pulsed such as the "quality switch" (Qs) laser working in the nanosecond range; both forms release very large amounts of energy over very short intervals

B. Nonspecific Coagulation

These lasers emit energy in the near infrared range and thus are able to penetrate up to 5 mm, but heat tissue in a nonspecific fashion. For example the cw Nd:YAG (neodymium-doped yttrium aluminium garnet) laser is often used to destroy large vascular malformations and tumors. The radiation is administered percutaneously, or in the case of deeper tumors, intraluminally, via a light-transmitting cannula.

C. Semi-selective Lasers

The semi-selective lasers emit in the blue-green to red range (depending on laser between 488 and 598 nm) and have pulse durations of 10–1000 ms and a pulse diameter of 0.1–3.0 mm. They are suited for the percutaneous treatment of small vessels, such as telangiectases, but are painful.

D. Selective Photothermolysis

Pulsed and Qs lasers employ photothermolysis. As the size of the field increases, the possible radiation time increases. Depending on the wavelength, pulsed and Qs lasers are well-suited for coagulation of tiny vessels, epilation of dark thick hairs (pulsed alexandrite), and removal of tattoos (Qs ruby). In hair removal, melanin is the target but the TRT is deliberately exceeded so that the hair follicles are destroyed. Cooling of tissue (such as by shooting a laser through an ice cube or special cooling medium) helps to reduce collateral damage.

E. Vaporization and Ablation

The cw CO_2 laser, the super-pulsed CO_2 laser, and the erbium (Er):YAG laser are most useful. In the focused mode, the energy is so high that the cw CO_2 laser can be used for cutting; in a defocused mode, the super-pulsed CO_2 laser is used to vaporize superficial structures such as tumors or warts. The Er:YAG laser quickly vaporizes small volumes of tissue and is ideal for superficial removal. These lasers form a laser plume or pyrolytic aerosol, which contains infectious viral particles if a wart is being treated. Complex vacuum evacuation systems are required.

> **Caution:** While melanocytic nevi can be removed with lasers, we are opposed to this approach. There is no histological control to ensure that partial treatment of a melanoma is not taking place. In addition, laser ablation scars are less acceptable than surgical excision scars.

F. Intense Pulsed Light

Intense pulsed light (IPL) is high-energy, polychromatic light that delivers considerable energy in a short time (0.5–100 ms) and is used for coagulating small vessels or for epilation. Its advantage over laser is that a much larger treatment field is possible, speeding up procedures like hair removal.

Laser Therapy

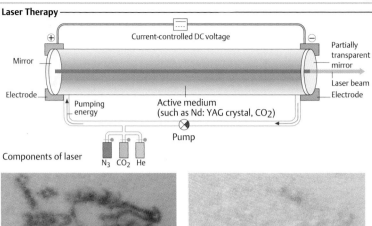

Components of laser

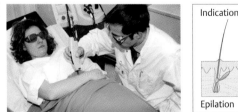

Tattoo before and after therapy

1. Nonspecific coagulation	cw CO_2 (10 600 nm) cw Nd:YAG (1064 nm)	– Deep penetration – Good coagulation/hemostasis – Risk of scars ↑
2. Semi-selective lasers	Argon (488, 514 nm) Copper vapor (578 nm) and others	– Coagulation of small vessels (telangiectases) – Painful
3. Selective photothermolysis	qs Ruby (694 nm) qs Alexandrite (755 nm) Pulsed dye (577–600 nm) fd Nd:YAG (532 nm)	– Destruction of melanin and tattoo pigments – Coagulation of smaller vessels
4. Vaporization and ablation	Er:YAG (2940 nm) Pulsed CO_2 (10 600 nm)	– Precise superficial ablation – No hemostasis – Used like dermabrasion for skin resurfacing

Types of lasers

A. Principles of Laser Therapy

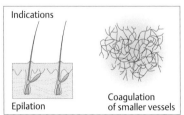

Indications

Epilation

Coagulation of smaller vessels

F. Intense Pulsed Light   Not monochromatic (not a laser)

A. General Aspects

Operative dermatology is an essential part of the specialty, for both diagnosis and therapy. The skin is readily accessible for diagnostic biopsies, which are easily and safely obtained. In addition, most skin tumors are amenable to surgical excision with anticipated cure.

Preoperative and perioperative management. The indications should be carefully considered. Operative planning, antisepsis, and perhaps prophylactic antibiotics and thrombosis should be addressed.

The responsible surgeon must counsel the patient within 24 hours of the operation, explaining the procedure and warning about all complications. This discussion should be documented. The patient can then give truly informed consent by signing an appropriate form along with the surgeon and a witness.

No matter how small the procedure is, it is important to ask about the following:

- allergies to local anesthetics, antibiotics, or other materials (tape, rubber)
- known infectious diseases (human immunodeficiency virus [HIV], hepatitis)
- metal in the body (endoprostheses, pacemakers, metal intrauterine device [IUD])—important when electrosurgical devices are used
- problems with earlier procedures (reactions to anesthetics, shock, keloid formation)
- problems with coagulation—is the patient on aspirin, warfarin, or heparin?

Anesthesia. The choice is based on the size and location of the planned procedure:

- cryoanesthesia with ethyl chloride spray can be used for lancing abscesses
- topical anesthesia with EMLA cream is useful in children for blood drawing and minor procedures (curetting mollusca)
- standard infiltration anesthesia
- tumescence anesthesia involves administering large amounts of highly diluted local anesthetics into the skin and subcutaneous tissue, providing regional anesthesia for larger procedures and liposuction
- regional blocks are useful for surgery on fingers and toes
- general anesthesia.

B. Operative Techniques

Biopsy. The most common dermatologic procedure is a diagnostic biopsy, which can be a punch, shave, or elliptical excision. The goal is to provide nontraumatized tissue for histological evaluation.

Superficial removal

- *Curettage* with a ring curette is useful for superficial lesions such as seborrheic and actinic keratoses.
- *Scissor excision* is a simple way to remove skin tags with a stalk.

■ Excisions

Complete excision, usually with a margin of safety, is the standard approach to removing tumors:

- small lesions are removed with a *spindle-shaped excision with primary closure*
- larger lesions or those on areas where the skin is not freely movable may be excised and then closed after tissue mobilization, by undermining the adjacent skin to allow easier closure
- in small, concave areas with a good blood supply, a wound can be left open to heal by secondary intention
- congenital nevi are often removed by *serial excision.* This is time-consuming but produces a better cosmetic result than flaps or grafts. A central spindle is removed, the defect closed primarily, and then after 6–9 months when the skin has stretched a bit, another spindle is excised. This is repeated until the lesion is completely removed
- cysts can be removed by making a small incision, then carefully expressing the cyst contents, and finally fishing out the empty cyst sack. The incision is then closed with a stitch or left open. The scar is much less noticeable than when the entire cyst is excised. If the cyst is inflamed or ruptured, it may be so adherent to the adjacent tissue that this approach is impossible
- lipomas can generally be extricated through a small incision, as they tend to be easily separated from the adjoining tissue even though they often have no capsule.

Caution: Lipomas on the forehead are often subfascial and then provide an unpleasant surprise—preoperative sonography is useful here.

— General Aspects and Techniques —

Preoperative checklist

○ Previous difficulties with anesthesia?
Allergies to:
  anesthetics?
  antibiotics?
  topical agents?
○ Infections (HIV, hepatitis)?
○ Metal in body?
○ Problems with keloids?
○ Taking anticoagulants (aspirin, warfarin)?

1. Preoperative and perioperative management

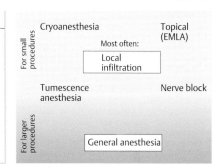

For small procedures

Cryoanesthesia   Topical (EMLA)

Most often:

| Local infiltration |

Tumescence anesthesia   Nerve block

For larger procedures

| General anesthesia |

2. Anesthesia

A. General Aspects

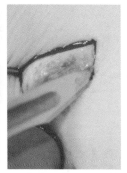

Punch biopsy

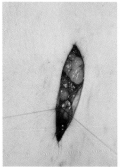

Curettage of seborrheic keratosis

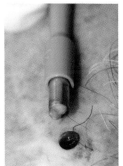

Spindle-shaped excision with subcutaneous butterfly closure (after Breuninger)

Types of excision

B. Operative Techniques

12 Operative Dermatology

■ Plastic-reconstructive Techniques

A variety of techniques are required to close defects after removal of larger lesions:

- a flap means that tissue is freed up and moved about a base to cover a defect. There are many different forms of flaps, which can be prepared and then *advanced, rotated or transposed* to produce a low-tension closure. It is crucial to retain the vascular and nerve supply to a flap so that the wound heals without necrosis, and postoperative sensory defects are avoided
- if it is impossible to close a defect with a flap, then a *skin graft* may be needed. Facial defects are usually closed with a *full-thickness skin graft*, which includes the entire dermis and does not shrink. The skin from behind the ear matches facial skin best, but other options include the groin and clavicle region
- if larger pieces of skin are needed, a *split-thickness skin graft* that includes only part of the dermis may be better. Here a dermatome is used to remove skin from the thigh or buttocks. The harvested graft is then incised in several sites for drainage, and attached. It tends not to match the recipient site and often remains depressed. The donor site also heals with a slight scar; it is simply covered with a nonadherent wound dressing
- when very large areas must be covered, such as when treating a burn patient, a split-thickness graft is cut in a special machine to produce a *mesh graft.* New skin grows into the uncovered spaces from the sides of the meshwork, but the results are not cosmetically elegant
- a final almost nonsurgical approach for burn patients is the application of skin substitutes, which may even involve cultured keratinocytes from the patient on an artificial dermal meshwork.

■ Special Operative Procedures

Several other special procedures are also performed in dermatologic practice:

- *vermilionectomy or lip shave*—the transitional epithelium of the lower lip can be removed; the usual indication is severe actinic damage. Then the exposed area can be covered with an advancement flap of mucosa from the inferior labial mucosa, or allowed to heal secondarily
- *circumcision*—the foreskin can be removed in cases of chronic balanitis or phimosis; in addition, circumcision is sometimes the most elegant way to remove a penile neoplasm
- *nail operations*—the Emmert procedure for ingrown nails involves excision of the lateral nail fold including a part of the nail matrix. Sometimes the entire nail plate must be removed prior to biopsying or excision of periungual or subungual tumors. As much as possible, the nail matrix should be spared or repaired to avoid postoperative nail dystrophy
- *amputation*—in Europe, some dermatologists may perform digital amputations for otherwise inoperable acral tumors
- traumatic tattoos from road accidents, black powder explosions, or firework accidents are best removed by prompt scrubbing with a firm brush. The eyes should always be checked by an ophthalmologist
- *lymph node biopsy*—may be required when lymphoma or metastasis is suspected
- *sentinel lymph node biopsy*—here the sentinel or first lymph node in the chain immediately draining a melanoma, thick squamous cell carcinoma or Merkel cell carcinoma is identified, removed, and microscopically evaluated (Ch. 24.3)
- *lymph node dissection (lymphadenectomy)*—in Europe, some dermatologists perform complete lymph node dissections for node chains involved with melanoma or squamous cell carcinoma.

— General Aspects and Techniques —

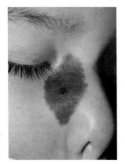
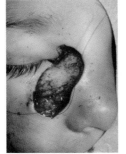
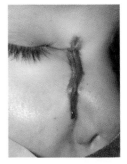

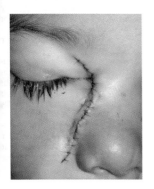
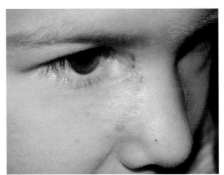

Staged serial excision of congenital melanocytic nevus

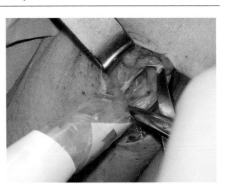

Injection of
radioactive
technetium
marker

Melanoma

Radioactive marking of
sentinel lymph node

Identification of sentinel lymph node with gamma-ray
counter

Special operative procedures

B. Operative Techniques

12 Operative Dermatology

Many individuals today are driven by a quest to look young and perfect. Individuals are no longer willing to live with wrinkles or age spots; if their bodies do not meet the aesthetic ideal, they are ready to be resculptured. In addition, an amazing variety of products are applied or ingested to retard cutaneous aging. While the field has some frivolous care providers and techniques, there are also many serious approaches to help individuals meet their expectations.

Caution: When performing purely cosmetic procedures, it is even more important to counsel the patient in detail, explain the expected improvements and risks, document the current situation with photographs, address the issue of costs, and then obtain signed informed consent!

A. Botulinum Toxin A

Botulinum toxin A is primarily used to treat facial mimicry wrinkles, especially on the glabella (frown lines) and lateral to the eyes (crows' feet), as well as nasolabial and perioral wrinkles. It is injected superficially under the skin or in the muscle of facial expression, and blocks neurotransmission to the muscle and thus makes contraction impossible for around 4 months. Once the effects have worn off, the procedure can be repeated. Many individuals receive regular treatments.

B. Fillers

When patients have deeper wrinkles that have been present for a long time, injection with fillers is usually chosen. A variety of agents can be injected in the superficial, middle or deep dermis to fill or elevate wrinkles. These are also used to make fuller lips and to correct scars. The principal distinction is between resorbable and nonresorbable (permanent) fillers. The latter contain, ideally, inert substances, but eventually all of them can lead to inflammation, abscesses, rejection, or migration of the material.

The resorbable fillers are easier to use and less risky because they are designed to be taken up by the dermal macrophages over months to years. The most commonly used agents are:
- hyaluronic acid
- collagen (modified in many ways)
- poly-L-lactic acid
- calcium hydroxyl apatite
- autologous fat (obtained by liposuction).

General risks for all fillers include: injection at the false level, foreign-body reaction, and allergic reaction to the ingredients.

C. Peeling

There are several methods for superficial removal of facial skin to improve wrinkles, pigmentary alternations, or acne scars, as discussed in the following sections. It is important to distinguish between the level of removal or destruction:
- *superficial peeling*—only the outer layers of the epidermis are removed; methods include mechanical abrasion with fine salt or aluminum crystals (microdermabrasion, lunchtime peel) or topical application of retinoids or α-hydroxy acids (such as lactic acid, mandelic acid, or glycolic acid). The latter can be used in low concentrations by the patient or applied in the office at high levels
- *medium peeling*—the entire epidermis is removed with trichloroacetic acid or other agents; healing usually takes about a week
- *deep peeling*—phenol mixtures are used to penetrate into the dermis. Healing takes weeks and the procedure is not often used in Europe.

Risks. With medium and deep peels, there is a risk of bacterial and viral infections, as well as scarring. There is likely to be postoperative pain and burning. Phenol is generally avoided because of the threat of percutaneous induction of cardiac arrhythmias.

D. Laser Skin Resurfacing

Lasers can be used to remove superficial layers of skin to carefully defined depths. They are effective for superficial wrinkles. The ultra pulsed CO_2 laser is often used; it also warms the tissue, causing coagulation and dermal shrinking, which may further reduce wrinkles.

The erbium:YAG laser is also ablative but causes less collateral damage. Both are used with computer-driven scanning patterns to ensure uniform coverage. Many new approaches are available, including a variety of nonablative lasers.

Risks. Viral or bacterial infections, alteration in pigment, scarring, keloids, milia. Ectropion of the lower lid is a risk with periorbital procedures, especially using a CO_2 laser.

Aesthetic Dermatology

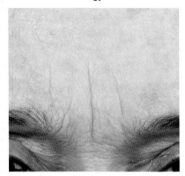
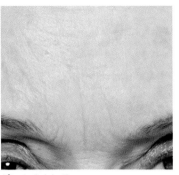

Before therapy
A. Botulinum Toxin A

After toxin injection

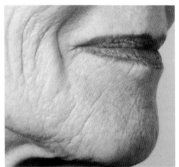
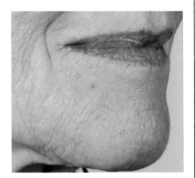

Before therapy
B. Fillers

After filler injection

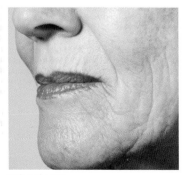
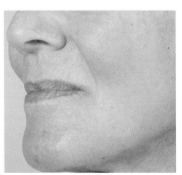

Before therapy
C. Peeling

After mid-level peeling

E. Dermabrasion

A fine diamond fraise is used to sand off the epidermis. Dermabrasion is most often used for acne scarring, especially on the cheek, chin, and perioral region. It is also used for pigmentary abnormalities and superficial to medium wrinkles. It is less helpful around the eyes.

Risks. These are the same as for laser treatment.

F. Lip Augmentation

Lips may be thickened with resorbable fillers such as hyaluronic acid, collagen, and fat. Other options include inserting Gore-Tex or silicone threads or small Plexiglas particles.

Risks. Infections, foreign body reactions, migration of foreign material.

G. Lifting

Classic face lifts involve excising excess skin and then advancing the remaining skin to achieve a tightened, but as natural as possible, look. Some areas are only partly amenable, such as the forehead, cheeks, neck, and eyelids. The abdominal skin, as well as that of the triceps and inner thigh areas can also be tightened.

H. Thermal Lifting

This new approach uses radiofrequency waves to treat superficial wrinkles. The epidermis is ice cooled, so that the waves heat the dermal collagen, causing shrinkage and smoothing. There is no healing time, as the epidermis remains intact. Another related approach is fractional photothermolysis where tiny columns of collagen are heated in a meticulous pattern designed to produce overall dermal tightening with little epithelial damage.

I. Liposuction

Areas of localized excessive fat, such as a double chin or fatty thighs can be improved by liposuction. Following tumescent anesthesia, the fat is removed with suction cannulas, some of which have tiny rotating cutting tips. The cannulas are inserted at multiple sites and the undesired fat removed. It can then be used for augmentation of facial wrinkles and folds.

Caution: The autologous fat must be injected on the day it is removed. Conservation of the material is not possible for medicolegal reasons.

J. Cosmetic Vein Surgery

Small varicosities and starburst veins are often removed for cosmetic indications. The veins can be destroyed with lasers, injected with sclerosing material, or excised through tiny incisions (miniphlebectomy). Larger varicosities especially when associated with chronic venous insufficiency, are usually treated by crossectomy and vein stripping, although foam sclerosing, intravascular laser destruction and radiofrequency destruction are also possible (Ch. 25.2). The keys to successful venous surgery are a precise phlebologic diagnosis and meticulous compression therapy postoperatively.

K. Plastic-reconstructive Surgery

The classic operations of plastic surgery such as lid correction (blepharoplasty), rhinoplasty and otoplasty are all performed not only by dermatologists but are also carried out by other specialists. There is considerable variation from country to country.

Plastic-reconstructive surgery may be required after burns, injuries, or removal of large or destructive tumors. Here dermatologic surgeons are more likely to be involved, especially after micrographic surgery has been performed for large basal cell carcinomas of the face. Depending on the site and nature of the defect, they may work together with plastic surgeons, ophthalmologists, and otorhinolaryngologists on the subsequent repair. Sometimes prostheses are required, to replace an eye or ear; here, collaboration with specialist centers is crucial.

The classical procedures of plastic cosmetic surgery such as corrections of the nose, ears, or breasts (enlargement or reduction) represent an area of overlap between dermatologic and plastic surgeons.

— **Aesthetic Dermatology** —

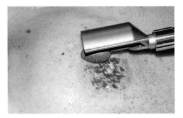
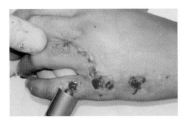

Treatment of acne scars and linear epidermal nevus
E. Dermabrasion

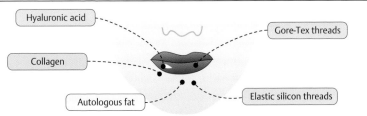

| Hyaluronic acid |
| Collagen |
| Autologous fat |
| Gore-Tex threads |
| Elastic silicon threads |

F. Lip Augmentation

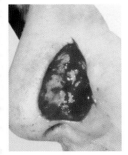
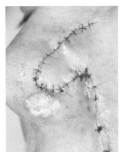
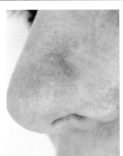

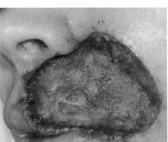
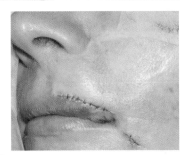

Excision of basal cell carcinoma and repair with flap
K. Plastic-reconstructive Surgery

IV Dermatologic Diseases

A. History

In dermatology, the history often seems unnecessary, such as when a patient presents with a solitary lesion that can be diagnosed at a glance (*Blickdiagnosis*). Nonetheless, a minimal history should be taken and expanded as the situation warrants.

> **Note:** It may seem absurd to take a history and enquire about cold sensitivity before freezing a wart but the patient could have cryoglobulinemia and develop an ulcer, or have cold urticaria and go into anaphylaxis. Always take a history!

1. History of present illness. The history should include the following:
- how lesions appeared at the start
- how long they have been present
- how they have changed
- whether pruritic or not
- systemic complaints
- exposures, occupation, travel
- any relation to light or physical stress
- what treatments have been tried.

> **Note:** Always ask about the use of over-the-counter medications or home remedies.

2. Family history. This should include:
- anyone with similar lesions
- others with other skin diseases
- predisposition to psoriasis, atopic dermatitis.

3. Past medical history. Ask about:
- medications
- underlying diseases.

> **Note:** The answers received to such a screening history determine the need for more detailed questions, more complete physical examination, and associated diagnostic procedures.

B. Symptoms

■ Pruritus

The most frequent dermatologic symptom is pruritus or itching (Ch. 14.10). It can be valuable to more precisely define the pruritus. For example, night-time pruritus is typical for scabies, while pruritus after a warm bath is a sign of polycythemia vera. Many dermatoses are typically pruritic; two common ones are atopic dermatitis and lichen planus. Others never itch—most notorious in this regard is syphilis. Pruritus may also reflect underlying disturbances or not have an obvious cause. Patients with pruritus may complain of sleep loss or inability to concentrate. They may scratch or rub their skin, inducing excoriations or even erosions and ulcers. Peculiarly, patients with atopic dermatitis scratch vigorously, but those with lichen planus only rub. Prurigo patients typically remove a lesion with their fingernail leaving a defect that scars.

■ Other Complaints

Other possible complaints include:
- pain (herpes simplex, zoster, vulvodynia)
- tenderness (many tumors are tender to touch or even painful. The acronym ANGEL (see opposite) is a helpful way to remember them)
- burning (some lesions are typically described as burning, for example dermatitis herpetiformis (Ch. 15.1)
- fever (infections, connective-tissue diseases).

C. Signs (Physical Findings)

Dermatology has developed a special language, almost a code, to facilitate the description of cutaneous findings. This difficult terminology is considered on the next page.

The lesion should always be assessed for the following properties:
- tenderness
- temperature
- consistency (firm, soft)
- mobile or fixed
- estimation of the depth or level of involvement (epidermis, dermis, subcutis).

> **Note:** Whenever possible, the entire integument should be examined. There are several reasons:
> - important clues regarding the presenting problem may be uncovered
> - a total body examination is an inexpensive and effective form of screening for skin cancer.
> - patients tend to hide the most worrisome lesions because they fear a grim diagnosis.

History and Symptoms

Pruritus, pain?

How long?

Where?

Light-exposed areas?

Worse at work?

Suspected triggers?

Travel-related?

Prior treatment?

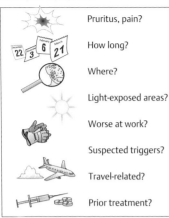

1. History of present illness
A. History

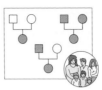

In the family
– Genetic diseases
– Psoriasis or atopic dermatitis
– Other skin diseases

2. Family history

Medications   Other diseases

3. Past medical history

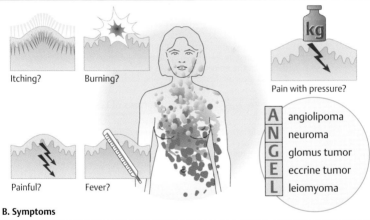

Itching?

Burning?

Pain with pressure?

Painful?

Fever?

A angiolipoma
N neuroma
G glomus tumor
E eccrine tumor
L leiomyoma

B. Symptoms

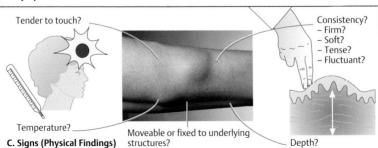

Tender to touch?

Temperature?

Moveable or fixed to underlying structures?

Consistency?
– Firm?
– Soft?
– Tense?
– Fluctuant?

Depth?

C. Signs (Physical Findings)

The first decision is to determine if a lesion is primary or secondary. Primary lesions are the initial manifestation of the disease, unaffected by the course of the disease or manipulation by the patient. Secondary lesions do show such changes.

A. Primary Lesions

1. Macule. This is a flat lesion, identified only by color change and *not palpable*. Large macules are sometimes called *patches*. The color can be caused by leakage of blood, changes in the blood flow, hemosiderin, melanin, or exogenous pigment.

> **Note:** A blind examiner cannot find a macule.

2. Papule. A raised lesion, usually defined as less than 1 cm in diameter. Larger similar lesions are *nodules*. A papule may consist of a thickened epidermis, dermis, or combination thereof. Subcutaneous space-occupying lesions are usually nodules.

3. Plaque. A flat-topped lesion larger than 10 mm in diameter; it is fancifully compared with a mesa in Southwest USA.

4. Vesicle. A fluid-filled lesion; when larger than 1 cm, it is usually designated as a *blister*. The site of fluid may be within the epidermis or subepidermal. It is either clear or hemorrhagic.

5. Pustule. A pus-filled vesicle; it can be primary (psoriasis) or secondary, when a vesicle becomes cloudy (impetigo).

6. Hive. Also known as *urtica* or *wheal*, this elevated lesion is caused by leakage of fluid from a vessel; it is usually pruritic and transient, lasting <24 hours.

> **Note:** Hive is both a primary lesion and also a diagnosis; the disease is then known as urticaria or hives.

B. Secondary Lesions

1. Scale. An abnormal accumulation of corneocytes, secondary to excessive epidermal turnover (psoriasis) or delayed shedding (some forms of ichthyosis), as well as repetitive trauma. Types include:
- psoriasiform—silvery
- pityriasiform—fine
- rupial—thick, coarse
- collarette—prominent at the periphery.

2. Crust. A surface coating consisting of dried serum, pus, or blood, sometimes with scale.

> **Note:** Always establish what lesion is beneath a crust. Sometimes it is a malignant tumor with overlying necrosis and crusts.

3. Erosion. A superficial loss of epidermis, caused by ruptured intraepidermal blister or slight trauma.

Excoriation. A defect in the epidermis, and often the dermis, induced by scratching or manipulation (not shown).

4. Fissure. A crack or split in the epidermis and dermis; fissures around circular orifices are known as *rhagades*.

5. Ulcer. A defect in the epidermis and dermis with impaired healing, caused by trauma, impaired vascular supply, tumors, and infections.

6. Atrophy. Thinning of the skin because of loss of dermis; epidermal atrophy is a microscopic finding.

7. Lichenification. A distinctive response to inflammation, leading to pronounced skin markings. Rubbing produces epidermal thickening with many small smooth papules, as in lichen simplex chronicus (Ch. 14.10) or atopic dermatitis (Ch. 14.4).

8. Sclerosis. Dermal scar-like induration, such as in morphea or systemic sclerosis (Ch. 17.4).

9. Scar. The site of repair of a dermal defect, scars may be hypertrophic (thickened), flat, or atrophic (depressed).

C. Features of Lesions

1. Description. Color, size, margin (well-defined or diffuse; scaly or not), consistency.

2. Number of Lesions. Solitary or multiple; if multiple, confluent or distinct?

3. Arrangement

Linear. There are two main linear patterns:
- *dermatomal*: following cutaneous sensory nerves, as in herpes zoster (Ch. 32.2)
- *lines of Blaschko*: following lines of embryonic skin development, as in epidermal nevi (Ch. 20.3).

Annular.
- Papules grouped in circular pattern, as in granuloma annulare (Ch. 17.7).

Herpetiform.
- Grouped vesicles, as in herpes simplex (Ch. 32.2).

Disseminated.
- Scattered lesions.

— Types of Lesions —

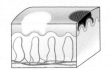

1. Macule

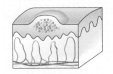

2. Papule ≤10 mm

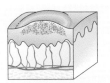

3. Plaque >10 mm

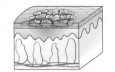

4. Vesicle ≤10 mm

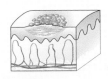

5. Pustule

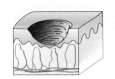

6. Hive

A. Primary Lesions

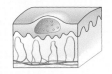

1. Scale

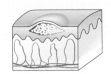

2. Crust

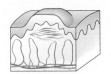

3. Erosion

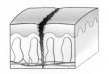

4. Rhagade, fissure

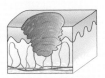

5. Ulcer

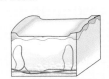

6. Atrophy

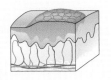

7. Lichenification

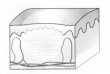

8. Sclerosis

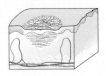

9. Scar

B. Secondary Lesions

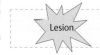

Lesion

Shape ?

Number ?

Color ?

Border ?

Distribution ?

C. Features of Lesions

13 Dermatologic Examination

A. Definition

Erythroderma is a diffuse redness or erythema of the skin, generally involving more than 95 % of the skin surface. It is not a disease but a clinical sign.

B. Pathophysiology

Erythroderma is the result of intense cutaneous inflammation, with marked vascular dilatation and increased cutaneous blood flow. Thus, there is an excessive cooling effect (transfer of warmth to environment), leading to chilling. The epidermal barrier is often breached, leading to scaling, desquamation, and then exudation of fluids. A similar process in the gut can cause protein-losing enteropathy.

C. Etiology

The causes of erythroderma vary greatly with the age of the patient. The most important causes are atopic dermatitis, psoriasis, systemic drug reactions, allergic contact dermatitis, cutaneous T-cell lymphoma, and pityriasis rubra pilaris. Thus, the single most important question for the patient is, *is there any history of preexisting skin diseases?*

D. Clinical Features

Not surprisingly, the predominant clinical finding is marked erythema. The skin is red, scaly, and often thickened. Desquamation or exfoliation is expected. The skin folds are often exaggerated. Nail changes typical for psoriasis or atopic dermatitis, or islands of sparing, so suggestive of pityriasis rubra pilaris, may provide clues to the underlying diagnosis. Both hair loss and shedding of nails may occur. Lymphadenopathy is also common, reflecting cutaneous secondary infections, immunologic reactions, and, in rare cases, cutaneous lymphoma. It may be very difficult to separate dermatopathic lymphadenopathy from a lymphoma. One of the most striking forms of erythroderma is Sézary syndrome—a form of cutaneous T-cell lymphoma with marked erythroderma, lymphadenopathy, and circulating atypical T lymphocytes.

Note: Patients with erythroderma are critically ill; they may have fever, chills, weight loss, malaise, and anorexia. The term *exfoliative erythroderma syndrome* is sometimes applied to acute erythroderma with systemic signs and symptoms.

E. Diagnostic Approach

- Ask about and search for preexisting skin disease, especially stigmata of atopic dermatitis or psoriasis.
- Take an extensive drug history; always enquire about antiseizure medications, hypoglycemic agents, nonsteroidal anti-inflammatory drugs (NSAIDS), and allopurinol.
- Examination of the hair and nails may provide useful clues, as they are less likely to be involved.
- Use skin biopsy to exclude lymphoma and perhaps identify other diseases.
- Take a complete blood count (CBC) and routine blood chemistry; check electrolytes and serum proteins.
- Check the peripheral blood for atypical lymphocytes (Sézary cells); generally, ≥ 20 % atypical T cells is taken as diagnostic.
- Use lymph node sonography and, if questions persist, perhaps lymph node biopsy. Yet it is sometimes impossible to distinguish between reactive and neoplastic T cells.

F. Therapy

Note: The most important point is to set the skin at rest; the analogy of having "broken skin" as others may have a "broken leg" is sometimes helpful for the patient. Erythroderma is potentially life-threatening and must be treated aggressively.

- Admission, bedrest, a room in which the temperature can be can be maintained at 22–24 °C.
- Careful attention to general physical status, nutrition, electrolytes.
- Initially bland topical therapy, especially if allergic contact dermatitis is still a possibility—options include soaking in a tub and generous application of emollients.
- Often a short burst of systemic corticosteroids is helpful, but avoid using corticosteroids if psoriasis is a likely diagnosis, and especially avoid embarking upon long-term therapy.
- As soon as possible, start disease-specific therapy, such as photochemotherapy or methotrexate for psoriasis or T-cell lymphoma, or retinoids for pityriasis rubra pilaris.

Note: In some patients, no cause for the erythroderma is found. They are best treated conservatively and regularly re-examined.

Erythroderma

Generalized inflammation

Increased peripheral blood flow ↑

Barrier function disturbed ⇩

Heat loss ↑ ⇩

Loss of fluids and proteins

Chills

B. Pathophysiology

Underlying causes

– Psoriasis
– Atopic dermatitis
– Drug reaction
– Cutaneous T-cell lymphoma
– Pityriasis rubra pilaris
– Allergic contact dermatitis

C. Etiology

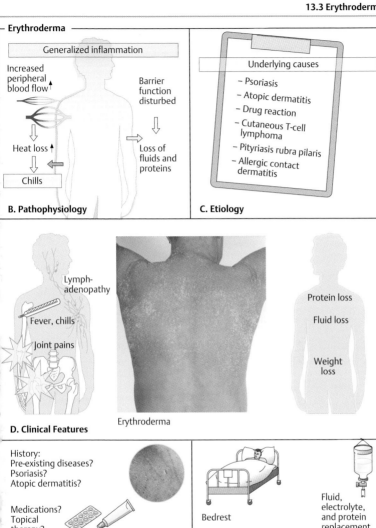

Lymphadenopathy

Fever, chills

Joint pains

Protein loss

Fluid loss

Weight loss

Erythroderma

D. Clinical Features

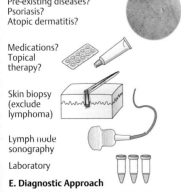

History:
Pre-existing diseases?
Psoriasis?
Atopic dermatitis?

Medications?
Topical therapy?

Skin biopsy (exclude lymphoma)

Lymph node sonography

Laboratory

E. Diagnostic Approach

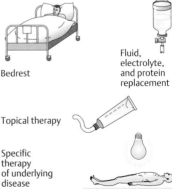

Bedrest

Fluid, electrolyte, and protein replacement

Topical therapy

Specific therapy of underlying disease

F. Therapy

Phototherapy

13 Dermatologic Examination

The terms dermatitis and eczema are almost interchangeable. Theoretically, dermatitis refers to acute disease, while eczema describes a more chronic process. We will generally use dermatitis in this book, but some diseases are, almost by tradition, always called eczema.

A. Epidemiology

Dermatitis is the most common reason for seeking dermatologic care in every age group; after musculoskeletal complaints, it is the second most common reason for visiting a general physician.

B. Clinical Features

In acute dermatitis, the skin is erythematous, edematous, and may blister in severe cases. In the flexures, as in atopic and diaper dermatitis, erosions are common. As the disease persists, the dermal inflammatory infiltrate tends to decrease, while the epidermis shows reactive proliferation of keratinocytes and spongiosis and then develops scales and later becomes lichenified, reflecting chronic rubbing. Accurately identifying the degree of acuity is essential for planning appropriate therapy.

C. Histopathology

Acute dermatitis features epidermal edema (spongiosis) damage to keratinocytes. The classical features of inflammation are reflected under the microscope:
- *rubor and calor*—dilated vessels
- *tumor*—inflammatory cells, spongiosis, blisters, scales, and crusts
- *dolor*—often pruritic, sometimes painful
- *functio laesa*—epidermal barrier damage with fluid loss, and increased infections.

Chronic dermatitis features epidermal reaction with thickening (acanthosis), dilated vessels, and perivascular lymphocytic infiltrates.

D. Differential Diagnosis

It is often very difficult to diagnose the type of dermatitis clinically. Many possible triggers (atopy, irritation, sensitization, dryness) all produce amazingly similar clinical changes.

Note: The best approach is a careful history and then observation of the pattern of distribution. Pay attention to sites of predilection such as flexures in atopy or sites that are typical for certain contact allergens.

Always consider the possibility of irritant or allergic contact dermatitis, since if a triggering agent is overlooked and not eliminated, therapy attempts are doomed to failure, especially if the patient is allergic to a topical medication that he continues to use.

Many disorders can present as dermatitis. Examples of disorders often misdiagnosed as dermatitis are briefly discussed next and considered in greater detail later.

■ Tinea and scabies

Always think of tinea when a lesion has an expanding border; KOH examination gives a quick answer. Scabies may be so excoriated that primary lesions are hard to find; always check the nipples, glands, and interdigital webs.

■ Carcinoma in situ

Superficial basal cell carcinoma, Bowen disease, and Paget disease can all mimic a clinically persistent dermatitis.

Caution: Always biopsy dermatitis that is localized and fails to respond to therapy.

■ Mycosis fungoides

Early lesions can be very subtle and hard to identify with certainty, even with histology.

E. Therapy

Note: The therapy of dermatitis must always be adjusted to the acuity of the disease. Often the choice of the vehicle is more important than the selection of the active ingredient.

■ 1. Acute dermatitis

Wet dressings, baths, nonocclusive vehicles like lotions or creams. No ointments. Water-based shake lotions are good for drying, while alcohol-based products burn too much. Mid-potency corticosteroids.

■ 2. Chronic dermatitis

Emollient creams and ointments, perhaps containing urea. If scales are prominent, keratolytics such as salicylic acid can be added. Stronger corticosteroids may be tried, but always consider steroid-sparing measures such as phototherapy or topical calcineurin inhibitors.

Dermatitis and Eczema

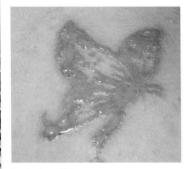

Acute dermatitis

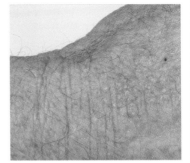

Chronic dermatitis with lichenification

B. Clinical Features

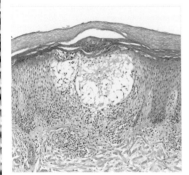

Acute dermatitis

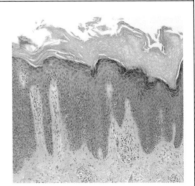

Chronic dermatitis

C. Histopathology

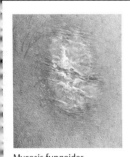

Mycosis fungoides
(cutaneous T-cell lymphoma)

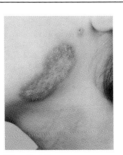

Tinea faciei

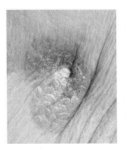

Bowen disease

D. Differential Diagnosis

IV Dermatologic Diseases

A. Definition

Allergic contact dermatitis (ACD) is a T-cell-mediated immune reaction against haptens or protein allergens.

B. Epidemiology

The rate of sensitization for common contact allergens is well established. They can be encountered as an occupational risk, during the course of daily life, or as a complication of topical medications.

C. Pathogenesis

The patient must have an initial exposure during which he or she becomes sensitized before allergic contact dermatitis is possible. The allergen must initially be directly applied to the skin or arrive via airborne spread. Under most conditions, sensitization occurs in skin areas damaged by irritant dermatitis such as irritant hand dermatitis or stasis dermatitis around a leg ulcer. It does not usually induce a toxic dermatitis, but instead elicits a T-cell-mediated immunologic memory, so that on later re-exposure, inflammation occurs. When allergic contact dermatitis appears to occur without prior exposure, the usual culprits are very widespread allergens (such as poison ivy) or sensitization by cross-reacting substances.

D. Clinical Features

When dermatitis is localized, allergic contact dermatitis should always be considered. Avoidance of the allergen leads to prompt improvement and a permanent cure.

The hands. These are the most common site, especially for occupational allergic contact dermatitis. Sensitization usually occurs on the background of cumulative-toxic dermatitis; thus, bands with chronic wet exposure (cement work, machinists, cooks, beauticians) are at special risk. Frequent hand washing and latex gloves put healthcare workers at risk. Gardeners may react to variety of allergens, such as geraniol in geraniums.

The face. Cosmetics and airborne agents are the most common causes. Patients using inhalation or aroma therapy have become a high-risk group. *Ficus benjamina* (weeping fig) has become a favorite room plant, but also a common airborne allergen. Dermatitis of the ears is usually from nickel allergy, induced during the process of ear piercing. Piercings in other sites, such as the umbilicus, may also induce dermatitis from nickel allergy.

The legs. About 30% of individuals with chronic venous insufficiency and venous leg ulcers develop allergic contact dermatitis, almost invariably to one or more of the medications they have used. Typical sensitizers include antibiotics, fragrances, and preservatives.

Intertriginous areas. In the groin and axillae, patients are often sensitized to fragrances or preservatives in personal hygiene items. Irritant contact dermatitis is far more common when these agents are improperly used.

Hematogenous allergic contact dermatitis. Once topical sensitization has occurred, patients can react dramatically when the same agent, often an antibiotic, is administered systemically. Often the reaction is limited to the axillae, groin, and buttocks, presumably because of exudation in sweat; this dramatic picture is known as baboon syndrome. Other patients develop widespread dermatitis, as well as systemic signs and symptoms.

Occupational issues. Young individuals in the first years of a high-risk profession are at special risk of becoming sensitized. This has been best established in young beauticians, as the combination of irritant dermatitis and frequent allergen exposure forms a vicious cycle. Other at-risk professions include healthcare workers, bakers, gardeners, machinists, and car mechanics. Many individuals have to give up their profession, requiring retraining at considerable societal expense. In some countries, preemployment screening is used to prevent patients with atopic dermatitis and similar diseases entering such professions. In most instances, proactive prophylactic treatment of atopic dermatitis is effective and more appropriate.

E. Diagnosis and Therapy

A high index of suspicion is required. Patch testing is used to confirm allergic contact dermatitis. A positive test must be interpreted against the background of the patient's findings and previous exposures.

The main treatment is avoiding the allergen. Topical corticosteroids usually suffice to control attacks; rarely short-term systemic use is required. The memory responses are designed to prevent infections and are usually so strong that even corticosteroids fail to control them if the allergen is not avoided or eliminated.

Allergic Contact Dermatitis

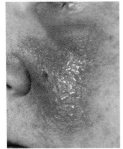

ACD to topical antibiotic

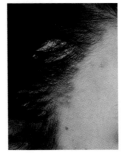

Allergy to hair dye

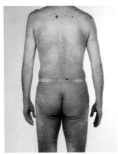

Baboon syndrome

D. Clinical Features

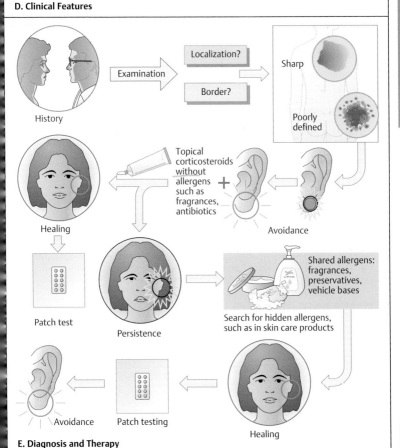

History

Examination → Localization? / Border? → Sharp / Poorly defined

Topical corticosteroids without allergens such as fragrances, antibiotics + Avoidance

Healing

Patch test

Persistence

Shared allergens: fragrances, preservatives, vehicle bases

Search for hidden allergens, such as in skin care products

Healing

Patch testing

Avoidance

E. Diagnosis and Therapy

14 Inflammatory Diseases of the Epidermis

145

A. Definition

External contact with irritating substances leads to toxic skin damage. Long-term low-level exposure to toxic substances causes cumulative-toxic dermatitis, often with lichenification.

B. Epidemiology

This is probably the most common human disease, if one considers occupational hand dermatitis, housewives' hands, and diaper dermatitis as its three most common manifestations.

C. Pathogenesis

Toxic dermatitis results when epidermal protective mechanisms are overwhelmed; in severe changes, the dermis is also involved. Triggers can be physical (trauma, radiation) or chemical. Depending on their intensity, they can cause proliferation, senescence, apoptosis, or necrosis of keratinocytes, as well as affecting Langerhans cells and melanocytes.

D. Clinical Features

■ Acute Irritant Dermatitis

This is characterized by sharply bordered erythematous lesions with edema, blisters, crusts, and scales. It may heal with hypo- or hyperpigmentation. Common examples include acute sunburn or acute hand dermatitis when soaps or disinfectants are trapped behind rubber gloves.

■ Subacute Irritant Dermatitis

A mixture of acute and chronic changes, so that blisters, crusts, and scales appear together, sometimes with early epidermal thickening.

■ Cumulative-toxic or Chronic Irritant Dermatitis

Epidermal repair with lichenification dominates. There may still be punctate erosions. Histologically, one sees incontinence of pigment and a lymphocytic perivascular infiltrate.

Note: Chronic irritant dermatitis predisposes the patient to allergic contact dermatitis, as it activates the immune system by alarming dendritic cells in the skin and lymph nodes, as well as facilitating their exchange of information with T cells in lymph nodes.

E. Therapy

Avoiding toxic agents is key. Topical corticosteroids should be used only in combination with disinfectants. Protective measures are essential to avoid recurrences.

F. Other Types of Dermatitis

■ Nummular Eczema

Nummular means coin shaped; patients have 1–5 cm round inflamed patches. Lesions often have blisters or yellow crusts, suggesting an infectious component, usually *Staphylococcus aureus*. Associated findings may include dry skin and chronic venous insufficiency; sometimes contact sensitization is identified. Topical corticosteroids are the mainstay, but work better if combined with systemic antibiotic therapy. Phototherapy is a useful adjunct. This therapy-resistant form of dermatitis should not be confused with nummular lesions in atopic dermatitis or the annular lesions of tinea.

■ Lichen Simplex Chronicus and Prurigo Nodularis

Endstage of chronic inflammation with pruritus-induced manipulation (Ch. 14.10)

■ Dyshidrotic Dermatitis

This is characterized by tiny pruritic blisters on the sides of the fingers; there are sometimes larger blisters on the palms of the hand and soles of the feet (pompholyx). While most cases are idiopathic, possible causes include atopic diathesis, fungal id reactions, contact dermatitis, and systemic allergic reactions to nickel. Heals with collarette scale (dyshidrosis lamellosa sicca). Worsens with smoking. Treatments include topical high-potency corticosteroids and photochemotherapy, as well as short bursts of systemic corticosteroids for flares.

■ Unexplained Dermatitis

Often the cause of dermatitis remains a mystery. Such patients should be patch tested, repeatedly questioned and re-examined, but treated symptomatically.

Note: Consider possibility of scabies or mites from pets or environment. 50 % of pruritus and dermatitis in pet owners can be explained in this way.

Irritant Contact Dermatitis and Other Types of Dermatitis

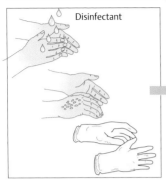
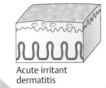

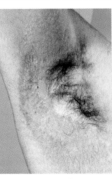

Disinfectant

Acute irritant dermatitis

Cumulative-toxic dermatitis

Innate immune system activated

Risk of sensitization ↑

C. Pathogenesis

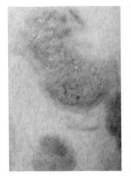

Acute irritant dermatitis

Cumulative-toxic dermatitis caused by antibacterial additive to detergent

D. Clinical Features

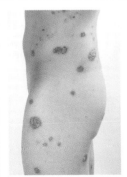
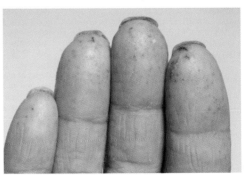

Nummular dermatitis

Dyshidrotic dermatitis

F. Other Types of Dermatitis

14 Inflammatory Diseases of the Epidermis

The atopic diseases include three major entities—atopic dermatitis, allergic rhinoconjunctivitis, and allergic asthma—whose pathophysiologic interactions are not completely understood. All three diseases share a tendency to elevated levels of total immunoglobulin (Ig)E, as well as IgE that is specific for protein allergens from pollens, house dust mites, and, less often, foodstuffs. The predisposition toward the three disorders is inherited together. The degree to which atopic dermatitis shares pathophysiologic features with the others is unclear. For example, almost half of all patients with atopic dermatitis have no serum evidence for IgE-mediated hypersensitivity.

A. Atopic Dermatitis

■ Epidemiology

There are four peaks of incidence; the largest is between 3 and 24 months (with 5%–10% of infants affected); others occur between 6 and 16 years, at the start of work, and after 60 years of age.

■ Pathogenesis

Four pathogenetic factors appear especially relevant. They are not mutually exclusive, but instead are interacting cofactors.

Impaired epidermal barrier. The impaired barrier seems to be the leading cause. It frequently results from mutations in filaggrin, a key protein of the cornified membrane, as well as by abnormalities in the epidermal lipids, which not only provide a barrier function but also influence keratinocyte differentiation. The skin is easily irritated and dries out readily. There are also defects in innate immunity and the T-cell response, as well as a propensity to over-respond with IgE. Filaggrin mutations are also a key feature of ichthyosis vulgaris, explaining the long-appreciated clinical overlap between the two common disorders.

> **Clinical correlate:** Clinical correlations include increased epidermal water loss and development of follicular keratoses. In addition, mice with genetic defects in epidermal filaggrins show a tendency to inflammation and dermatis resembling atopic dermatitis.

Impaired innate immunity. The second key aspect is defects in innate immunity. Atopic patients produce reduced amounts of defensins on their epidermis and in their sweat. Defensins are small cysteine-rich cationic proteins found in vertebrates and invertebrates. They are active against bacteria, fungi, and viruses.

Infection with *Staphylococcus aureus*. The combined dysfunction of the epidermal barrier and the lack of defensins may explain why 95% of atopic individuals are colonized with *Staphylococcus aureus*.

Altered Immunity. There are elevated skin and serum levels of IgE, as well as activated T cells and dendritic cells laden with IgE in the skin. The latter can effectively stimulate T cells, helping recruit allergen-specific T cells to the skin and thus initiate an autoimmune response.

■ Clinical Features

Infant/young child. After 3 months, babies are likely to present by scratching their pruritic skin and developing thick crusted scales on their scalp (cradle cap). They may then develop an exudative dermatitis with urticarial plaques, crusts, scales, and excoriations, usually favoring the head and extremities. Diaper dermatitis is very common. Superinfection is often the dominant feature, necessitating a combined anti-inflammatory/antimicrobial therapy. Up to 90% show marked spontaneous improvement between 2 and 3 years of age.

School age/puberty. Often the atopic child flares again, this time showing a predisposition for the flexures, although generalized disease may develop. The initial lesions are erythematous papules and vesicles; then there is a rapid transition to chronic dermatitis, with excoriations and lichenification being the most prominent finding. Typical sites are the antecubital and popliteal fossae, as well as the neck. Superinfections are once again a problem. There is often spontaneous clearing at puberty.

Onset of work. Atopic patients carry a lifelong burden of being more sensitive to irritants. This makes it imperative that they are trained to protect against exposure to possible toxic agents. They should be counseled to use continuous skin therapy if they enter high-risk professions such as beauticians, machinists, or healthcare workers. Instead of developing a proactive hyperkeratotic response, they tend to get cumulative-toxic dermatitis. They are also very sensitive to wool, but generally learn for themselves to avoid this fabric.

Atopic Dermatitis, Allergic Rhinitis, and Asthma

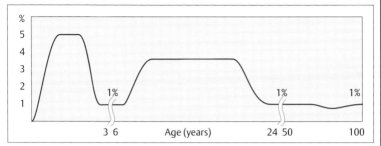

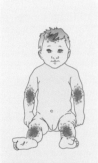

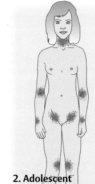

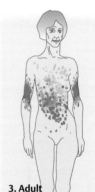

1. Infant/small child
Diffuse distribution especially head, arms, legs

2. Adolescent
Marked flexural involvement: neck, popliteal and antecubital fossae, backs of hands and feet

3. Adult
Primarily involvement of trunk and arms

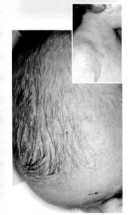

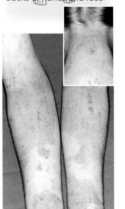

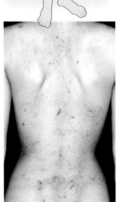

A. Atopic Dermatitis

Adults. Most adults have only a tendency to be more susceptible to irritants. The prevalence of active atopic dermatitis in adults is under 1%. Nonetheless, there are several adults who have only hand, eyelid, or neck dermatitis as a reflection of their atopic tendency. Others may have marked cheilitis.

Seniors. There is another peak flare late in life, often with a totally different clinical picture. Patients present with pruritus and prurigo nodules. The clinical picture is dominated by single or grouped erythematous papules and nodules with central excoriations. This form is often associated with severe, almost intractable, pruritus, may have eosinophilia, and is much more difficult to manage than the exudative or lichenified forms.

■ Therapy

Therapy must take into consideration the abnormal barrier function with a tendency to dryness, the likelihood of superinfection with *S. aureus*, and the excessive T-cell–mediated immune response. The dramatic response of almost all patients to topical corticosteroids, and the resolution of infections under such therapy, demonstrate the essential role of inflammation in both dermatitis and superinfection.

The mainstay of treatment is suppressing inflammation with topical corticosteroids, coupled with disinfectants like triclosan. In severe cases, the steroids can be alternated with calcineurin inhibitors like pimecrolimus or tacrolimus. Long-term topical corticosteroids must be avoided; the side effects are considerable, especially in children, although a whole generation of safer agents is now available.

Topical antibiotics sound attractive but should be avoided because of the risks of antibiotic resistance, which contributes to resistant strains in the community, and sensitization, which then means the patient can no longer use that class of antibiotics systemically. They should be replaced by disinfectants.

Perhaps most crucial is continuous skin care with emollients to address the permanent problem of dry skin. Products containing 5%–12% urea are humectants, helping maintain water in the stratum corneum. They also help corticosteroids to penetrate. Urea burns on application in acute dermatitis, making it hard to use in infants.

In severe flares, systemic penicillinase-resistant antibiotics that are effective against *S. aureus* are indicated. Infections with herpes simplex require systemic antiviral agents, to avoid widespread skin disease and protect against the development of herpetic keratitis and even herpetic meningoencephalitis.

Sometimes all these measures fail to control atopic dermatitis. In such instances, the diagnosis should be reviewed, as well as the therapy, and especially the patient or parents' compliance. Other alternatives include phototherapy; ultraviolet (UV)B 311 nm is generally preferred for children, while psoralen plus UVA (PUVA) is an option in adults. Immunosuppressive agents such as azathioprine are also effective, but are associated with potential side effects. Azathioprine is used at 100–150 mg daily. The regimen should be stopped only after the patient has been clear for a long period of time; otherwise relapses are the rule.

> **Note:** Prompt and aggressive management of atopic dermatitis may halt the "atopic march"—the progression to allergic rhinoconjunctivitis and/or asthma.

B. Allergic Rhinoconjunctivitis

Allergic rhinoconjunctivitis, better known as hay fever, is the most common atopic disorder with a prevalence of around 20%. The peak onset is during adolescence, but the disease generally persists for many years. Of all the atopic manifestations, it is most tightly linked with specific IgE antibodies and positive type I prick test reactions against protein aero-allergens. The most important allergens are early blooming shrubs and trees, grasses, and weeds; in Europe, grains such as rye are important, while in the USA the most important allergen is ragweed (*Ambrosia artemisifolia*), as well as pine pollens. Nonseasonal allergens include house dust mites, cat hairs, and rodents.

■ Clinical Features

Allergic rhinoconjunctivitis presents with weeping red eyes, a runny nose, sneezing, or a combination thereof. Symptoms start within minutes of allergen exposure. Surprisingly, recurrent exposure to modest or high levels of allergens leads to clinical problems, while continuous exposure to high levels of allergen may lead to a suppression of the symptoms. For example, many individuals with cat-hair allergy first begin to have problems when they no longer have a cat in the home and have only occasional exposure. This explains why getting rid of a pet frequently does not help solve the problem.

— Atopic Dermatitis, Allergic Rhinitis, and Asthma —

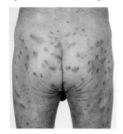 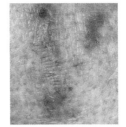 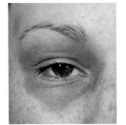

Prurigo nodules   Prurigo nodule   Lid dermatitis

Late manifestations

UV therapy; not combined with calcineurin inhibitors

Systemic immunomodulation (azathioprine)

Topical corticosteroids   and/or calcineurin inhibitors
Systemic antibiotics, antiviral agents as needed

Basic therapy   Humectant creams/ointments (5%–12% urea) + disinfectants as needed

Therapy

A. Atopic Dermatitis

Hay fever

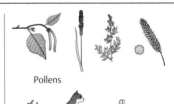

Pollens

20% of the population

House dust mite, cat hair, other small pets

13.   20.
Age (years)

Prevalence   Common allergens

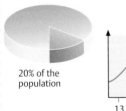 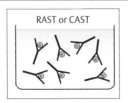 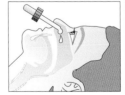

RAST or CAST

Positive prick test to aeroallergen   Specific IgE   Nasal provocation

Diagnostic approach

B. Allergic Rhinoconjunctivitis

IV Dermatologic Diseases

■ **Diagnostic Approach**

The suspected allergies can be confirmed with prick or intracutaneous testing, as well as determination of the specific IgE levels with a radio-allergosorbent test (RAST) or cellular allergen stimulation test (CAST). The clinical findings, in-vivo tests and in-vitro tests must all be correlated to determine which allergen is truly causing the problems.

■ **Therapy**

The mainstays of therapy are antihistamines (oral, nose sprays, eye drops), and perhaps corticosteroid nose sprays. The symptoms can usually be well controlled if the treatment is started before allergen exposure, or before the season begins. If this is not the case, specific immunotherapy over 3–5 years may provide longer-lasting relief. Subcutaneous injection of the responsible allergen in increasing doses over years leads to satisfactory protection in some 70% of patients. Sublingual immunotherapy (SLIT) has recently become available for some allergens and may be effective, but perhaps not as good as injections. There are good data showing that treating allergic rhinoconjunctivitis reduces the likelihood of developing allergic asthma.

C. Asthma

Asthma is a chronic inflammatory disease of the lower airways. About one-third of cases are caused by classic type I allergens (extrinsic asthma), by hyper-reactive airways (instrinsic—associated with infections, medications, additives, emotional triggers), and by a combination of both. Up to 10% of children and 5% of adults suffer from the disease.

■ **Clinical Features**

The main clinical triad is coughing, shortness of breath, and wheezing. Although patients have the feeling that they are getting no air, the real problem is with expiration, so that the lungs are overinflated. The cause is generally reversible bronchoconstriction, associated with thickened mucus, airway edema, and hypertrophy of the airway smooth muscle cells. These effects are primarily caused by CD4+ T cells producing interleukin (IL)-4 and IL-13; mediators such as tumor necrosis factor (TNF) aggravate the problem; they are so important that TNF antagonists can be helpful in asthma.

Asthma attacks can be triggered by external triggers (specific allergens, cold, smoke, medications [aspirin], and exercise) or appear in the early morning hours (3:00 am to 6:00 am), as the tone of the bronchial smooth muscles is primarily regulated by the parasympathetic nervous system.

■ **Diagnostic Approach**

Of the three atopic disorders, asthma correlates best with the total IgE level. After history, prick testing, and IgE measurements (total and specific), the next steps are pulmonary function and bronchial provocation testing. If the forced expiratory volume in 1 second (FEV_1) indicates that bronchial obstruction is present, it is important to determine whether or not it is reversible. If no primary obstruction is found, then allergens or other triggers that are inducing transient obstruction should be sought.

■ **Therapy**

Treatment must be adjusted to the severity of disease. Pharmacologic management is usually divided into obtaining quick relief during attacks and providing long-term control to avoid attacks. In general, inhaler therapy is preferred to deliver active ingredients to the bronchi and avoid (or minimize) systemic side effects. For immediate relief, short-term β_2-adrenergic agonists are inhaled. Long-term prophylactic control involves inhaled corticosteroids, mast cell stabilizers, or long-acting β_2-agonists, as well as oral leukotriene receptor antagonists and, rarely, oral corticosteroids or β_2-agonists. Avoidance of allergens or other triggers is also valuable, and breathing training is often useful.

Atopic Dermatitis, Allergic Rhinitis, and Asthma

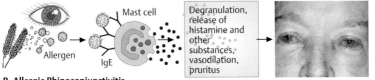

Allergen → Mast cell → IgE → Degranulation, release of histamine and other substances, vasodilation, pruritus

B. Allergic Rhinoconjunctivitis

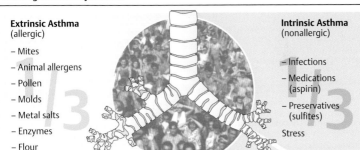

Extrinsic Asthma
(allergic)

– Mites
– Animal allergens
– Pollen
– Molds
– Metal salts
– Enzymes
– Flour

Intrinsic Asthma
(nonallergic)

– Infections
– Medications (aspirin)
– Preservatives (sulfites)

Stress

Mixed form

Etiology

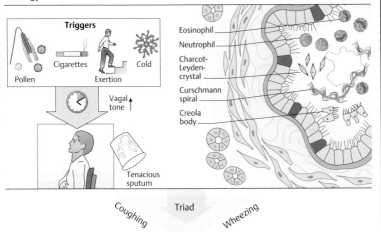

Triggers

Pollen Cigarettes Exertion Cold

Vagal tone ↑

Tenacious sputum

Eosinophil
Neutrophil
Charcot-Leyden-crystal
Curschmann spiral
Creola body

Coughing Triad Wheezing

Shortness of breath

Clinical features

Avoid allergens   Avoid noxious inhalants   Avoid broncho-constrictors

Therapy based on severity:
- Corticosteroids
- β₂ sympathomimetic agents
- Leukotriene antagonists
- Theophylline

Therapy

C. Asthma

14 Inflammatory Diseases of the Epidermis

A. Epidemiology and Subtypes

Psoriasis is an inflammatory disease with increased proliferation and impaired differentiation of keratinocytes. It affects 2%–3% of the population. Of this group, about 10% have arthritis, and in 3%–5% of them it is severe. There is a genetic predisposition to psoriasis, with around 60% concordance in identical twins. A trigger is required to produce the disease—either a local stimulus to proliferation or activation of oligoclonal T cells. About two-thirds of patients have type I psoriasis with a positive family history, peak onset at 20 years of age, and tendency to severe skin disease and arthritis. The disease first appears after a streptococcal infection in 90% of these patients. The other one-third have type II psoriasis, typically starting after 40 years of age, without a family history, and usually more localized. Psoriasis is also now appreciated to be an intimate part of the metabolic syndrome, associated with hypertension, diabetes mellitus, and coronary artery disease. The persistent immune stimulation may thus have wide-reaching effects.

B. Pathogenesis

The risk of type I psoriasis is especially high when the patient has a human leukocyte antigen (HLA) pattern Cw6, B13, Bw57, and DR7. The disease starts with the influx of interferon (IFN)-γ-producing T_{H1} cells and IL-17-producing T_{H17} cells. The most common initial trigger is a streptococcal infection. Medications that increase the T_{H1}/T_{H17} response aggravate psoriasis. They include IFN-α, β-blockers, lithium, and chloroquine. Although the data clearly suggest that psoriasis can be induced and maintained by IL-23-producing antigen-presenting cells (APCs) and a T_{H1}/T_{H17} response, there is also good evidence that local cell damage, such as persistent rubbing or injury, can trigger psoriasis in loco. This is known as the Köbner phenomenon, where a nonspecific trigger produces reaction, most likely driven by TNF. In some psoriasis patients, the keratinocytes show abnormalities in the AP1- or nuclear factor kappa B (NFκB) signal cascades. Thus it seems likely that psoriasis is a disturbance in keratinocyte proliferation that can be elicited indirectly by T_{H1}/T_{H17} cells, IL-23 and TNF, or directly by physical stimuli.

C. Histopathology

The epidermis is acanthotic and features elongated rete ridges. Over the tips of the papillary dermis, it is paradoxically thinned. The dilated and vertically elongated papillary vessels can be seen as blood-filled points when scale is peeled away (Auspitz sign). Epidermal differentiation is incomplete with the granular layer missing, and parakeratosis (retained nuclei in stratum corneum). The dermis contains activated mast cells, dendritic cells, T cells, and neutrophils; the latter migrate into the epidermis and form Munro micro-abscesses, small sterile accumulations.

D. Clinical Features

The sites of involvement, severity, and frequency of recurrence all determine the pattern of psoriasis. Involvement of the scalp, face, hands, or nails is very troublesome for patients, as is widespread or pustular disease. Few diseases negatively influence the patient's quality of life more than psoriasis; it is as troublesome and disabling as coronary artery disease or chronic pulmonary disease.

The hallmark of psoriasis is sharply delineated erythematous plaques with silvery scale. Blisters never form, but the exocytosis of neutrophils may lead to pustules. The pustule may develop on erythematous skin or in established lesions. On the palms and soles, the thickened stratum corneum tends to contain the pustules, which become confluent and larger.

Note: When considering the diagnosis of psoriasis, always check the scalp, gluteal cleft, and nails for possible clues.

■ Guttate Psoriasis

Almost always triggered by streptococci, this form presents as papules and small plaques that are usually less than 3 cm but cover the entire body. It is common in children, in whom it may be confused with pityriasis rosea or pityriasis lichenoides et varioliformis acuta. The lesions respond well to vitamin D analogs, anthralin, and UVB.

■ Chronic Plaque Psoriasis

The most common locations are the knees, elbows, and sacral areas—sites of trauma. There is usually prominent scaling. This form does not respond well to vitamin D analogs and UVB, and is better treated with vitamin D analogs combined with corticosteroids, anthralin (perhaps along with phototherapy), or PUVA therapy.

Psoriasis

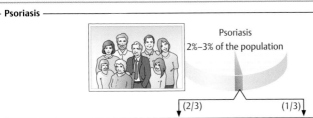

Psoriasis
2%–3% of the population

(2/3)   (1/3)

	Type I	Type II
Family history	HLA positive (Cw6, B13, Bw57, DR7)	None
First appearance	~20 years	> 40 years
Trigger	Often streptococcal infection	?
Distribution	Often guttate	Usually localized
Arthritis	More common	Less common

A. Epidemiology and Subtypes

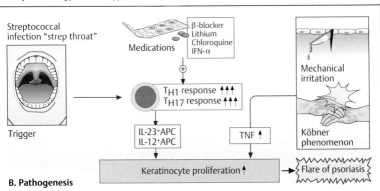

Streptococcal
infection "strep throat"

Medications

β-blocker
Lithium
Chloroquine
IFN-α

⊕

$T_{H}1$ response ↑↑↑
$T_{H}17$ response ↑↑↑

Trigger

IL-23⁺APC
IL-12⁺APC

TNF ↑

Mechanical
irritation

Köbner
phenomenon

Keratinocyte proliferation ↑

Flare of psoriasis

B. Pathogenesis

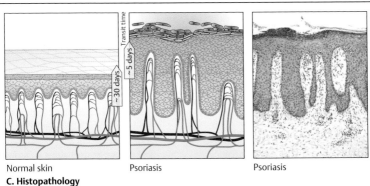

Transit time
~5 days
~30 days

Normal skin   Psoriasis   Psoriasis

C. Histopathology

■ Inverse Psoriasis

In the axillary and inguinal folds, trauma, and usually obesity, combine to produce maceration and rubbing. The lesions here lack significant scale and appear as erythematous almost glistening patches. The area must be made less moist (careful drying with hair dryer, weight loss); then the lesions usually respond well to vitamin D analogs in a gel.

■ Palmoplantar Psoriasis

The thickened stratum corneum leads to more prominent pustules, which are often associated with hyperkeratotic plaques. Treatment is difficult because medications penetrate poorly. Combinations of anthralin and PUVA, or vitamin D analogs and corticosteroids may be effective; systemic therapy is frequently needed.

■ Pustular Psoriasis

This is the maximum variant of an acute psoriatic eruption, with the microscopic migration of neutrophils in the epidermis transformed into a macroscopic phenomenon. The pustules can be localized, or generalized when the trigger is systemic, such as when systemic corticosteroids are used to treat psoriasis and then stopped. This risk is just one reason why corticosteroids are not used systemically in psoriasis. The pustules usually appear in patients with a previous history of psoriasis, but sometimes appear de novo on erythematous skin. Pustular psoriasis is potentially fatal, as patients have severe metabolic problems. They require methotrexate or PUVA immediately.

■ Psoriatic Erythroderma

Psoriasis is one of the most common reasons for erythroderma (Ch. 13.3). Here the disease covers more than 95% of the body surface, with marked protein and fluid loss. Either methotrexate or PUVA is usually required.

■ Nail Psoriasis

The classic nail findings are pits, oil spots, and distal onycholysis with subungual debris. Sometimes the nail plate has pustules (acrodermatitis Hallopeau). Even when only one finger is involved, the patient can be severely disabled. Topical therapy is extremely difficult and most patients end up on systemic measures, often TNF antagonists.

■ Psoriatic Arthritis

While many psoriasis patients have spondylopathies on imaging or have mild and variable arthritic complaints, 3%–5% have mutilating disease, typically affecting the interphalangeal joints. The swollen fingers are often called sausage fingers. Sacroiliitis or a picture like rheumatoid arthritis with large joint involvement is less common. Methotrexate appears to delay the disease progression, while the TNF antagonists seem to arrest it. Fumaric acid esters may also be helpful.

■ Other Variants

Seborrheic dermatitis and reactive arthritis (Ch. 14.6) are considered variants of psoriasis. HIV/AIDS patients often have all three disorders, sometimes appearing abruptly.

E. Course

Psoriasis is a chronic relapsing disease, active over decades, and usually a lifelong problem. Thus, when planning therapy for younger patients, not only must the effectiveness and ease of use be considered, but also long-term side effects and cumulative toxicity. About 30% of patients have >10% of the body surface affected; 5%–10% (0.2% of general population) have widespread and severe disease.

F. Therapy

There are three basic ways to approach the disease—topical, systemic, and phototherapy. Topical agents include vitamin D analogs (often together with topical corticosteroids), which help mild disease and can be combined with phototherapy or systemic agents. Anthralin is very effective, but messy and only practical for inpatients. Phototherapy options include UVB for guttate psoriasis and UVB 311 nm or PUVA for plaque psoriasis. The most important systemic agents are methotrexate (15–20 mg weekly) and fumaric acid esters in Germany. TNF and IL-12/IL-23p40 antagonists are reserved for severe cases because they are strongly immunosuppressive; they can be used with methotrexate and are often required for nail involvement or psoriatic arthritis. Alitretinoin, a systemic retinoid, may be helpful for palmoplantar disease. Ciclosporin is effective for rapid control, but fraught with side effects, and cannot be used along with phototherapy. It should be limited to rare indications like pregnancy.

Psoriasis

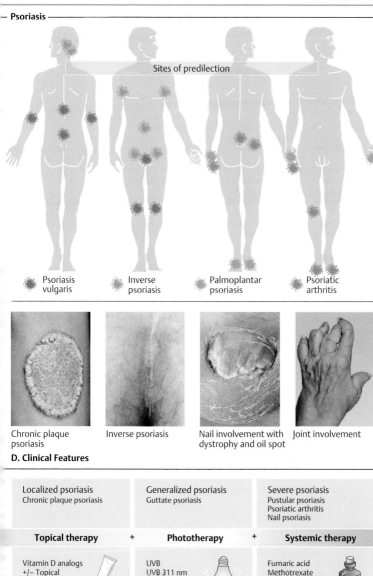

Sites of predilection

Psoriasis vulgaris

Inverse psoriasis

Palmoplantar psoriasis

Psoriatic arthritis

Chronic plaque psoriasis

Inverse psoriasis

Nail involvement with dystrophy and oil spot

Joint involvement

D. Clinical Features

Localized psoriasis	Generalized psoriasis	Severe psoriasis
Chronic plaque psoriasis	Guttate psoriasis	Pustular psoriasis Psoriatic arthritis Nail psoriasis

Topical therapy +	**Phototherapy** +	**Systemic therapy**
Vitamin D analogs +/– Topical corticosteroids	UVB UVB 311 nm PUVA + systemic therapy (fumaric acid, methotrexate)	Fumaric acid Methotrexate TNF antagonists IL-12/IL-23-p40 antagonists

F. Therapy

Seborrheic dermatitis and reactive arthritis share many similarities with psoriasis. Some schools of dermatology include them as psoriasis variants. HIV/AIDS has shown us how they interact and appear in same patient. Sebopsoriasis is a term that has sometimes been used to describe patients with overlapping features.

A. Seborrheic Dermatitis

Epidemiology. Seborrheic dermatitis is an extremely common disorder with peaks in infants and the elderly.

Pathogenesis. The pathogenesis is multifactorial; *Malassezia furfur* is clearly important in infants, and immune status is also key; there are also neurological factors, as patients with Parkinson disease have severe seborrheic dermatitis.

Clinical features. Sharply bordered erythema with greasy yellow scales are always present, with a typical distribution pattern involving the scalp (especially anterior hairline), external auditory canal, retroauricular fold, nasolabial fold, eyebrows, and eyelashes. Some regard dandruff as mild seborrheic dermatitis. In severe cases, patients may have multiple nummular lesions on the neck and trunk (petaloid seborrheic dermatitis). There is no clear distinction from psoriasis.

Histology. The subacute dermatitis shows acanthosis and parakeratosis, as in psoriasis.

Differential diagnosis. In adults, it overlaps with psoriasis. Petaloid seborrheic dermatitis resembles pityriasis rosea. External ear canal disease is usually misdiagnosed as otomycosis. Retroauricular and nasolabial disease mimics allergic contact dermatitis to glass frames.

Course. Seborrheic dermatitis has a chronic course, is usually easy to control, and impossible to cure.

Therapy. Shampoos (imidazoles, zinc pyrithione, selenium sulfide) are used for scalp involvement, and topical low-potency corticosteroids, vitamin D analogs, or imidazoles for the rest of the skin.

B. Reactive Arthritis

Epidemiology. This is an uncommon disorder, also known as Reiter syndrome[1], associated with HLA-B27. It is much more common in HIV/AIDS patients (up to 10%).

Pathogenesis. It is triggered by variety of gastrointestinal infections (classically *Shigella, Salmonella,* or *Yersinia*), as well as chlamydial urethritis.

Clinical features. The classic triad was:
- urethritis
- arthritis
- conjunctivitis.

However, today more cases are associated with gut disease. Skin findings include:
- *keratoderma blennorrhagicum*—a type of pustular psoriasis of the palms and soles
- *circinate balanitis*—sharply circumscribed annular erythema with a white border on the glans or labia minora.

The arthritis starts an enthesopathy, involving tendons at their sites of insertion, most often on the feet (Achilles tendonitis, plantar fasciitis). Large joints are affected, as in psoriatic arthritis. Iridocyclitis is also common.

Histology. The histology is identical to pustular psoriasis.

Differential diagnosis. Psoriasis and psoriatic arthritis, as well as other forms of reactive arthritis (especially that with inflammatory bowel disease).

Course. The course is highly variable; some resolve rapidly; in others, it is a lifelong problem.

Therapy. If an infectious trigger is suspected or urethritis present, doxycycline for the patient (and partner) is first-line therapy. Arthritis usually responds to NSAIDs. Depending on the severity of the skin and joint disease, methotrexate or TNF antagonists are the treatments of choice.

---

[1] Hans Reiter has fallen into disrepute because of his medical activities during the Nazi regime.

— Seborrheic Dermatitis and Reactive Arthritis —

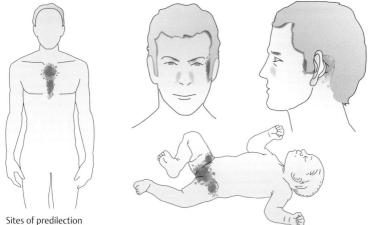

Sites of predilection

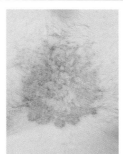
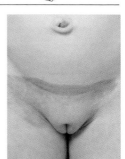

Clinical features
A. Seborrheic Dermatitis

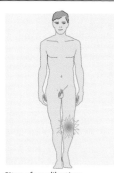
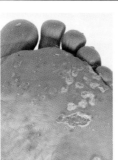
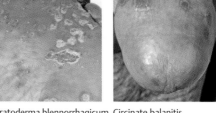

Sites of predilection   Keratoderma blennorrhagicum   Circinate balanitis
B. Reactive Arthritis

14 Inflammatory Diseases of the Epidermis

159

Pityriasis means "having fine or branlike scale." These diseases share nothing other than a name and a tendency to scale.

A. Pityriasis Lichenoides

Two diseases are grouped together here:
- pityriasis lichenoides et varioliformis acuta (PLEVA or Mucha–Habermann disease)
- pityriasis lichenoides chronica.

Epidemiology. PLEVA is relatively common.
Pathogenesis. Although a viral cause has long been suspected, no good candidates have been identified.
Clinical features. There is a sudden onset of numerous hemorrhagic macules and papules with central scale, which are surprisingly asymptomatic. PLEVA develops necrotic areas. Patients typically complain that they look terrible but feel fine. Rare cases may ulcerate and have systemic findings.
Histology. The prototype of lymphocytic vasculitis with hemorrhage, massive exocytosis of activated lymphocytes, and epidermal damage. Wedge-shaped dermal infiltrate extends deeply.
Differential diagnosis. Guttate psoriasis and pityriasis rosea are differential diagnoses, but are never hemorrhagic. If it is persistent or there are few lesions, consider lymphomatoid papulosis.
Course. Most cases resolve spontaneously; some evolve into less-inflamed persistent macules with an adherent scale (pityriasis lichenoides chronica) and are very therapy resistant.
Therapy. Treatment is topical corticosteroids if pruritic; systemic macrolides or tetracyclines for months; also UV therapy, especially for pityriasis lichenoides chronica.

B. Pityriasis Rosea

Epidemiology. Almost everyone has pityriasis rosea once; it is extremely common.
Pathogenesis. The cause is unknown. It is considered a skin reaction to a systemic infection; many viruses have been suspected but none well proven. Gold salts may produce a very similar eruption.
Clinical features. It has a striking clinical picture with oval erythematous or pale macules and almost atrophic patches with a collarette (peripheral) scale. There is often an initial larger lesion—herald patch—which is frequently mistaken for nummular dermatitis or tinea corporis. Then many lesions develop, often with a Christmas tree pattern on the trunk,

and the diagnosis becomes clear. In white individuals, the face and limbs are usually spared, but in black individuals, these distal sites are often affected with postinflammatory hypopigmentation *(inverse pityriasis rosea)*. It is almost never pruritic.
Histology. Histology is rarely specific, but focal areas of spongiosis and parakeratosis may suggest the diagnosis.
Differential diagnosis. Secondary syphilis can be identical. Pityriasis lichenoides chronica and guttate psoriasis may be similar but lack the pattern and herald patch.

> **Caution:** If any question exists or if the patient is pregnant, do syphilis serology.

Course. Patients recover rapidly, usually over 3–6 weeks, and recurrences are uncommon.
Therapy. Avoid drying or irritating measures. Topical antipruritics usually suffice; topical corticosteroids can be tried; UVB is a useful adjunct.

C. Pityriasis Rubra Pilaris

Epidemiology. This is uncommon; both adult and juvenile forms exist.
Pathogenesis. The pathogenesis is unknown but it is not related to psoriasis.
Clinical features. Early cases are notoriously difficult to diagnose, often presenting as hand or scalp erythema with fine (pityriasiforme) scale. Later findings are distinctive, with salmon-colored plaques, follicular keratotic papules, diffuse palmoplantar Keratoderma and dramatic areas of sparing *(nappes claires)*.
Histology. Histology is surprisingly nonspecific in view of the dramatic clinical picture. Hyperkeratosis is seen, with parakeratosis around follicles.
Differential diagnosis. It is often confused with psoriasis or atopic dermatitis. When papular, it also resembles lichen planus.
Course. This can evolve into erythroderma. In adults it tends to be chronic; in children, it usually resolves over 1 year.
Therapy. Topical corticosteroids are often tried but give little benefit. Systemic retinoids (≤ 20 mg daily) are the usual choice; a short burst of systemic corticosteroids may speed improvement. Ciclosporin for 3–4 months or even longer may induce prolonged remission. Phototherapy is poorly tolerated and best avoided. TNF antagonists may help, even in refractory cases.

Pityriasis Lichenoides, Pityriasis Rosea, and Pityriasis Rubra Pilaris

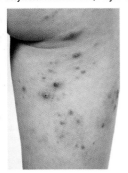
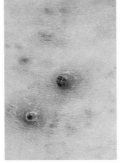
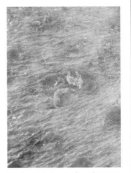

Pityriasis lichenoides et varioliformis acuta

Pityriasis lichenoides chronica

A. Pityriasis Lichenoides

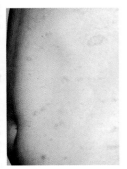
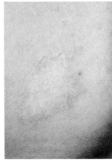
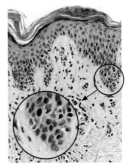

Christmas tree pattern

Herald patch

Focal spongiosis and parakeratosis

B. Pityriasis Rosea

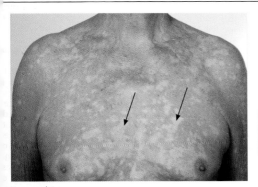
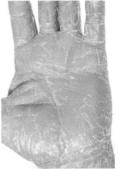

Nappes claires

Palmoplantar hyperkeratosis

C. Pityriasis Rubra Pilaris

14 Inflammatory Diseases of the Epidermis

Lichen planus (LP) is an inflammatory T-cell-mediated disease of the skin and mucosa, which involves the dermal–epidermal junction (DEJ).

A. Pathogenesis

LP is primarily a disease of cytotoxic CD8+ T cells. The immune response could be directed against antigens of hepatitis C or human herpes virus 8, as these viruses appear connected with LP, especially oral LP. In addition, when hepatitis C is treated via immunostimulation with IFN-α, LP can severely flare. On the mucosa, LP can also represent a contact reaction to dental metals.

B. Clinical Features

LP is primarily an adult disease with an incidence of 0.25%–1.0%. The clinical manifestations are quite variable. Hallmark lesions are polygonal circumscribed violaceous flat-topped papules, which favor the inner aspects of the wrist. Acute LP can be exanthematous with macular lesions and it is intensely pruritic. Another typical finding is a lacy white network on the surface of the papules, reflecting hypergranulosis. On the oral mucosa, these lines are easier to see and called Wickham striae.

The papules can appear anywhere on the body and may be follicular, annular, or linear. If the epidermal repair reaction dominates, then LP can become hyperkeratotic (especially when follicular) or even verrucous (on the shins and soles of the feet). LP frequently appears in scars or sites of trauma; this induction by trauma is known as the Koebner phenomenon. In oral and genital lesions, the destruction usually dominates over the repair, so they tend to be ulcerated. On the scalp, LP damages follicles causing scarring alopecia. It also causes nail thinning, longitudinal ridging, and trachyonychia (20-nail dystrophy). Permanent scarring of the nail bed also occurs in the form of wing-shaped dystrophy (pterygium).

C. Histology

The histological hallmark is a linear band of T cells along the basement membrane. This pattern, no matter where it is seen, is called lichenoid or interface dermatitis, as the DEJ is damaged and partially obliterated. There is often orthohyperkeratosis with focal, wedge-shaped hypergranulosis. Epidermal damage is seen in the form of focal destruction (sawtooth rete ridges) and keratinocytic apoptosis (eosinophilic cells known as colloid or Civatte bodies). If the infiltrate is massive, then blisters or erosions can be seen, as well as destruction of hair follicles. Such lesions heal with pigment incontinence, where melanin drops into the dermis and is taken up by macrophages. Deposits of IgM, IgG, and complement can be seen at the DEJ and in Civatte bodies, as well as fibrin about the dermal vessels.

D. Differential Diagnosis

The usual challenge is to separate LP from a lichenoid drug reaction. Clinically, the overlap may be minimal, but histologically the two disorders are quite similar. Lichenoid graft versus host disease (GVHD) is identical, but the clinical setting is totally different. In the mouth, LP closely remembers lupus erythematosus, pemphigus vulgaris, or an erosive contact mucositis to metals. On the scalp, the main challenge is to separate LP from lupus erythematosus and other scarring alopecias.

E. Course

Acute LP is often self-limited; 75% resolve over 18 months. The oral, genital, scalp, and nail forms are chronic. Oral and genital LP carries a small but definite risk of malignant change.

F. Therapy

Standard therapy is topical corticosteroids to suppress the T-cell response; topical calcineurin inhibitors can also be used, sometimes in combination. Both PUVA and systemic retinoids (isotretinoin 10 mg daily, or alitretinoin) also help. Rarely, systemic corticosteroids are needed to suppress severe flares.

G. Variants

Lichen nitidus features tiny 2 mm ivory papules that are closely grouped. Some patients have both LP and lichen nitidus.

Erythema dyschromicum perstans, or *ashy dermatosis*, presents as a variant seen primarily in patients of Hispanic-American-Indian origin. The inflammatory phase is not recognized; the patients present with postinflammatory pigmentary changes, with abundant melanin in the dermal macrophages. There is no good treatment.

Lichen Planus

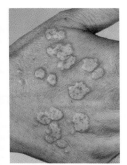

Polygonal papules with Wickham striae

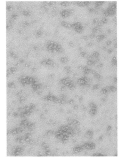

Disseminated lichen planus

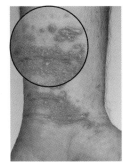

Confluent polygonal papules in typical location

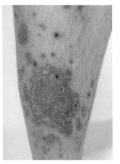

Verrucous lichen planus on the shin

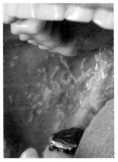

Wickham striae on oral mucosa

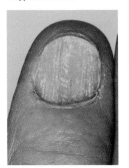

Trachyonychia

B. Clinical Features

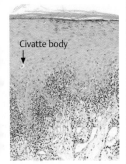

Civatte body

Interface dermatitis with saw-tooth epidermis

C. Histology

Lichen nitidus

G. Variants

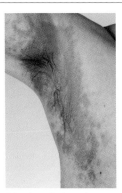

Ashy dermatosis

Graft versus host disease (GVHD) is an immunologic reaction that can develop following allogeneic bone marrow or stem cell transplantation. In GVHD, the donor T cells react against the recipient tissues. GVHD is divided into acute GVHD for the first 99 days and then chronic GVHD from day 100.

A. Pathogenesis

After a bone marrow transplant, T-cell-mediated inflammation commonly develops against HLA antigens, minor antigens like the HY gene products of men if the donor was a woman, and microbes. These processes dominate the early stage of the disease. As the immune system is gradually reconstituted, there is also a prominent reaction against infectious agents, which often leads to significant damage to the involved organs. For this reason, tissues rich in microbes such as the oral and intestinal mucosa are early targets.

In the skin, the early lesions of GVHD are very similar to a viral exanthem and may be a reaction against human herpes virus 6. Cutaneous GVHD then becomes lichenoid, perhaps reflecting incomplete control of the virus or bacteria; the attempt to control infectious agents may blend imperceptibly with graft rejection. With the exception of sclerodermiform GHVD, where B cells may also be important, all aspects are primarily T-cell dependent. Donor T cells react directly against the host antigens.

B. Clinical Features

Early acute GVHD features painful mucosal erosions and edematous macules and papules, often starting on the hands or in the flexures at the beginning of immune reconstitution. They can coalesce forming large patches and plaques. Severe disease may advance to erythroderma. After about day 30, lichenoid papules begin to appear; they are identical in every way to lichen planus and mimic many of its variations. Scaring lichenoid inflammation of the nails is very common.

After day 100, chronic GVHD begins, typically with firm edema of the wrists and hands, which is the first sign of sclerodermiform changes. It is associated with systemic eosinophilia and can advance to diffuse pansclerosis, with virtually the entire integument involved.

C. Histopathology

The microscopic features vary with the stage of the disease. Acute, lichenoid and sclerodermiform patterns can be identified. In the acute phase, as the graft takes at around day 20, the dominant change is epidermal damage with apoptosis of keratinocytes, dermal edema, and infiltration of T cells around the vessels. By day 30, lichenoid changes can be seen, as the CD8+ T cells have started to collect along the DEJ, as in lichen planus. The cells focally pass through the basement membrane and damage individual keratinocytes (satellite cell necrosis). Often the epidermal damage is extensive, leading to blisters and erosions, especially on the oral mucosa. The sclerodermiform phase features dermal edema with chronic inflammation; the infiltrate contains T cells, eosinophils, and plasma cells; it evolves into a cell-poor collagen-rich homogenous dermal pattern that is identical to scleroderma.

D. Course

The prognosis for acute GVHD is good, except for the most severe forms. Lichenoid GVHD can generally be controlled with immunosuppressive agents. Chronic GVHD is unpredictable but its severe forms have around a 25% 5-year survival.

E. Therapy

Acute GVHD is usually self-limited. The lichenoid form can be controlled with immunosuppressive regimens, mainly ciclosporin A. Combined systemic immunosuppression is usually needed for chronic GVHD, but is not always effective. Both the lichenoid and sclerodermiform variants also respond to photochemotherapy, perhaps best combined with low dose retinoids (isotretinoin 10 mg daily). Extracorporeal photophoresis also appears effective. In the mouth, topical calcineurin inhibitors are usually helpful.

Graft Versus Host Disease

Classification	Grade	Clinical and histological criteria
Subclinical	I	No clinical signs of GVHD but positive histology
Limited	II	1. Localized skin disease and/or 2. Liver dysfunction

Extensive	III	1. Generalized skin disease or
		2. Localized skin disease and/or liver dysfunction plus:
		    a. liver biopsy showing chronic aggressive hepatitis, confluent necrosis or cirrhosis
		    b. eye involvement (Schirmer test <5 mm)
		    c. biopsy-proven involvement of minor salivary gland
		    d. involvement of other target organs (gut, lungs)

Clinical-pathological classification of chronic GVHD

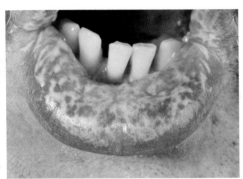

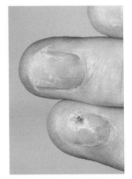

Lichenoid GVHD of lips

Scarring lichenoid nail damage

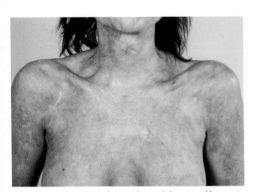

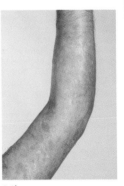

Sclerodermoid GVHD; sclerotic skin with hypo- and hyperpigmentation

B. Clinical Features

A. Pruritus

Pruritus or itching is the most common cutaneous symptom. Patients with pruritus may complain of sleep loss or inability to concentrate. They may scratch or rub their skin, inducing excoriations or even erosions and ulcers.

The first step is to decide whether skin lesions are present or not (pruritus sine materia).

The common pruritic skin diseases include atopic dermatitis, lichen planus, arthropod assault, and urticaria. More subtle causes are xerosis, mastocytosis, dermatitis herpetiformis, early bullous pemphigoid, and Grover disease.

When no skin findings are present, a systemic cause should be sought, such as:

- hepatic disease, especially with cholestasis
- malignancies, most commonly Hodgkin lymphoma and polycythemia vera
- endstage renal disease
- diabetes mellitus
- thyroid disease
- pregnancy (Ch. 28.2)
- HIV infection
- drug reactions.

Note: When no cutaneous or systemic disease is identified, the diagnosis is idiopathic pruritus, but one should still keep looking for a possible cause, which frequently is xerosis.

B. Localized Pruritus

Among the most difficult therapeutic challenges are localized forms of pruritus. Notalgia paresthetica is localized intrascapular pruritus, sometimes associated with sensory nerve entrapment. Damage to keratinocytes by chronic scratching may lead to localized amyloidosis (Ch. 27.1). Pruritus ani may also be caused by improper hygiene, pinworms, or ingestion of spicy foods. Both pruritus vulvae and scroti are more common in atopic patients, but usually have a significant psychological component and are difficult to treat. Both diabetes mellitus and iron deficiency may also play a role in anogenital pruritus.

C. Prurigo

Prurigo is a general term for the combination of pruritus and scratch-induced skin lesions. Variants include:

1. *prurigo simplex*—excoriated papules and nodules, usually following arthropod assault
2. *lichen simplex chronicus*—a localized area of lichenification (exaggerated skin markings usually on the nape or top of the foot, a result of chronic rubbing
3. *prurigo nodularis*—dome-shaped papules that are the result of chronic scratching and manipulation, usually on the arms. They are often centered on the hair follicles, sometimes associated with enlarged or abnormal cutaneous nerves. Prurigo nodularis is often seen in chronic renal disease. Perforating disease of renal dialysis is closely related. It may be a manifestation of atopic dermatitis in older patients.

D. Therapy

If an underlying cutaneous or systemic disease is found, it should be treated aggressively.

Topical corticosteroids are useful for inflammatory lesions, such as lichen planus, and for acute excoriations. Polidocanol or other topical anesthetics, as well as distracters such as menthol, can be helpful. Topical antihistamines are available, but efficacy has not been shown and they carry a risk of allergic contact dermatitis. The calcineurin inhibitors are effective antipruritic agents, as is topical capsaicin, which depletes neuropeptides in peripheral nerves. Extensive lubrication is required for dry skin.

Localized lesions such as lichen simplex chronicus and prurigo nodularis respond well to corticosteroids under occlusion or intralesional triamcinolone acetonide (3–5 mg/mL in local anesthetic). Cryotherapy may be a useful adjunct. Thalidomide is occasionally used for severe prurigo nodularis.

More standard systemic measures include antihistamines (surprisingly ineffective, underlining that histamine is not the sole mediator) and opiate receptor antagonists, whose exact role is still being defined. Tranquilizers or sedating antihistamines should be prescribed for those with difficulty sleeping. Renal pruritus responds to broad-spectrum UVB light or activated charcoal, while hepatic pruritus can be treated with ursodeoxycholic acid or cholestyramine. Psychosomatic counseling will benefit many patients, teaching them to deal with their pruritus.

Pruritus and Prurigo

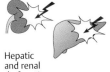

Hepatic
and renal
dysfunction

Medications

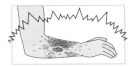

Blood
sugar ↑

Thyroid
disease

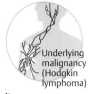
Underlying
malignancy
(Hodgkin
lymphoma)

HIV/AIDS

Pregnancy

A. Pruritus

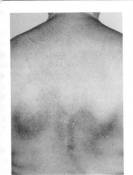

Notalgia paraesthetica

B. Localized Pruritus

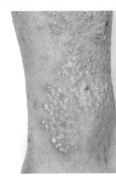

Lichen simplex chronicus

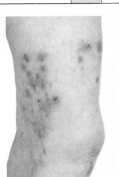

Prurigo nodularis with
excoriations

C. Prurigo

Antipruritic
topical
agents

Menthol
Capsaicin
Polidocanol

Anti-
inflammatory
topical
agents

Calcineurin
inhibitors
Corticosteroids

D. Therapy

Basic therapy with
urea-containing creams

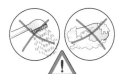
Avoid
irritation and
excessive
dryness

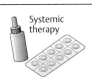
Systemic
therapy

Antihistamines
Opiate antagonists
for hepatic
pruritus

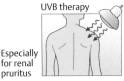
UVB therapy

Especially
for renal
pruritus

IV Dermatologic Diseases

A. Epidemiology

Pemphigus vulgaris, pemphigus foliaceus, and paraneoplastic pemphigus all feature acantholysis (disassociation of keratinocytes) mediated by autoantibodies. The incidence is 0.7–5.0:100 000 yearly, but much higher (15–30) in Jewish populations. While pemphigus can appear at any age, the peak age of onset is 50–60 years. Pemphigus vulgaris is the most common form, except in Finland, Tunisia, and Brazil where pemphigus foliaceus is more common.

B. Pathogenesis

Most often, IgG antibodies against desmoglein 1 (pemphigus foliaceus) or 3 (pemphigus vulgaris) are responsible. Less often, IgA antibodies against desmoglein 1 or 3 as well as desmocollin 1, and, in paraneoplastic pemphigus, IgG antibodies against a variety of intercellular molecules including desmoplakins, are responsible. The cause is an immune response dominated by T cells that are desmoglein specific and produce IL-4. These cells then induce B cells which produce antibodies against the desmogleins.

Desmoglein 3 is crucial for cell adhesion in the oral mucosa and is found in the lower layers of the epidermis, while desmoglein 1 is almost only present in the skin and most expressed in the upper layers. Thus pemphigus foliaceus never involves the mucosa and has superficial erosions, while pemphigus vulgaris often presents with oral disease and may have full-thickness acantholysis. There may then be epitope spreading in pemphigus vulgaris, with development of antibodies against desmoglein 1 that are almost always needed for skin disease. Both penicillamine and captopril can trigger drug-induced pemphigus.

C. Clinical Features

Pemphigus foliaceus usually presents with poorly healing erosions and crusts on the head and trunk. The endemic form is known as fogo selvagem and is seen in areas of Brazil where civilization encroaches on the habitat, suggesting an arthropod vector. Pemphigus vulgaris presents with either oral erosions or denuded blisters in areas of trauma or maceration. Intact blisters are very short lived (in comparison to pemphigoid). Why lesions appear in certain sites is unclear, as the autoantibodies are diffusely distributed in the skin. If a pemphigus vulgaris lesion heals spontaneously, it may become vegetating in the flexures (pemphigus vegetans) or even verrucous. Paraneoplastic pemphigus features prominent oral involvement, widespread blisters, and marked resistance to therapy. IgA pemphigus may present with subcorneal pustules; it is almost always associated with an underlying tumor, often hematopoietic. *Sneddon-Wilkinson disease* (subcorneal pustular dermatosis) may be a variant of IgA pemphigus.

Pemphigus erythematosus represents an overlap between pemphigus foliaceus and lupus erythematosus, with typical clinical and immunological findings for both diseases.

D. Histopathology and Immunofluorescence

An intact blister features marked acantholysis with keratinocytes floating in an intraepidermal space. Denuded lesions may show just a single layer of keratinocytes adherent to the basement membrane (tombstone effect). Pemphigus foliaceus has superficial acantholysis. Both feature a minimal inflammatory infiltrate. The diagnosis is confirmed by the identification on direct immunofluorescence of IgG antibodies against desmoglein 1 or 3 between the keratinocytes. The same antibodies against desmoglein 1 or 3 can be identified in serum with enzyme-linked immunosorbent assay (ELISA); their titers correlate with disease activity.

E. Course

Before the advent of corticosteroids, pemphigus vulgaris was fatal within 2 years. Today it is a controllable chronic disease, with patients at risk for complications of therapy. Pemphigus foliaceus has a milder course; paraneoplastic pemphigus is invariably fatal, often because of the underlying malignancy or lung complications.

F. Therapy

The starting point is always systemic corticosteroids (prednisolone 1–2 mg/kg daily) and an immunosuppressive agent (azathioprine 150 mg daily or mycophenolate mofetil 2g daily). With improvement, the prednisolone is slowly tapered over months to 5 mg daily, and perhaps further tapered if all antibodies disappear. Those patients who respond quickly have a normal life expectancy. If the disease fails to respond, options include intravenous immunoglobulins, corticosteroid pulse therapy, plasmapheresis, anti-CD 20 (anti-B cell) antibodies, and cyclophosphamide.

─ Pemphigus ─

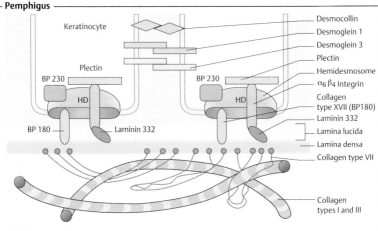

Keratinocyte

Plectin

BP 230

HD

BP 180 ── ── Laminin 332

Desmocollin
Desmoglein 1
Desmoglein 3
Plectin
Hemidesmosome
$\alpha_6\ \beta_4$ Integrin
Collagen type XVII (BP180)
Laminin 332
Lamina lucida
Lamina densa
Collagen type VII

BP 230

HD

Collagen types I and III

B. Pathogenesis

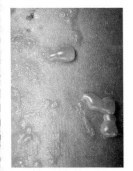

Pemphigus vulgaris

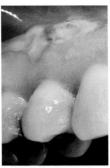

Oral pemphigus vulgaris

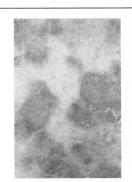

Pemphigus foliaceus

C. Clinical Features

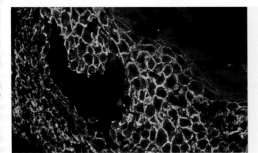

Intraepidermal blister. Direct immunofluorescence shows net-like pattern of IgG (yellow) attaching to desmoglein 3 and outlining the individual cells

Direct immunofluorescence of pemphigus vulgaris

D. Histopathology and Immunofluorescence

The pemphigoid group includes three diseases all characterized by autoantibody-mediated inflammation at the dermal–epidermal junction (DEJ): bullous pemphigoid (BP), cicatricial pemphigoid (CP), and epidermolysis bullosa acquisita (EBA).

A. Pathogenesis

The usual cause is immunoglobulin (Ig)G antibodies against molecules in the hemidesmosome, which anchor keratinocytes to the basement membrane (nonscarring) or anchor the basement membrane to the dermis (then often scarring). In BP, the primary antibodies are directed against the extracellular domains of type XVII collagen (BP180) and secondarily against an intracellular plakin (BP230). Both molecules anchor keratinocytes to the basement membrane. In linear IgA disease, the antibodies recognize an N-terminal of BP180. In CP, the antibodies are against laminin 332, α6β4-integrin (ocular form) or C-terminal components of BP180, all involved in the basement membrane and its connections to the dermis. In EBA, the antibodies are against type VII collagen, the main component of the anchoring fibrils in the papillary dermis.

Antibody binding alone does not cause the problem; antibody-initiated inflammation mediated by mast cells and complement is the key factor. The blood and tissue eosinophilia often lead to intense pruritus, which may precede the other disease manifestations by weeks.

B. Clinical Features

■ Bullous Pemphigoid

BP usually affects individuals aged over 60 years, and is relatively common, with an incidence of 6–10:100 000. It is uncommon in children and young adults and incidence increases with age. BP often starts with pruritus and then excoriated urticarial papules, without a hint of blister formation or lichenification. Thus BP should be considered in any older individual with therapy-resistant "eczema." The disease may be present for weeks or even months before blisters appear. They are stable, often become quite large, contain enough fluid to show a fluid level, and almost never involve mucosal surfaces. They may become hemorrhagic because of their proximity to the vessels of the dermal papillae. *Herpes gestationis* is a variant of BP, which occurs during pregnancy.

■ Linear IgA Dermatosis

Fine stable blisters appear, often arranged in a grouped (herpetiform) or rosette fashion, generally with little inflammation. The disease is uncommon, but often affects children and young adults. In children, there may often be facial involvement but with erythematous papules rather than distinct blisters.

■ Cicatricial Pemphigoid

Also known as mucosal pemphigoid, this variant affects the ocular, oral, or genital mucosa with relatively asymptomatic inflammation that slowly leads to scarring. Ocular involvement may progress to blindness. Fewer than one-third of patients have skin involvement.

■ Brunsting–Perry Pemphigoid

These patients have CP of the head and neck without mucosal disease, caused by antibodies against laminin 332. They have erosions with crusts; blisters are occasionally seen at the periphery. Scarring alopecia may develop; it is not related to the follicles and is more eroded than other forms (Ch. 26.4). Fewer than 10% of patients develop widespread disease.

■ Epidermolysis Bullosa Acquisita

This rare disorder may be associated with chronic inflammatory diseases such as Crohn disease. Patients with lupus erythematosus may also develop bullous disease with the same pattern as EBA. It often presents in areas of trauma, with a mixture of firm vesicles, blisters, erosions, and scars. Some patients closely resemble BP, while others are confused with porphyria cutanea tarda but have negative porphyrin studies. While the entire pemphigoid group can heal with milia, they are most common in EBA.

Pemphigoid Diseases and Dermatitis Herpetiformis

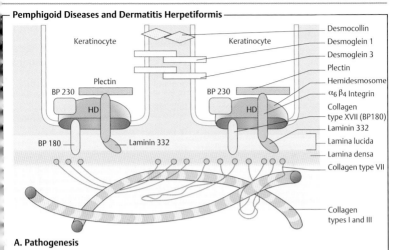

	Desmocollin
	Desmoglein 1
	Desmoglein 3
	Plectin
	Hemidesmosome
	$\alpha_6 \beta_4$ Integrin
	Collagen type XVII (BP180)
	Laminin 332
	Lamina lucida
	Lamina densa
	Collagen type VII
	Collagen types I and III

Labels within diagram: Keratinocyte, Keratinocyte, Plectin, BP 230, HD, BP 230, HD, BP 180, Laminin 332

A. Pathogenesis

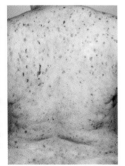

Bullous pemphigoid with excoriated papules and plaques

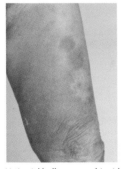

Urticarial bullous pemphigoid

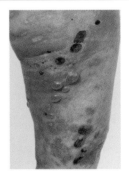

Bullous pemphigoid with stable blisters, some hemorrhagic, on an urticarial background

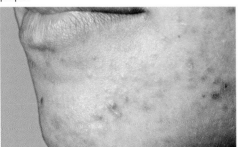

Linear IgA disease with blisters and papules

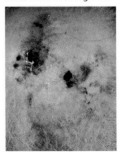

Brunsting–Perry pemphigoid

B. Clinical Features

C. Histopathology and Immunofluorescence

BP is dominated by large blisters at the DEJ. There is no acantholysis; the inflammatory infiltrate is usually rich in eosinophils. Direct immunofluorescence shows complement, IgG and, less often, IgA (linear IgA dermatosis—LAD) along the DEJ. EBA can be separated from BP using indirect immunofluorescence on salt-split skin, where antibodies against type VII collagen in the upper dermis can be found. Enzyme-linked immunosorbent assay (ELISA) studies and immunoelectromicroscopy also help.

D. Course

BP can usually be controlled, but immunosuppressive therapy is required for years. LAD is also usually controllable. In contrast, CP frequently does not respond and advances to blindness or genital strictures. EBA is also notoriously hard to treat.

E. Therapy

Therapy always starts with systemic corticosteroids (prednisolone 1–2 mg/kg daily) and an immunosuppressive agent (azathioprine 150 mg daily or mycophenolate mofetil 2.0 g daily). Once healing has occurred, the prednisolone is tapered to 5 mg daily, while the adjunctive therapy is maintained. Further reduction should only be tried if antibody levels drop to zero. Sometimes therapy can be discontinued after several years. If the disease fails to respond, options include intravenous immunoglobulins, corticosteroid pulse therapy, plasmapheresis, anti-CD 20 (anti-B-cell) antibodies, and cyclophosphamide.

In patients with mild BP or severe comorbidities, high-potency topical steroids can be combined with systemic anti-inflammatory therapy with tetracyclines or antihistamines. Topical steroids are also preferred for treatment during pregnancy, but systemic corticosteroids and azathioprine can be used, working with the obstetrician.

LAD is treated like dermatitis herpetiformis. EBA is very refractory and generally requires aggressive immunosuppression and adjunctive measures such as plasmapheresis or perhaps anti-CD 20 antibodies.

In the scarring forms, high-potency topical corticosteroids should always be additionally employed, as they may reduce local inflammation and ameliorate scarring and milia formation.

F. Dermatitis Herpetiformis

■ Epidemiology

Dermatitis herpetiformis (DH) or Duhring disease shows great regional variation in frequency. In Europe it has an incidence of 1–3:100 000 and a prevalence of >50:100 000 demonstrating its chronicity.

■ Pathogenesis

DH is caused by IgA antibodies against skin and tissue transglutaminases. Specific human leukocyte antigen (HLA) patterns favor the development of DH. There is also an association with gluten-sensitive enteropathy. About 90% of DH patients have bowel changes on biopsy, although they usually do not have clinical symptoms. They have a small risk of developing intestinal lymphoma. DH can be provoked by gluten or halogens.

■ Clinical Features

The hallmark of DH is intense pruritus; the sensation is often described as burning, rather than itching. Usually all that one sees is excoriations; sometimes multiple grouped vesicles can be seen; their grouping led to the term "herpetiformis," but there is no relation to herpes viruses. Mucosal surfaces are not affected. Children with DH may have tiny punctate palmar hemorrhages.

■ Histopathology

The hallmark feature is neutrophilic abscesses in the papillary dermis, with tiny areas of separation at the DEJ. Eosinophils may be present. This diagnosis is confirmed by direct immunofluorescence on a biopsy of perilesional skin (as the IgA antibodies are rapidly degraded in the active lesions), which reveals granular deposits of IgA in the papillary tips. Antibodies against skin or tissue transglutaminase as well as gluten may be measured.

■ Therapy

All patients should be on a gluten-free diet which will reduce their need for medications and perhaps lower their lymphoma risk. They should avoid halogenated compounds, which can trigger the disease. DH responds well to dapsone 50–100 mg daily; rarely, up to 200 mg is required, but then hemolysis is often a problem. The older sulfonamide, sulfapyridine, is also effective, but not widely available.

— Pemphigoid Diseases and Dermatitis Herpetiformis —

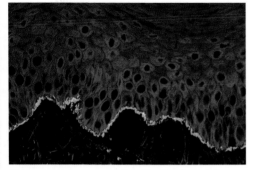

Direct immunofluorescence: deposits of IgG (green) along the basement membrane zone

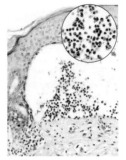

Subepidermal blister rich in eosinophils in bullous pemphigoid

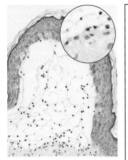

Subepidermal blister with neutrophils in linear IgA dermatosis

C. Histopathology and Immunofluorescence

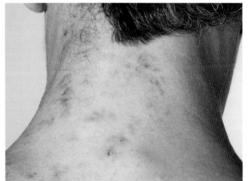

Grouped papules, vesicles, and erosions

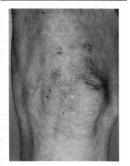

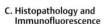

Grouped papules, vesicles, and erosions on the elbow

F. Dermatitis Herpetiformis

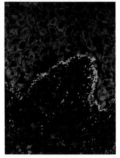

Granular IgA deposits in the tip of a dermal papilla

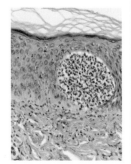

Collection of neutrophils in the tip of a dermal papilla

15 Inflammatory Diseases of the Dermal–Epidermal Junction

A. Definition

Epidermolysis bullosa (EB) is a group of disorders, not a single disease, all featuring mechanically unstable or fragile skin because of genetic defects in the complex structures of the basement membrane zone.

B. Pathogenesis

Three broad groups of EB have traditionally been identified:

- EB simplex (EBS) (epidermolytic blisters)
- Junctional EB (JEB) (junctional blisters)
- Dystrophic EB (DEB) (dermolytic blisters).

Related structures such as the hair, nails, teeth, and mucosa may be involved. In addition, since many other organs also have junctions joining epithelial and connective tissue, there is a possibility of systemic involvement. Some types of epidermolysis bullosa are associated with pyloric atresia, esophageal stenosis, and even muscular dystrophy. EB is a rare disease, with an incidence of roughly 1 : 100 000 in Caucasian populations. Most forms are inherited in an autosomal dominant fashion with mutations in structural genes.

C. Clinical Features

Clinically, all forms of EB look similar, with fragile skin so that slight trauma produces blisters or erosions. The skin may heal with pigmentary changes, milia, or scarring.

EBS. This is a defect in the basal keratinocytes. Damage is superficial and generally nonscarring. Patients have defects in keratin 5 and 14, found in the basal keratinocytes. The mildest form is EBS Weber–Cockayne; these patients tend to only develop blisters with some degree of trauma, such as playing sports or taking long hikes. Other forms may have more generalized disease (EBS Köbner), or a herpetiform pattern with marked blistering at birth (EBS Dowling–Meara). Keratin 5 (and perhaps 14) is also involved in transfer of melanin to keratinocytes, so some forms of EBS have mottled pigmentation. Hyperhidrosis and palmoplantar keratoderma can be associated.

Patients with a defect in plectin, a protein that binds keratin filaments to hemidesmosomes, may have generalized EBS with scarring, as well as muscular dystrophy or pyloric stenosis.

JEB. This is a defect in junctional proteins, and is usually nonscarring. The most severe form is JEB Herlitz, which was formerly known as EB letalis, not leaving much to the imagination.

Patients have defects in laminin and tend to develop widespread, poorly healing erosions, with fluid loss and infections, often leading to death in the first two years of life. In contrast, JEB nonHerlitz (also known as generalized atrophic bullous epidermolysis [GA-BEB]) is caused by mutations in BP180 (now known as collagen XVII), and is characterized by widespread blisters, alopecia, and nail and dental problems but a less severe course. Patients with JEB and pyloric atresia usually have mutations in α6β4 integrin.

DEB. This is a defect in the upper papillary dermis; there is always scarring, with an increased risk of developing cutaneous malignancies. The most severe form is autosomal-recessive DEB (RDEB) (Hallopeau-Siemens); patients have two abnormal collagen VII molecules and very fragile skin. They develop widespread erosions, mucosal fragility with prominent esophageal disease, constipation secondary to perianal disease, and the peculiar mitten formation where the skin of the digits heals together (syndactyly). These patients have a 20-fold increased risk of squamous cell carcinoma in such regions. In autosomal-dominant DEB (DDEB) (Cockayne-Touraine-Pasini), only one collagen VII molecule is abnormal. These patient have less fragile skin, do not have syndactyly and have a much lower risk of developing squamous cell carcinoma.

D. Therapy

There is no specific therapy for any form of EB Because some forms are so devastating, there is intensive research looking for methods of gene transfer or stem cell therapy, with the aim of providing the patient with a normal gene to synthesize the missing protein.

Supportive care is an emotional, physical and financial burden for the parents and later the patient. Special training in how to manage EB is available at some reference centers Avoidance of trauma and careful gentle dressing of blisters are the mainstays, along with prompt attention to infection and systemic problems. The syndactyly can be corrected surgically.

Epidermolysis Bullosa

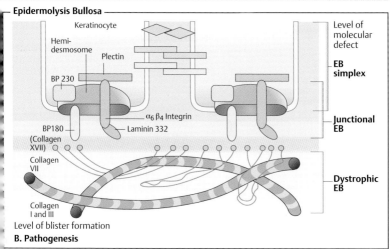

Level of molecular defect

EB simplex

Junctional EB

Dystrophic EB

Keratinocyte

Hemi-desmosome

Plectin

BP 230

$\alpha_6\beta_4$ Integrin

BP180 (Collagen XVII)

Laminin 332

Collagen VII

Collagen I and III

Level of blister formation

B. Pathogenesis

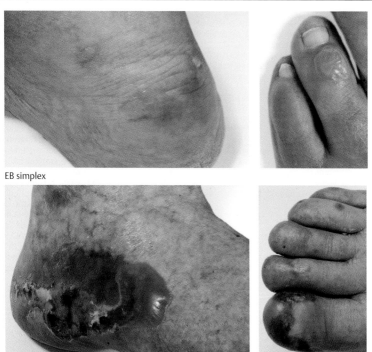

EB simplex

Dystrophic EB

C. Clinical Features

Urticaria and angioedema affect 25% of people at least once. Their maximal variant is anaphylaxis, which is life-threatening.

A. Pathogenesis

Urticaria is the result of vasodilation with serum extravasation and then edema. In the upper airways, the same reaction leads to hypersecretion, in the lower airways to bronchospasm, and in the gut to colicky contractions.

Urticaria is triggered by the release of mediators from mast cells. This release can be triggered by allergic, pseudoallergic, toxic, and physical mechanisms. In addition, mast cell function is regulated by epinephrine and acetylcholine from the autonomic nervous system and substance P from neurons. Other important regulators include angiotensin-converting enzyme (ACE) and C 1 inactivators.

Urticaria is *allergic* when specific antigens (hymenoptera toxin, penicillin, many others) cross-link specific IgE antibodies attached to mast cells. *Pseudoallergic* describes the release of mast cell mediators after exposure to foods or medications but without the presence of specific immunoglobulin (Ig)E antibodies. Endogenous or exogenous substances such as opiates, codeine, or complement proteins (C_3a, C_5a) can alter the sensitivity of mast cells to both stimuli.

Hives (also known as wheals or urticae) are primarily the result of histamine release. Other mediators such as prostaglandins, leukotrienes, and cytokines such as interleukin (IL)-8 or tumor necrosis factor (TNF) are also involved. In autoimmune urticaria, the trigger is autoantibodies directed against IgE. This great variety explains the modest effect of antihistamines in some patients, although most are controlled with combined H_1–H_2 antihistamines.

B. Clinical Features

Urticaria. Hives are intensely pruritic, appear suddenly, and may be solitary, localized, or generalized. Lesions vary in diameter, from 1–2 mm to covering the entire back. The individual lesions last <24 hours. When individual lesions (not the attack) persist ≥24 hours, the possibility of urticarial vasculitis should be considered, which may be associated with autoimmune disorders and is identified with a biopsy.

Often urticaria occurs once, lasts a few days, and disappears. An acute attack is still very uncomfortable and can be associated with respiratory or cardiovascular signs and symptoms.

Less often, urticaria recurs or persists. The time course can be used to subdivide:
- acute and acute recurrent urticaria—attack <6 weeks
- chronic urticaria—attack >6 weeks; this means hives every day for >6 weeks.

The clinical features and triggers vary with age. In children, foodstuffs are likely triggers, while in adults they are uncommon. Chronic urticaria is likely to have pseudoallergic triggers (like aspirin), reflect an underlying infection (usually intestinal worms or chronic rhinosinusitis), or have an autoimmune basis.

Physical urticaria is a special type of chronic urticaria, elicited by a variety of physical traumas. Causes include rubbing (factitial *urticaria* or *dermatographism*), persistent mechanical pressure, such as the prolonged sitting of a truck driver or even walking (*pressure urticaria*), temperature changes (*cold and heat urticaria*), ultraviolet (UV) or visible light (*solar urticaria*), sweating (*cholinergic urticaria* usually with tiny punctate hives), emotional stress (*adrenergic urticaria*), and even water, such as after showering (*aquagenic urticaria*).

Contact urticaria results from exposure to toxins that cause the release of histamine. Most common are arthropod assaults and contact with stinging nettles (*Urtica dioica*), the source of the name urticaria. Some allergens such as natural latex may cause allergic contact urticaria after sensitization.

Two rare form of urticaria are:
- *Schnitzler syndrome*—caused by an inflammasome defect, with urticarial vasculitis, fever, arthralgias, and IgM gammopathy
- *Muckle–Wells syndrome*—a familial inflammasome defect with urticaria, fever, deafness, and later renal amyloidosis with nephropathy.

Angioedema. This is deep urticaria of the skin or more often mucosa; sometimes free-standing and sometimes in association with urticaria. It may be allergic, drug induced (ACE inhibitors) or hereditary, involving defects in C 1 esterase inhibitor. It can last >24 hours and be life-threatening if it involves the space around the upper airways.

Anaphylaxis. This is the maximal variant of urticaria, which can occur after repeated exposure to an allergen or pseudoallergen, or sometimes as a singular event. There is maximal body-wide mast cell degranulation leading to vasodilation and bronchoconstriction and then to anaphylactic shock, which is life threatening. Typical allergic triggers are hymenoptera toxin and penicillin.

Urticaria, Angioedema, and Anaphylaxis

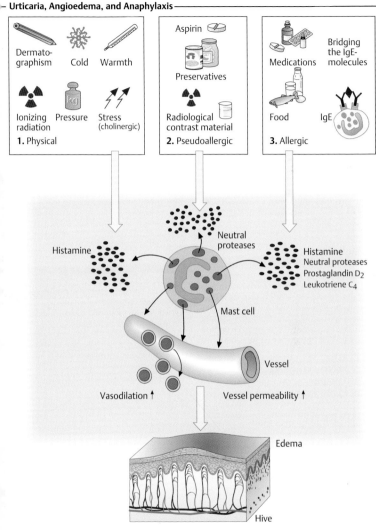

Dermato-graphism   Cold   Warmth

Ionizing radiation   Pressure   Stress (cholinergic)
1. Physical

Aspirin

Preservatives

Radiological contrast material
2. Pseudoallergic

Medications   Bridging the IgE-molecules

Food   IgE
3. Allergic

Neutral proteases

Histamine

Histamine
Neutral proteases
Prostaglandin D$_2$
Leukotriene C$_4$

Mast cell

Vessel

Vasodilation ↑   Vessel permeability ↑

Edema

Hive

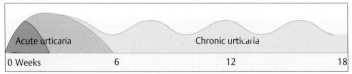

Acute urticaria   Chronic urticaria

0 Weeks   6   12   18

A. Pathogenesis

Oral allergy syndrome (OAS). Individuals with type I allergies to birch, hazelnut, and other pollens can react to carrots, celery root, apples, hazelnuts, stone fruits (drupes), herbs, and spices. Patients typically report a burning sensation of the tongue or lips. The key allergen responsible for most reactions is Bet v1 from birch pollen that cross reacts with raw apples. Less common is *protein contact urticaria* from contact with fish or vegetable juices.

C. Histopathology

A biopsy from urticaria is not dramatic—in contrast to the clinical appearance. There is edema with scattered neutrophils and eosinophils. Vessels may be dilated or compressed by the edema. Urticarial vasculitis has typical leukocytoclastic vasculitis with vessel wall damage, exocytosis of erythrocytes, fragmented neutrophils, and fibrin deposits.

D. Diagnostic Approach

The history is crucial—the patient must be encouraged to try and identify triggering factors. Questions should address the possibility of physical urticaria. Mast cell disease (Ch. 23.2) may present with urticaria, but because of excess mast cells rather than abnormal stimulation; it can be excluded by physical examination, biopsy or measuring serum mast cell tryptase.

Acute urticaria is generally not investigated; studies are only needed when a trigger such as hymenoptera toxin or penicillin is suspected, as these can be associated with later anaphylaxis.

Acute recurrent urticaria is frequently clarified with a history, as a possible trigger (food, medication, activity) can be identified. One should not forget to enquire about mucosal contacts, such as toothpaste, latex condoms, or even semen. A diary should be kept documenting everything with mucosal contact—medications (prescription and over-the-counter; asking directly about aspirin and nonsteroidal anti-inflammatory drugs [NSAIDs]), all foodstuffs including spices, drinks (tonic water), and even chewing gum.

Even with extensive investigations, chronic urticaria often remains idiopathic and is difficult to cure. Physical urticaria can be excluded with a variety of standard tests (Ch. 8.2), which are discussed in advanced texts and require specialized equipment. Intestinal parasites and chronic rhinosinusitis should be excluded. The diagnosis of autoimmune urticaria is not

standardized, but patients do react with hives to an intracutaneous injection of their own serum.

Angioedema has the same causes as urticaria, but is also commonly triggered by ACE inhibitors. Hereditary angioedema requires specialized testing. In anaphylaxis, the cause is rarely a mystery, but it should be confirmed, so that a medication can be avoided or hyposensitization performed for hymenoptera toxin sensitivity.

E. Therapy

Both urticaria and angioedema should first be treated with nonsedating H_1 antihistamines (desloratidine, cetirizine, fexofenadine). In chronic urticaria, the dose can be increased to four times the usual starting dose. If the response is poor, an H_2 antihistamine or leukotriene antagonist (montelukast) can be added. Systemic corticosteroids are only indicated for acute emergency usage.

Note: Anaphylaxis is treated with the standard ABCD measures—airway, breathing. circulation, and drugs. Patients at risk for recurrent anaphylaxis should be given an emergency set, which ideally contains auto-injectable epinephrine (adrenalin), corticosteroids, and antihistamines. Once the acute emergency has passed, then it is essential to discover the trigger and institute avoidance measures, or, in the case of hymenoptera sensitivity, start desensitization.

Urticaria, Angioedema, and Anaphylaxis

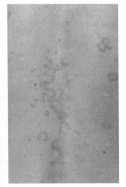

Urticaria

Hive or wheal

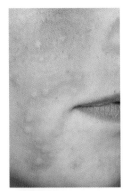

Cold urticaria

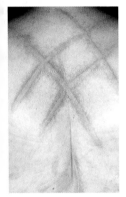

Dermatographism

Contact urticaria from caterpillar hairs

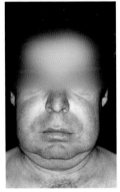

Angioedema

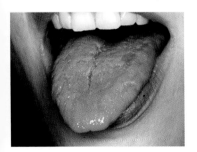

Oral allergy syndrome, mild case

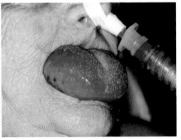

Oral allergy syndrome, severe case

B. Clinical Features

IV Dermatologic Diseases

A. Erythema Multiforme

Erythema multiforme (EM) is a reaction pattern with typical target-shaped or iris lesions.
Pathogenesis. Almost all cases of recurrent EM are caused by recurrent oral herpes simplex infections; genital herpes infections rarely trigger the reaction. One-time cases are often caused by other infectious agents such as mycoplasma and tend to be more severe.
Clinical features. Classic EM is also known as EM minor. Typical lesions are erythematous macules on the back of the hands, forearms, knees, elbows, palms of the hands, and soles of the feet. Within 1–2 days, the macules have expanded to 1–2 cm in diameter, with a central area of hemorrhage, blistering, and necrosis surrounded by a band of cyanosis and then peripheral erythema—producing a target or iris effect. Post-herpetic EM often features erosions on the lips; it can be hard to distinguish between the herpetic changes and the later EM lesions.

In EM majus, mucosal lesions predominate. Oral mucosal involvement is common, ranging from small aphthae to large erosions. There may be genital or ocular involvement. The latter is sometimes referred to as Stevens–Johnson syndrome (Ch. 29.1).
Histopathology. There is interface dermatitis, with a lymphocytic perivascular inflammation and epidermal necrosis. Initially there may be only basal layer damage but later the changes are full thickness.
Differential diagnosis. Drugs, especially sulfonamides, tend to cause EM-like reactions (Ch. 29.1).
Therapy. Acute disease is treated symptomatically with topical corticosteroids. Severe disease can be suppressed with systemic corticosteroids but this may allow an underlying infection to flare. Recurrent EM is treated with antiviral agents—either long-term prophylaxis or short-term therapy at the first sign of herpetic lesions. Even patients with recurrent EM and no history of herpetic lesions tend to improve, suggesting they have subclinical recurrent herpes.

B. Figurate Erythemas

There is a long list of diseases that all present with expanding annular or polycyclic erythematous and sometimes scaly lesions. They have no pathogenetic relationship, but instead a wide variety of causes.
Erythema migrans. This is the most common figurate erythema in Europe, characterized by a slowly expanding erythematosus ring caused by *Borrelia burgdorferi* (Ch. 33.4).
Erythema annulare centrifugum (EAC). This presents as erythematous plaque, which then slowly expands. Peripheral scale is found on the trailing edge of the lesion, pointing toward the pale center. Causes include infections, tumors, food allergies, and drugs. The familiar form is *erythema gyratum perstans*. The deep form of EAC is most often lupus tumidus (Ch. 17.5).
Erythema gyratum repens. This is a paraneoplastic marker, with rapidly advancing erythema and scale resembling the grain of wood (Ch. 27.9).
Necrolytic migratory erythema. This is a paraneoplastic marker, with acral and genital erythematous plaques and erosions with fine scaling. It is associated with glucagonoma (Ch. 27.9).
Others
- Annular lupus erythematosus and Rowell syndrome (EM-like lupus erythematosus) (Ch. 17.5)
- Annular psoriasis
- Annular Sjögren syndrome
- Erythema marginatum (rheumatic fever)

C. Nodose Erythemas

These lesions present as red-brown plaques or nodules. The only common representative is erythema nodosum, the most common form of panniculitis (Ch. 18.1). Another is granuloma faciale, which is rich in eosinophils (Ch. 17.6).
Sweet syndrome. Also known as acute febrile neutrophilic dermatosis, patients present with fever, elevated erythrocyte sedimentation rate (ESR), and pseudopustular erythematous nodules. Often the trigger is unknown, but infections, underlying myeloid leukemia, and drug reactions have been implicated. Histology shows an extensive neutrophilic infiltrate with marked edema and sometimes vasculitis. The disease responds rapidly to systemic corticosteroids.
Erythema elevatum et diutinum. Form of chronic vasculitis, sometimes associated with hematological disorders or HIV. Presents with red-brown nodules on extensor surfaces, especially over joints of hands. Histopathology shows marked perivascular fibrosis and little active inflammation. Some patients respond to dapsone.

— Erythema Multiforme, Figurate Erythemas, and Nodose Erythemas

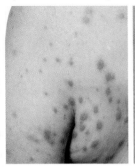 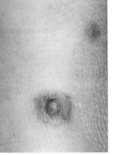 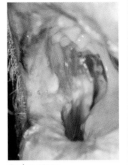

Edematous targetlike plaques

Oral erosions

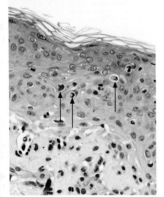

Interface dermatitis with necrotic keratinocytes (arrows)

A. Erythema Multiforme

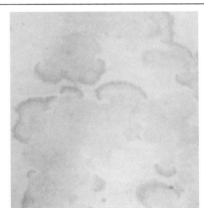

Erythema annulare centrifugum

B. Figurate Erythemas

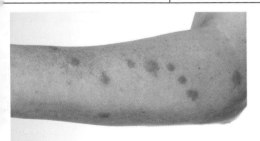 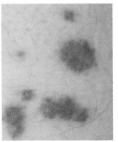

Sweet syndrome; erythematous nodules and plaques with pseudopustules

Sweet syndrome: close-up view

C. Nodose Erythemas

Dermatomyositis is an autoimmune disease that primarily affects the skin and striated muscles. In adults, it is a potential paraneoplastic marker for an underlying malignancy.

A. Pathogenesis

Dermatomyositis is an autoimmune disease mediated by CD8+ T cells. Paradoxically, it is more likely to be associated with major histocompatibility complex (MHC) class II/human leukocyte antigen (HLA)-DR genotypes than with MHC class I/HLA-A, B types. Although over 90% of patients have a positive antinuclear antibodies (ANA) test, specific antibodies against Jo1, Mi2, mRNP or PM-Scl are less common (±30%). Dermatomyositis is presumably antigen triggered as a model for molecular mimicry. It is associated with other autoimmune diseases, numerous viral infections, and in some 30% of adults with an underlying carcinoma, most often involving the female urogenital tract or the gastrointestinal tract.

B. Clinical Features

The incidence is 2–7:100 000, with women affected six times more often than men. The disease can predominantly affect either the skin or the muscles, although usually both are obviously involved. It is usually divided into three groups: juvenile dermatomyositis and adult dermatomyositis with and without associated malignancy.

All forms have photosensitivity with *poikiloderma* (atrophy, telangiectases, hyper- and hypopigmentation) on the face, around the eyes, and on the backs of the fingers. This evolves into edematous slightly livid plaques, such as the almost pathognomonic heliotrope eyelids; sometimes the patients look as if they had been crying. Gottron papules may develop over the interphalangeal joints, as a hyperkeratotic response to the inflammation. They are circumscribed livid papules. The nail folds are hyperkeratotic and, when examined with capillary microscopy, the vessels are enlarged, coiled, and associated with tiny hemorrhages.

The myositis especially affects the triceps and quadriceps muscles, as well as the proximal muscles of the thigh. The patients may have difficulty holding their arms up, combing their hair, or arising from a chair. Sometimes the pharyngeal muscles are affected, interfering with swallowing and breathing. Perhaps 10% have *dermatomyositis sine myositis*—that is, no muscle findings.

The best laboratory tests to assess muscle involvement are muscle creatinine kinase (CK) and aldolase. Their levels can be used to follow therapy. Muscle biopsy may be used to confirm diagnosis.

Children often develop severe calcinosis affecting the skin, subcutaneous tissues, and muscles. The extensor surfaces of the extremities are most often affected. Other complications include pulmonary fibrosis and myocarditis, which is often associated with conduction defects.

C. Histopathology

There is epidermal atrophy with degeneration of the basal layer keratinocytes producing vacuolar interface dermatitis. There is a sparse lymphocytic infiltrate. Gottron papules tend to show acanthosis and a dense lichenoid infiltrate. Thus, under the microscope, dermatomyositis appears very similar to lupus erythematosus.

A muscle biopsy shows an admixture of atrophy, apoptosis, regeneration, and hypertrophy of fibers. CD8+ T cells surround and infiltrate the muscle fibers.

D. Differential Diagnosis

Polymyositis–scleroderma overlap syndrome may also feature calcinosis and pulmonary involvement. About 10% of patients with dermatomyositis have overlaps with lupus erythematosus, rheumatoid arthritis, or other autoimmune diseases. Polymyositis and inclusion body myositis have no skin findings.

E. Course

The disease may be chronic or resolve after 2–3 years. If an underlying tumor can be cured, the dermatomyositis usually disappears rapidly. In children, the calcinosis clouds the outlook; prompt treatment and extensive physical therapy are crucial.

F. Therapy

Initial therapy should be prednisolone 1 mg/kg daily with low-dose methotrexate or azathioprine 150 mg daily. If there is prominent muscle involvement or slow response, high-dose intravenous immunoglobulins are rapidly effective and help protect against myosin-induced renal damage.

Dermatomyositis

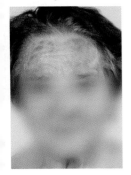

Edematous erythematous facial patches

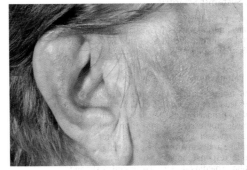

Facial erythema and poikiloderma

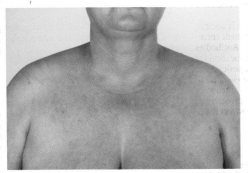

Diffuse erythematous patches on the trunk

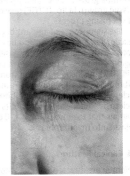

Heliotrope eyelids

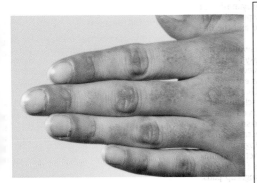

Erythematous papules with atrophy over the joints (Gottron papules) and nail fold hyperkeratosis with hemorrhage

B. Clinical Features

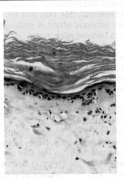

Atrophic epidermis with interface dermatitis

C. Histopathology

A. Systemic Sclerosis

Systemic sclerosis (SSc) affects the skin and many internal organs. It is usually divided into acral or limited form (lSSc) and diffuse form (dSSc). Scleroderma is a synonym.

■ Pathogenesis

The major feature is the deposition of increased amounts of extracellular matrix molecules, primarily collagen. SSc results from slowly progressive inflammation which first causes vessel spasm, and then later vessel damage and scarring. A helper T cell (T_{H2}) immune response appears involved as eosinophilia (mediated by IL-4/IL-5/IL-13) and plasma cells dominate at the start. Then transforming growth factor (TGF)-β and connective tissue growth factor (CTGF) take over and drive a sclerosing process.

The significance of autoantibodies is unclear, except for anti-Scl70 antibodies which correlate with pulmonary disease. Antibodies against platelet-derived growth factor receptor (PDGFR) push the transition from pericytes to fibroblasts. PDGFR and $PDGF_1$ are elevated in sclerotic areas, and PDGF inhibitors ameliorate sclerosis. Endothelin transmits prosclerotic signals that together with TGF-β convert fibroblasts into myofibroblasts.

■ Clinical Features

Women are affected 15 times more often than men. The population incidence is 7:100 000. Patients with lSSc usually present with *Raynaud syndrome* (white fingers from digital vasospasm and ischemia, followed by cyanosis and hyperemia). lSSc may first be suspected when the ischemic phase is prolonged and the fingers become edematous.

Some patients present with a swollen limb, often after physical activity. Biopsy reveals extensive infiltration of eosinophils even into the fascia. This situation is known as eosinophilic fasciitis or Shulman syndrome (Ch. 17.6).

There is a slow transition to a sclerotic form where the skin in the beginning is edematous, then smooth, tight, and finally too small for the tissues it must enclose. Telangiectases almost invariably develop. Next, dermatogenous contractures occur, as the skin restricts joint motion. Punctate fingertip necrosis (rat-bite ulcers), loss of substance of the fingertip pads, and shortening of the distal phalanx with nail damage follow. Subcutaneous calcification may also result (Thiebièrge–Weissenbach syndrome).

With time, the sclerosis gradually moves proximally at a variable rate. The mouth becomes tightened and expressionless, while frenular sclerosis limits tongue mobility. About 90% have GI involvement, usually affecting the esophagus, with stenosis and loss of peristalsis interfering with the passage of food. The lungs may be initially inflamed but progress to fibrosis and pulmonary hypertension, which can be disabling. The heart may show cor pulmonale or interstitial myocardial fibrosis. The most feared complication is malignant hypertension coupled with rapidly progressive renal failure, accounting for 50% of fatalities. Blood pressure should be monitored carefully and treated aggressively with ACE inhibitors.

A variant of lSSc is *CREST syndrome* (calcinosis, Raynaud phenomenon, esophageal involvement, sclerodactyly, telangiectases) with anticentromere antibodies.

In contrast, dSSc is less common, affects men as often as women, and often features anti-Scl70 antibodies. It typically starts on the trunk with edematous changes that rapidly progress to pansclerosis with multiple systemic problems and a poor prognosis.

■ Histopathology

Early lesions show swelling of collagen fiber and an infiltrate of CD4+ T cells, plasma cells and eosinophils around vessels. This inflammatory stage evolves into a sclerotic form with few cells and thickened collagen bundles running parallel to the epidermis. Adnexal structures, vessels, and subcutaneous fat are gradually trapped and then slowly atrophy.

■ Differential Diagnosis

Polymyositis–scleroderma overlap also features calcinosis and pulmonary fibrosis. Sclerodermiform GVHD is almost identical clinically. The many causes of pseudoscleroderma should be considered and include eosinophilia–myalgia syndrome (contaminated tryptophan), toxic oil syndrome, bleomycin fibrosis, nephrogenic systemic fibrosis in renal dialysis (triggered by gadolinium), scleredema, scleromyxedema, and diabetic stiff skin.

■ Course

Patients with dSSc may die within months from heart or renal disease, while those with lSSc have impaired quality of life but scarcely altered life expectancy.

IV Dermatologic Diseases

Systemic Sclerosis, Morphea, and Lichen Sclerosus et Atrophicus

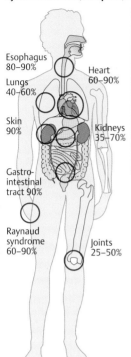

Esophagus
80–90%

Heart
60–90%

Lungs
40–60%

Skin
90%

Kidneys
35–70%

Gastro-
intestinal
tract 90%

Raynaud
syndrome
60–90%

Joints
25–50%

Common manifestations

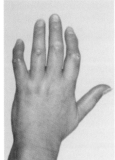

Microstomia, loss of expression, telangiectases

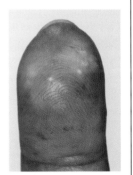

Typical perioral radial folds

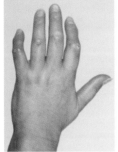

Acrosclerosis, pointed fingers (Madonna fingers), and dermatogenous contractures

Calcinosis

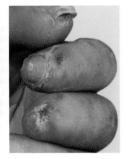

Scarring inflammation of the distal digits with nail loss and hyperkeratosis of the nail fold

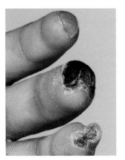

Fingertip necrosis with shortening of the digits and hyperkeratosis

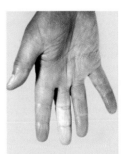

Raynaud syndrome

A. Systemic Sclerosis

IV Dermatologic Diseases

■ **Therapy**

Every patient needs optimized physical therapy. Medical intervention is directed to:

- control inflammation with corticosteroids, methotrexate, azathioprine, cyclophosphamide, and other agents
- reduce fibrosis with bath psoralen plus UVA (PUVA) or UVA$_1$
- inhibit platelet aggregation
- vasodilatation with prostaglandins or endothelin antagonists such as bosentan or sildenafil.

B. Morphea

Morphea features only cutaneous sclerosis without systemic involvement.

Pathogenesis. Tissue accumulation of activated B cells, as well as tissue and occasionally blood eosinophilia is seen. Only the linear variant has ANA. This suggests that T_{H2}-driven inflammation initiates the disease. A possible role for *Borrelia burgdorferi* has been excluded.

Clinical features. Classic morphea starts as a red-violet macule or patch that spreads with central sclerosis and peripheral *lilac ring*. Linear morphea typically involves a limb and may lead to atrophy, scarring and involvement of underlying fascia, muscles and bones with contractures. Linear morphea of the scalp and forehead is known as *en coup de sabre*. Hemifacial atrophy *(Parry–Romberg syndrome)* damages subcutaneous structures and bones. *Atrophoderma of Pasini and Pierini* is very superficial morphea of the trunk with little inflammation. The maximal variant is disabling pansclerotic morphea, affecting almost the entire integument with contractures, ulcers, and disfigurement. Patients thus resemble those with dSSc but have no systemic involvement.

Histopathology. Identical to SSc.

Differential diagnosis. Early morphea resembles erythema migrans. There are overlaps between morphea and LSA. Disabling pansclerotic morphea must be separated from dSSc.

Course. Classic morphea is usually self-limited, burning out after 3–5 years. The sclerosis may improve. The variants are more persistent. Linear morphea produces contractures and impaired bone growth in 10% of patients.

Therapy. In addition to physical therapy, both bath PUVA and UVA$_1$ are effective in arresting sclerosis. Early lesions may respond to high-potency topical corticosteroids. Methotrexate is reserved for severely affected patients.

C. Lichen Sclerosus et Atrophicus

Clinical features. Lichen sclerosus et atrophicus (LSA) can affect the skin or mucosa. Children often have atrophic white mucosal lesions which cause strictures, such as phimosis and vulvovaginal atrophy. The skin is fragile, so that hemorrhage, blisters, and erosions may develop. The process may persist into adulthood or start later. In adults, penile involvement is known as balanitis xerotica obliterans, and vulvar involvement as kraurosis vulvae.

On the trunk, porcelain atrophic plaques up to 1–2 cm in size are seen, which may become confluent. There is often an inflammatory reaction at the periphery.

Histopathology. Initially there is subepidermal edema with a sparse T-cell infiltrate. The epidermis is atrophic and may be separated from the dermis by blisters or hemorrhage. The collagen has a peculiar pale homogenous appearance, which is pathognomonic; elastic fibers are lost. Antibodies against extracellular matrix protein-1 (ECM-1) are found in most cases.

Differential diagnosis. Morphea, lichen planus, and, in girls, sexual abuse when erosions or hemorrhage is present.

Course. LSA usually resolves in children and young adults. Genital LSA in adults is a rare precursor for squamous cell carcinoma.

Therapy. High-potency topical corticosteroids over months often heal LSA. Calcineurin inhibitors are also helpful. Circumcision may be required.

Systemic Sclerosis, Morphea, and Lichen Sclerosus et Atrophicus

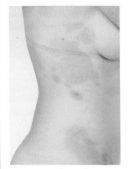

Disseminated morphea

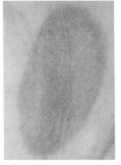

Inflammatory stage with lilac ring

Postinflammatory hyperpigmentation in resolved morphea

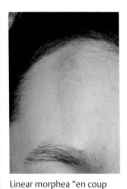

Linear morphea "en coup de saber"

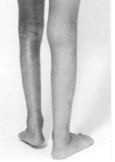

Linear morphea with shortening of the affected leg

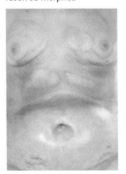

Disabling pansclerotic morphea

B. Morphea

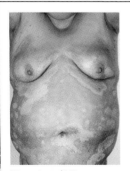

Disseminated LSA

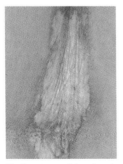

Confluent porcelain-colored papules and plaques

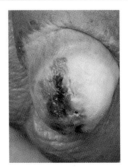

Bullous LSA with hemorrhage

C. Lichen Sclerosus et Atrophicus

17 Inflammatory Diseases of the Dermis

187

Lupus erythematosus (LE) includes three entities with only minimal overlap but the same pathogenesis and morphology:
- cutaneous or discoid LE (CDLE)
- subacute cutaneous LE (SCLE)
- systemic LE (SLE).

All three usually involve the skin (SLE occasionally does not) and can be triggered by UV radiation.

■ Pathogenesis

LE features a derangement in cell death and removal of dead cells. The complement abnormalities seen in SLE and the antinuclear antibodies (ANA) fit into this concept. The nuclear glycoproteins and nucleic acids of inadequately scavenged cells stimulate a specific immune response via toll-like receptors. The UV sensitivity also fits, as the UV-induced damage creates abnormal antigens for presentation such as Ro, which seems to be coupled with photosensitivity. Numerous medications, including some chemotherapy regimens, also induce cell damage and generate abnormal antigens that can trigger an immune response.

A. Chronic Cutaneous or Discoid Lupus Erythematosus

■ Clinical Features

CDLE is the most common form (incidence 0.05%) and primarily limited to the skin. The primary lesions are coin-shaped or discoid plaques involving the face and neck. The lesions are erythematous, may have diffuse fine adherent follicular scales (follicular plugging), and heal with central atrophy. Sometimes erosions develop. Hypo- or hyperpigmentation is common, as well as a slightly raised border. Scarred lesions may flare several weeks after repeated UV exposure. LE is one of the most common causes of scarring alopecia (Ch. 26.4). When the arms, legs, or trunk are involved, the term of disseminated discoid LE is used.

Another common manifestation is *lupus tumidus*, which has doughy erythematous plaques and nodules, usually in UV-exposed areas, such as the cheeks, nose, or nape. Histology shows extensive deposits of mucin. A related disorder may be reticulated erythematous mucinosis *(REM syndrome)*, which features lacy erythematous mid-truncal papules that coalesce into plaques with extensive dermal mucin Both these types of LE may resolve spontaneously without scarring.

Mucosal involvement usually suggests SLE, although the lower lip is frequently affected in CDLE. *Lupus panniculitis* or *lupus profundus* involves subcutaneous fat, usually with overlying discoid changes, but sometimes beneath normal skin. It may also appear in SLE. *Chilblain lupus* has erythematous plaques of the nose, ears, and fingers, mimicking pernio. Hypertrophic CDLE is often mistaken for a squamous cell carcinoma and is notoriously hard to treat.

Transition to SLE occurs in < 5% of cases, somewhat more often with disseminated disease. Illogically, CDLE is one of the criteria for the diagnosis of SLE.

■ Histopathology

The microscopic picture exactly reflects the clinical findings. There is follicular plugging and an atrophic epidermis with apoptotic keratinocytes, especially in the basal layer. The basement membrane is markedly thickened, while the dermis has lymphocytic infiltrates, especially around vessels and adnexal structures, and often mucin. Over time, the adnexal structures are destroyed. In lupus tumidus, the infiltrates produce a picture of pseudolymphoma and the mucin is abundant. Lupus panniculitis is usually rich in plasma cells. The immunoglobulins along the basement membrane are the result of nonspecific deposition but can be indentified with direct immunofluorescence *(lupus band test)*.

B. Subacute Cutaneous Lupus Erythematosus

■ Clinical Features

SCLE is most clearly connected to UV exposure. The lesions appear only in sun-exposed skin, such as the face, arms, décolleté, or upper back. The transition to normal sun-protected skin is sharp. The lesions may be sharply bordered erythematous flat plaques with prominent fine scale and erosions, or annular with an active erythematous border and collarette scale. While SCLE rarely scars, it often leads to hypo- or hyperpigmentation. SCLE, especially the annular form, occasionally overlaps with Sjögren syndrome, with dry eyes and mouth. SCLE is strongly associated with anti-Ro (SS-A; 75%–90%) and anti-La (SS-B; 30%–40%) antibodies, as is Sjögren syndrome. In contrast to CDLE, SCLE evolves into SLE in 10%–15% of patients, usually with renal or central nervous system (CNS) disease. Nonetheless, the course tends to be relatively mild.

Lupus Erythematosus

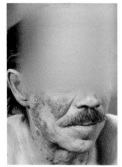

Chronic discoid lupus erythematosus

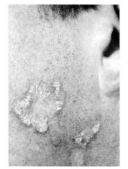

Hyperkeratotic rim with central healing

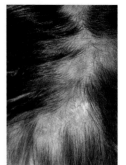

Scarring alopecia

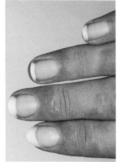

Chilblain lupus

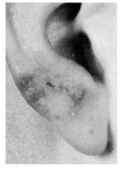

Lupus tumidus

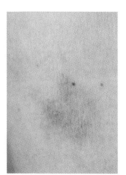

Lupus panniculitis

A. Chronic Cutaneous or Discoid Lupus Erythematosus

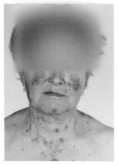

Facial and trunk involvement

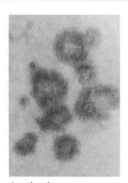

Annular plaques

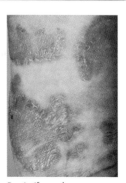

Psoriasiform plaques

B. Subacute Cutaneous Lupus Erythematosus

17 Inflammatory Diseases of the Dermis

189

IV Dermatologic Diseases

> **Caution:** Pregnant patients with SCLE can transfer anti-Ro antibodies transplacentally causing neonatal LE with transient skin changes but often a permanent and dangerous atrioventricular (AV) block.

■ Histopathology

The picture is similar to CDLE but less severe, with little scarring. The epidermal damage may be greater with more prominent apoptotic cells, reflecting the importance of photodamage. The epidermis is atrophic and once again there is a dermal lymphocytic infiltrate, which may be bandlike and edging toward the epidermis (interface dermatitis). The basement membrane may show patchy thickening with periodic acid–Schiff (PAS) stain.

C. Systemic Lupus Erythematosus

■ Clinical Features

The classic cutaneous change in SLE is acute cutaneous LE, with an acute erythema in sun-exposed areas, especially over the nose and cheeks, producing a "butterfly rash." Such patients are likely to have SLE and require prompt evaluation. Sunburn, rosacea, and polymorphic light eruption must be excluded; rosacea (Ch. 26.2) may cause confusion, as it affects older patients who are likely to have a low titer but not clinically relevant ANA. Sometimes acute SLE presents with EM-like lesions (*Rowell syndrome*).

Patients presenting with a butterfly rash may suddenly become quite ill. The organs most likely to be involved are the skin, kidneys, and blood. Thus, a careful examination, urinalysis, and complete blood count (CBC) get one started quickly in the right direction. In addition, ANA and anti-dsDNA antibodies should initially be checked. The page opposite gives more details.

Renal disease causes the most problems and must be monitored closely. The exact therapy depends on the type of renal damage, so a renal biopsy is generally required. Almost every organ can be affected; other common problems are non-destructive arthritis, pleuritis, pericarditis (ECG), and CNS disease.

Several medications may induce LE. The most notorious are procainamide (20% of users) and hydralazine (10%). Skin changes are rare; typical problems are pericarditis and pleuritis. Typically, antihistone antibodies and ANA are found, but not dsDNA antibodies.

■ Histopathology

Acute LE shows dermal edema, a sparse lymphocytic infiltrate, and usually prominent keratinocyte damage with apoptosis or hydropic degeneration. The basement membrane has usually not had time to thicken.

D. Course

The course of the disease is highly variable. Prior to corticosteroids, SLE was usually rapidly fatal. Today most aspects can be controlled but the overall prognosis depends on which internal organs are involved and how well they, especially the kidneys, respond to therapy.

E. Therapy

The mainstays of therapy are anti-inflammatory therapy and avoiding exposure to UV irradiation. Initial topical therapy for CDLE and SCLE consists of corticosteroids or calcineurin inhibitors. If the skin changes cannot be controlled topically, then the next step is antimalarial drugs (hydroxychloroquine 200–400 mg daily or chloroquine 125–250 mg daily), sometimes in combination with quinacrine 100 mg daily. Short bursts of systemic corticosteroids are a reasonable way to control the disease more rapidly. If all this fails, then immunosuppressive therapy with azathioprine, mycophenolate mofetil, or thalidomide may be required.

In SLE, the course of therapy is generally determined by what is required for the most severe of its life-threatening systemic manifestations. In general, if lupus nephritis is present its treatment takes precedence. Typical approaches include corticosteroid or cyclophosphamide pulse therapy for initial control. Later, corticosteroids may be combined with azathioprine or mycophenolate mofetil. Patients with systemic disease and minimal cutaneous findings should still use sunscreens religiously.

New approaches to systemic therapy include high-dose intravenous immunoglobulins while anti-CD20-mediated depletion of B cells surprisingly failed to show efficacy.

Lupus Erythematosus

History
Physical examination
- Skin findings
- Joints
- Lymphadenopathy

Laboratory
- Urine
- CBC
- ANA (dsDNA)
- Blood urea nitrogen (BUN), creatinine
- ESR
- Complement (C3, C4)

Diagnostic approach

- Butterfly rash
- Discoid lesions
- Photosensitivity
- Oral ulcer
- Arthritis, arthralgias
- Serositis (pleuritis, pericarditis)
- Nephritis
- CNS disorder
- Hematologic disorder
- Immunologic disorder (autoantibodies, [dsDNA], antiphospholipid [APL])
- Antinuclear antibodies (ANA)

American College of Rheumatology (ACR) criteria

Clinical findings	ANA
SLE, titers correlate with clinical activity	dsDNA
SCLE, neonatal LE, SLE, Sjögren syndrome	Ro (SS-A), La (SS-B)
Drug-induced LE	Histone
Antiphospholipid syndrome (thrombi, miscarriages)	APL

Important autoantibodies

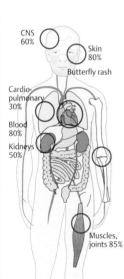

CNS 60%
Skin 80%
Butterfly rash
Cardio-pulmonary 30%
Blood 80%
Kidneys 50%
Muscles, joints 85%
Fever, malaise 90%

Common manifestations

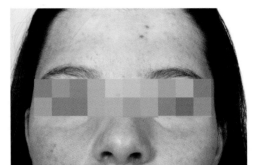

Butterfly rash

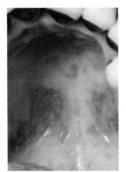

Annular erythema

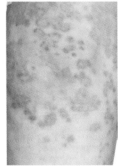

Oral erosions

C. Systemic Lupus Erythematosus

Eosinophilia in the blood (> 5 %; > 0.4×10^3/μL absolute count) or tissues is seen in many disorders. Physiologic eosinophilia may develop at the end of severe infectious diseases. It is typical for infections with extracellular parasites, whose removal requires eosinophils. A pathogenetic role is ascribed to eosinophils in allergic diseases, especially allergic asthma and allergic rhinoconjunctivitis. Other diseases where these cells are common include autoimmune diseases (common in bullous pemphigoid), drug reactions, and GVHD. Finally there is a heterogenous group of uncommon disorders in which eosinophilia is the only unifying factor.

A. Hypereosinophilic Syndrome

This systemic disease typically starts between 20 and 50 years of age and is defined as the presence of an eosinophil count ≥ 1500/μL for > 6 months without an explanation and with organ involvement. Two possible causes are a clonal T-cell proliferation producing IL-5, which drives eosinophil production, and a fusion gene (*PDGFRA-FIP1L 1*) on chromosome 4 that is sensitive to tyrosinase kinase inhibitors.

While all organs can have eosinophilic infiltrates, the main problems arise with the heart, great vessels, and CNS. Some patients develop eosinophilic leukemia. The skin features persistent urticarial papules and plaques, which are firmer and persist longer than ordinary urticaria. On biopsy, they may show leukocytoclastic vasculitis with eosinophilia. *Hypereosinophilic dermatitis* is a forme fruste of hypereosinophilic syndrome, with only skin involvement. The skin lesions are very difficult to treat and respond best to PUVA; depending on the cause, the systemic problems may respond to anti-IL-5 or tyrosine kinase inhibitors.

B. Eosinophilic Cellulitis

Also known as *Wells syndrome*, this disease goes through two clinical phases. The first is edematous erythematous plaques, which may resemble cellulitis, erysipelas, or early morphea. In the subsequent course, urticarial plaques, pruritic papules, or blisters appear. Eosinophilic cellulitis may be associated with fever, arthralgias, and facial nerve palsy. Histologically, there are dermal infiltrates of macrophages and eosinophils surrounding areas of collagen necrosis. These changes have fancifully been called "flame figures." Eosinophilic cellulitis responds rapidly to systemic corticosteroids.

C. Eosinophilic Fasciitis

Eosinophilic fasciitis or *Shulman syndrome* starts as an erythematous warm painful swelling with marked blood and tissue eosinophilia and an elevated ESR. Often a limb is affected, sometimes after strenuous physical activity. A distinctive physical finding is the "negative vein sign"; the cutaneous veins appear depressed as the area around them swells. The course shares many similarities with systemic sclerosis as the area becomes sclerotic, but some patients resolve after a few months and others have other underlying diseases. Sometimes, medications may cause a similar picture. Initially one may think of angioedema, erysipelas, or a localized severe reaction to an immunization. It may be challenging to exclude streptococcal necrotizing fasciitis, as it often starts without fever. Occasionally, eosinophilic fasciitis appears at the onset of chronic GVHD, with symmetrical involvement of the extremities; here it almost invariably becomes sclerotic. The histologic picture gives a rapid answer. A deep biopsy must be obtained, sampling the fascia which is dramatically thickened and full of eosinophils. The acute phase often responds well to systemic corticosteroids; subsequently low-dose isotretinoin and PUVA or methotrexate are indicated.

D. Granuloma Faciale

Also known as eosinophilic granuloma, these lesions represent a late stage of unique cutaneous vasculitis. They present as firm dome-shaped red-brown papules and nodules, almost always on the face. The infiltrate shows numerous eosinophils as well as chronic vascular changes. Sometimes there is associated upper airway disease known as eosinophilic angiocentric fibrosis. Intralesional corticosteroids appear to be the best approach; no reliable therapy is known.

E. Eosinophilic Pustular Folliculitis

This uncommon disease presents in two ways. Patients with human immunodeficiency virus/acquired immune deficiency syndrome (HIV/AIDS) have numerous intensely pruritic papules, most common on the trunk, which on biopsy show pustules laden with eosinophils. In Ofuji disease, the pruritic papules and papulopustules are combined with edematous plaques, usually affecting the face. Both disorders may have eosinophilia. Photochemotherapy appears to be the best treatment.

Diseases with Eosinophilia

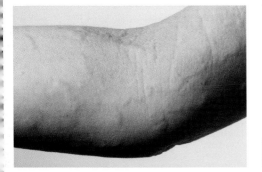

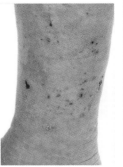

Urticarial papules and plaques
A. Hypereosinophilic Syndrome

Excoriated papules

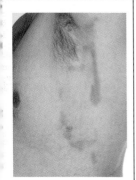

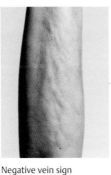

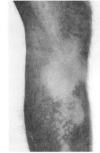

Negative vein sign

Diffuse sclerosis

C. Eosinophilic Fasciitis

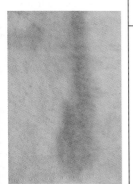

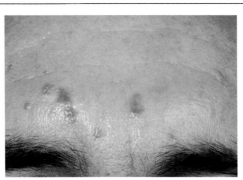

Erythematous,
edematous patches
B. Eosinophilic Cellulitis

Red-brown nodules
D. Granuloma Faciale

A. Sarcoidosis

Sarcoidosis is a systemic disease that features noncaseating granulomas. In white individuals, the incidence is 10:100 000, while in African-Americans it is 50:100 000 with a lifetime risk of 1%–2%.

■ Pathogenesis

Sarcoidosis is triggered by interferon (IFN)-γ-producing T_{H1} cells, but the stimulus to which these cells are responding remains a great medical mystery. While an infectious cause has long been suspected, no microbes have been unequivocally identified. T_{H1} cells produce inflammation by inducing TNF-producing macrophages. It is likely that TNF antagonists improve sarcoidosis without provoking disseminated infections, which further argues against an infectious cause.

■ Clinical Features

Sarcoidosis can affect every organ. Those most commonly affected are the lungs and mediastinum, but the skin in involved in 50%. The lupoid or apple jelly sign on diascopy is typical for many skin lesions, such as with cutaneous tuberculosis. The skin lesions are divided as follows:

Maculopapular sarcoidosis. Multiple pinhead to pea-sized blue-red papules in the face and proximal extremities. It often resolves with postinflammatory hyperpigmentation.

Subcutaneous sarcoidosis. Firm subcutaneous nodules; the overlying skin may have a blue sheen.

Plaque sarcoidosis. Exanthematous eruption of coin-shaped red-brown flat or slightly raised plaques. It is most likely to be associated with involvement of the lymph nodes and spleen.

Lupus pernio. Firm red-brown nodules on the distal surfaces such as the nose, ears, cheeks, earlobes, and fingers. It, too, is often associated with systemic involvement.

Scar sarcoidosis.
Papules in scars or areas of trauma.

> **Note:** Sarcoidosis must always be excluded in patients presenting with erythema nodosum (Ch. 18.1); it is one of the most common triggers of this type of panniculitis.

Special variants of sarcoidosis include:
- *Löfgren syndrome*—ill patient with fever, malaise, arthritis, erythema nodosum, and bilateral hilar lymphadenopathy
- *Mikulicz syndrome*—swelling of the salivary or lacrimal glands
- *Heerfordt syndrome*—a triad of facial nerve palsy, parotid swelling, and iridocyclitis, sometimes with CNS findings
- *Parinaud syndrome*—conjunctivitis with papillary nodules, lacrimal gland involvement, and ipsilateral lymphadenopathy.

■ Diagnostic Approach

The first step in the evaluation should be a chest x-ray. If there is lung involvement, then pulmonary function testing and bronchoalveolar lavage are the next steps. The serum ACE level is usually elevated and may be useful in diagnosis and monitoring. Serum calcium levels are not useful for diagnosis, but should be monitored to avoid complications. ECG is useful to exclude atrial or ventricular granulomas. Multidisciplinary care is the rule, not the exception.

■ Histopathology

In the dermis, there are sharply defined granulomas with activated macrophages, epithelioid cells, and multinucleated giant cells. The surrounding lymphocytic infiltrate is sparse (naked granulomas). There is no caseation.

> **Note:** Sarcoidal granulomas frequently contain foreign bodies, as sarcoidosis patients react more strongly to a variety of foreign objects. Thus, the presence of a foreign body in a granuloma does not exclude sarcoidosis.

■ Differential Diagnosis

The differential diagnosis encompasses virtually all of internal medicine. A wide variety of infectious diseases including mycobacterial and fungal infections can mimic or overlap with sarcoidosis and must be excluded.

■ Course

The course is highly variable, but there is >50% spontaneous resolution.

■ Therapy

Corticosteroids are the mainstay of therapy. Methotrexate is the best choice for severe cutaneous and systemic disease. There is little experience with other anti-inflammatory agents, although TNF antagonists offer promise.

– Noninfectious Granulomatous Diseases

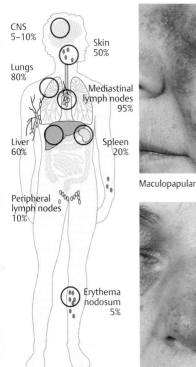

CNS
5–10%

Skin
50%

Lungs
80%

Mediastinal
lymph nodes
95%

Liver
60%

Spleen
20%

Peripheral
lymph nodes
10%

Erythema
nodosum
5%

Common manifestations

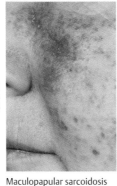

Maculopapular sarcoidosis

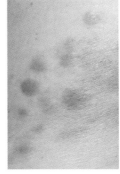

Plaque-type sarcoidosis

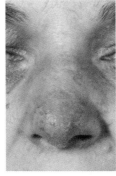

Lupus pernio

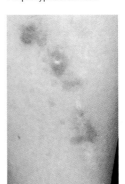

Scar sarcoidosis

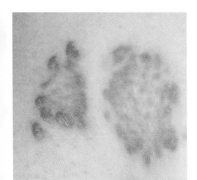

Annular sarcoidosis

A. Sarcoidosis

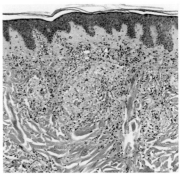

Noncaseating granulomas with few
surrounding lymphocytes (naked or sarcoidal
granuloma)

B. Granuloma Annulare

Granuloma annulare (GA) is a common granulomatous disease of the skin and subcutis, whose cause is unknown.

Clinical features. The classic lesion is a ring of blue-pink papules surrounding an area of central atrophy, often on the back of the hand or foot. There are many variants including disseminated papules, subcutaneous nodules, and large flat red-brown facial plaques with actinically damaged collagen (annular elastolytic granuloma).

Histopathology. The key finding is a palisading granuloma, as an area of necrotic collagen and mucin (*necrobiosis*) is surrounded by a ring of macrophages and lymphocytes.

Differential diagnosis. The classic lesions in children are usually missed as tinea. Subcutaneous lesions are identical to rheumatoid nodules.

Course. Most cases resolve spontaneously after years.

Therapy. Usually none, or corticosteroids under occlusion or intralesionally. For more severe cases, bath PUVA, systemic retinoids, or fumaric acid are used.

C. Necrobiosis Lipoidica (NL)

Pathogenesis. NL is an atrophic granulomatous disease of unknown cause. While some patients (10%–20%) have diabetes mellitus, the relationship is unclear. For this reason, the old name of *necrobiosis lipoidica diabeticorum* is avoided.

Clinical features. NL begins as a yellow-red macule or patch with prominent telangiectases, typically on the shins, but occasionally on sun-exposed skin. The lesion expands to produce a large easily injured atrophic plaque with slightly elevated wall. Because of the site, trauma is common and ulcers are quick to develop but slow to heal.

Histopathology. Once again, palisading granulomas are seen, often extending into the subcutis. There may be more vascular involvement than in GA.

Differential diagnosis. Morphea (clinically) and GA (histologically).

Course. Chronic disease with little tendency to improve, with or without treatment.

Therapy. Topical corticosteroids under occlusion. Prompt wound care for ulcers. Systemic clofazimine occasionally helps.

D. Rheumatoid Nodule

Clinical features. Rheumatoid nodules are the most common extra-articular finding in rheumatoid arthritis (RA), affecting 25% of patients. Firm subcutaneous nodules ranging in size from few millimeters to several centimeters, usually on the elbow or over the radius, often are just annoying, but can ulcerate and then be problematic. Rheumatoid nodulosis is a benign RA variant; methotrexate can trigger multiple tiny nodules.

Histopathology. Virtually identical to subcutaneous GA, but perhaps with more fibrin.

Differential diagnosis. In children, deep GA. In adults, gouty tophi, Heberden nodes of osteoarthritis.

> **Note:** Subcutaneous GA is far more common than rheumatoid nodule in children. Never diagnose rheumatoid arthritis in this age group without other evidence.

Therapy. Watchful waiting unless very painful or ulcerated; then excision.

E. Foreign Body Granuloma

Pathogenesis. A long list of foreign objects can induce an immune response when introduced into the skin.

Clinical features. Firm or edematous papules and nodules in sites of trauma, whether a splinter, road trauma, or sites of injection or fillers in aesthetic dermatology.

Histopathology. There is a variety of patterns but a foreign body can usually be seen with polarization.

> **Note:** Examine all granulomas with polarization to exclude the presence of a foreign body.

Therapy. If possible, excision. If the reaction is too widespread, topical anti-inflammatory measures should be used.

Noninfectious Granulomatous Diseases

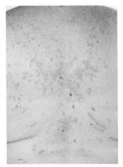 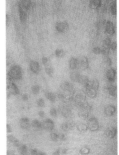 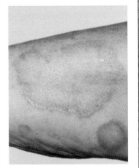

Disseminated papules   Multiple annular papules   Annular plaques

B. Granuloma Annulare

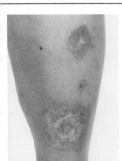 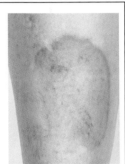 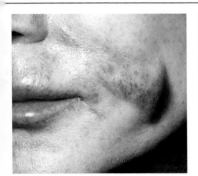

Atrophic telangiectatic scars

C. Necrobiosis Lipoidica

D. Rheumatoid Nodule

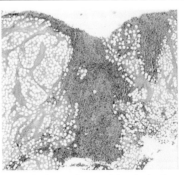

Foreign body granuloma following injection of filler

E. Foreign Body Granuloma

Foreign body granuloma with hundreds of small round uniform clear spaces reflecting filler material

A. Overview

Fat is a simple tissue with a homogenous structure and reacts in a limited number of ways to a variety of insults, such as trauma, microbes, noxious substances, metabolic products, or enzymes.

■ Clinical Features

Panniculitis presents as subcutaneous nodules, often red or red-brown and tender. The most common site is below the knees, but it can occur anywhere.

Note: Panniculitis above the knees should raise the possibility of systemic causes.

■ Histopathology

There are two basic patterns:

- *septal* with inflammation primarily confined to fibrous septae between lobules of fat
- *lobular* (inflammation centered in fat lobules).

There are often overlaps between two forms. Other features may include:

- *vasculitis* involving the deep dermal plexus and septa
- *saponification*—fat may dissolve; clue to pancreatic disease with release of enzymes
- *foreign body reaction*—suggests factitial panniculitis (injection into fat)

B. Clinical Types

Erythema nodosum. Only common form. Triggers are infections (streptococci, yersinia, deep fungi), hormones (pregnancy, contraceptives), and sarcoidosis. Presents with distinctive red-brown bruises on shins, usually painful. Prototype of septal panniculitis. Therapy with NSAID, support hose; usually resolves spontaneously. Treat any suspected triggering infection.

Note: Erythema nodosum never ulcerates. If a lesion is ulcerated, look for a different diagnosis. Although it is usually idiopathic, erythema nodosum may be a marker for systemic diseases such as sarcoidosis or Crohn disease. In Southwestern USA, coccidiomycosis is a common trigger. Always take a travel history!

Nodular vasculitis. Idiopathic or possibly tuberculid (*erythema induratum*); check for TB history (Ch. 33.5). Painful persistent nodules usually on calf. Tendency to recur with cold weather. Histology shows lobar panniculitis with vasculitis. Anti-TB therapy; if no evidence for TB, then systemic corticosteroids.

Metabolic panniculitis. Lesions typically above the knees or even on the trunk. Oily liquid may drain spontaneously or on biopsy.

Note: Always check for pancreatitis or pancreatic tumor, as well as α_1-antitrypsin deficiency (with risk of emphysema).

Connective-tissue panniculitis. Lupus profundus is the most common (Ch. 17.5). It is also seen with dermatomyositis, systemic sclerosis, and rheumatoid arthritis.

Trauma. Both physical trauma and cold may damage fat, causing inflammation. Cold panniculitis is often on hips of female equestrians.

Artifact. Fat is a favorite site for injection of foreign substances (urine, feces), illicit drugs, and other foreign substances.

Newborn. Fat necrosis secondary to trauma or cold injury (placing newborn on cold surface) is self-limited; sometimes it is complicated by hypercalcemia. *Sclerema neonatorum* is far more extensive fat necrosis in sick infants, and is potentially fatal.

Note: Be suspicious of self-induced panniculitis; always check biopsy for foreign material.

C. Lipoatrophy and Lipodystrophy

The only other clinical problem is loss of fat—known as lipoatrophy or lipodystrophy.

Localized. Follows injection of corticosteroids, insulin, or idiopathic (semicircular on thighs). Hemifacial atrophy is a deep morphea that also damages subcutaneous fat and bone (Ch. 17.4).

Generalized. Many different genetic forms, some associated with renal disease, malignancies, and insulin resistance. Patients look muscular because of fat loss.

HIV-associated. Poorly explained loss of facial and extremity fat with increased truncal fat; it is unclear if it is caused by human immunodeficiency virus (HIV) alone or by interaction with protease inhibitors (Ch. 37.1).

Panniculitis

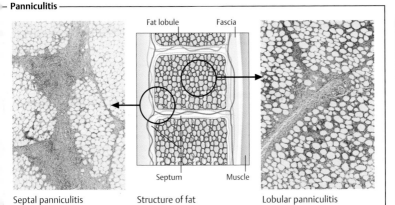

Fat lobule Fascia

Septum Muscle

Septal panniculitis Structure of fat Lobular panniculitis

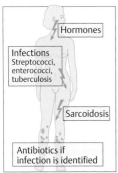

Hormones

Infections
Streptococci,
enterococci,
tuberculosis

Sarcoidosis

Antibiotics if
infection is identified

Erythema nodosum

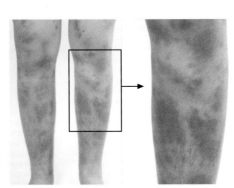

Erythema nodosum with bruiselike nodules

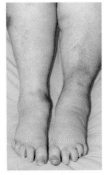

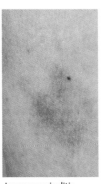

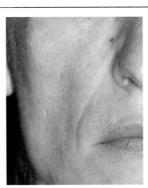

Nodular vasculitis Lupus panniculitis Lipodystrophy in HIV/AIDS

B. Clinical Types **C. Lipoatrophy and Lipodystrophy**

The synthesis of collagen and elastic fibers, as well as ground substance, is complex (Ch. 2.3) with many opportunities for errors. There are many rare disorders with inherited defects in connective-tissue production.

A. Ehlers–Danlos Syndrome

Ehlers–Danlos syndrome (EDS) is not a single disease, but rather a group of disorders with skin, joint, and in some instances skeletal and cardiovascular defects. The following types are identified:

Classical. Autosomal dominant. Mutations in type V collagen, type I collagen, and tenascin. Patients have hyperextensible joints and easily stretched skin; a typical finding is gaping scars (*molluscoid pseudotumors*), marked striae and frequent extensive bruises. Gorlin sign is the ability to touch the nose with the tongue. Joints are easily dislocated and may develop arthritis. Mitral valve prolapse, scoliosis, anal prolapse, hiatus hernia, and cervical insufficiency are possible systemic complications.

Hypermobile. Autosomal dominant. Marked joint hypermotility but relatively mild skin findings. The genetic defect is unknown.

Vascular. Autosomal dominant. Mutation in type III collagen. The skin is thin and easily bruised, with prominent vascular patterns. There is no joint or skin hyperextensibility. There is considerable risk of varicosities and aneurysms, as well as ruptured vessels and viscera, with reduced life expectancy. Some patients have acrogeria with premature aging, including marked wrinkling and facial atrophy.

Kyphoscoliosis. Autosomal recessive. Mutation in collagen I. Hypermobile joints, muscular hypotonia, and progressive scoliosis, present at birth. Marfanoid habitus, fragile skin, and sclerae with risk of rupture of the ocular bulb.

Arthroclasia. Autosomal dominant. Mutation in lysyl hydroxylase. Extreme joint hypermobility with recurrent subluxations.

Dermatosparaxis Type. Autosomal recessive. Mutations in N-terminal procollagen-I-peptidase. Overlap with cutis laxa with marked skin fragility.

■ Therapy

There is no effective therapy. Management consists of trying to avoid or control complications.

B. Marfan Syndrome

This is a defect in fibrillin, inherited in an autosomal dominant fashion with an incidence of 1:5000. Mutations in the fibrillin 1 gene lead to skeletal, cardiovascular, and ocular abnormalities. Patients are often tall with an elongated face and disproportionately long limbs (*arachnodactyly*) and are at considerable risk for aortic and visceral rupture. They often require aortic replacement surgery. Joint hypermotility is seen, with resultant orthopedic problems. Also, an easily displaced lens often leads to impaired sight. Cutaneous findings include prominent striae, elastosis perforans serpiginosa, and hyperextensibility.

Mutations in the fibrillin 2 gene cause congenital contractural arachnodactyly with Marfanoid habitus but marked contractures and crumpled ears.

C. Cutis Laxa

This is a group of rare disorders with various defects in elastin synthesis and variable patterns of inheritance. The most striking clinical feature is droopy skin (*basset hound look*) so that patients appear much older than their stated age. The autosomal dominant form primarily has skin changes while the autosomal recessive form has skin and systemic involvement with cardiovascular, pulmonary, and musculoskeletal problems secondary to loss of elastic fibers. It may also be acquired following variety of inflammatory skin diseases.

D. Pseudoxanthoma Elasticum

This is a rare defect in the MRP6 protein, a member of the ATP-binding cassette (ABC) family of proteins primarily expressed in liver and kidney. It is usually inherited in an autosomal recessive fashion. Puzzlingly, the main problems are with abnormal calcification of elastic fibers in the eyes, vessels, and skin. A classic cutaneous finding is *chicken skin* with subtle yellow plaques in the flexures. Skin biopsy shows disrupted elastin fibers, which are strikingly positive for calcium with von Kossa stain. The main vascular problems are gastrointestinal hemorrhage, myocardial infarction, and strokes. The eyes have *angioid streaks* (tears in the Bruch membrane); 60%–70% have impaired vision by the fourth decade. There is no therapy, but patients should avoid risk factors for vascular disease (smoking, elevated lipids, overweight).

Rare acquired forms are limited to the skin and associated with trauma, topical exposure to calcium salts, or medications.

Disorders of Collagen and Elastin

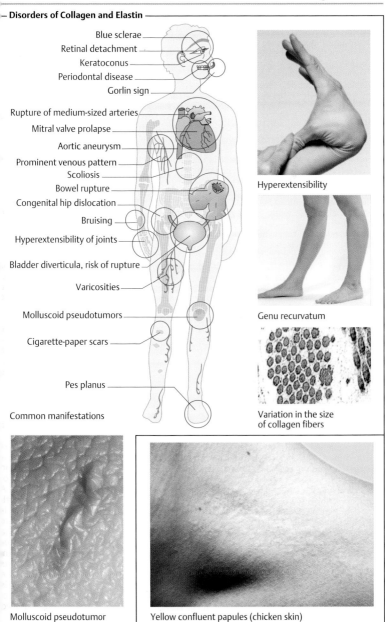

Blue sclerae
Retinal detachment
Keratoconus
Periodontal disease
Gorlin sign
Rupture of medium-sized arteries
Mitral valve prolapse
Aortic aneurysm
Prominent venous pattern
Scoliosis
Bowel rupture
Congenital hip dislocation
Bruising
Hyperextensibility of joints
Bladder diverticula, risk of rupture
Varicosities
Molluscoid pseudotumors
Cigarette-paper scars
Pes planus

Common manifestations

Hyperextensibility

Genu recurvatum

Variation in the size
of collagen fibers

Molluscoid pseudotumor
A. Ehlers–Danlos Syndrome

Yellow confluent papules (chicken skin)
D. Pseudoxanthoma Elasticum

The disorders of keratinization include diffuse disorders (ichthyosis), localized conditions (palmoplantar keratoderma), those distributed in a mosaic pattern (epidermal nevi), and sometimes also solitary acquired lesions such as epidermolytic acanthoma. In addition, milder ichthyosis can be a secondary phenomenon associated with a variety of disorders.

A. Ichthyoses

The ichthyoses are widespread disorders featuring prominent scales. There are many different types with varying pathogenesis and clinical features. They may be divided into two types:
- defects in keratin or intercellular substances (lipids, filaggrin) limited to the skin
- metabolic disease with involvement of other organs.

Ichthyosis vulgaris. This is the only common ichthyosis, with an incidence of 1:300. There is a defect in filaggrin, so scales are retained (retention hyperkeratosis). It appears during the first year of life. Patients have diffuse pale polygonal scales, typically sparing the flexural areas; it is often associated with atopic dermatitis.

X-linked ichthyosis. This only occurs in males; patients have dirty thick scales and also corneal defects (50%) and cryptorchism (20%). It is associated with steroid sulfatase deficiency and premature delivery in carrier females.

Lamellar ichthyosis. There are several forms, with mutations in transglutaminase, lipoxygenase, and other genes. It is likely to present as *collodion baby* with large sheets of scales and fissures at birth. The flexures, face, and scalp are generally involved. There is also a risk of ectropion and sweat gland occlusion, causing heat intolerance. The most common type is inherited in an autosomal-recessive manner with mutation in transglutaminase and thus a defect in the cornified envelope. Some collodion babies resolve entirely.

Harlequin ichthyosis. Extremely thick armor-like scales are present at birth and it is often fatal in infancy. There is a massive defect in keratinization caused by mutations in ABCA12, an ATP-binding cassette protein.

Congenital bullous ichthyosiform erythroderma. Patients have bullae at birth, later develop thick scales and spiny hyperkeratoses; plaques appear velvety. Caused by mutations in keratins 1 or 10, inherited in autosomal dominant fashion. Clumps of keratin with vacuolar degeneration produce the typical histologic picture (*epidermolytic hyperkeratosis*).

Acquired ichthyosis. Caused by drugs interfering with lipid metabolism (nicotinic acid), underlying tumors, sarcoidosis, and malnutrition.

■ Therapy

There is no curative therapy available:
- *topical*: keratolytic agents (lactic acid 5%–10%), humectants (urea 5%–12%), or lubrication
- *systemic*: systemic retinoids are helpful for severe cases, but are required for life.

B. Palmoplantar Keratodermas

These are disorders with mutations in keratin or other genes expressed in the palmoplantar skin.

Vörner type. This type is the most common; it is caused by mutations in keratin 1 or 9, the main components of the palmoplantar stratum corneum. Patients have thick noninflamed plaques that do not extend onto the lateral aspects of the extremities. Histology shows *epidermolytic hyperkeratosis*.

Greither type. This is a classic transgredien. type with gradual progression from the palms of the hands and soles of the feet to the sides and backs of the hands and feet, as well as the ankles, knees, and elbows.

Mal de Meleda. Patients are most commonly from an isolated population on the Adriatic island Meleda; it is a transgrediens type of keratoderma, with neonatal erythema, then hyperkeratosis, hyperhidrosis, and nail dystrophies. There is sometimes perioral and perinasal disease. It is caused by mutations in *SLURP1*.

Pachyonychia congenita. This is a palmoplantar keratoderma, with thickened nails, and hyperkeratotic plaques on the knees and elbows. Patients with mutations in keratin 6 or 16 have oral leukoplakia, while those with keratin 17 mutations do not, as this keratin is not expressed on oral mucosa.

Striate type. These linear keratoses start in 1st or 2nd decade and are usually associated with mutations in desmoglein or desmocollin.

Howel–Evans syndrome. Early onset of palmoplantar keratoderma and leukokeratosis of oral mucosa is associated with almost 100% risk of esophageal carcinoma in adult life.

■ Therapy

Therapy is the same as for ichthyosis; mechanical debridement (sanding) is also used.

Disorders of Keratinization

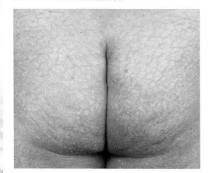

Ichthyosis vulgaris

Ichthyosis vulgaris with fissures and scaling

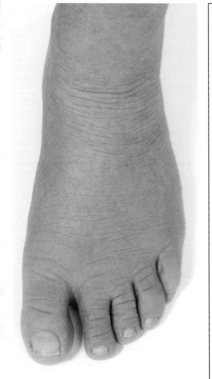

Congenital bullous ichthyosiform erythroderma

A. Ichthyoses

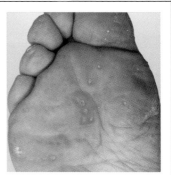

Vörner type

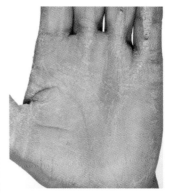

Striate type

B. Palmoplantar Keratodermas

C. Dyskeratotic-acantholytic Disorders

Two relatively common genodermatoses feature both abnormal keratinization and loss of adhesion between keratinocytes (acantholysis).

Note: Both involve mutations in calcium pumps, showing the importance of this ion for normal epidermal function.

■ Darier Disease

Mutation in the *ATP2A2* gene, coding for a calcium pump protein. It is inherited in autosomal dominant fashion with an incidence of 1:30 000.

Clinical Features. The presentation is pruritic brown follicular plugs that are most common in seborrheic areas, warty papules of the hands (*acrokeratosis verruciformis Hopf*), dystrophic nails, and cobblestoning of the oral mucosa. Patients are susceptible to secondary infections, such as widespread herpes simplex. It is also worsened by ultraviolet (UV) light.

Histopathology. Dyskeratosis with modest acantholysis; a hallmark is individual cell keratinization (*corps ronds* and *grains*).

Therapy. Topical or systemic retinoids, disinfectants or antibiotics for secondary infections.

■ Hailey–Hailey disease

Mutation in another calcium transport gene, *ATP2C1*. It is also inherited in an autosomal dominant way, with an incidence of 1:20 000–30 000.

Clinical Features. It favors intertriginous areas, showing maceration with fissures (*dusty road drying out after rain*), and it often waxes and wanes in severity. Patients have problems with secondary bacterial infections and disseminated herpes simplex.

Histopathology. Acantholysis (*dilapidated brick wall*) with little dyskeratosis. It was formerly called *familial chronic benign pemphigus* because of acantholysis but there is no relationship to autoimmune pemphigus.

Therapy. Topical or systemic retinoids, disinfectants, or antibiotics for secondary infections. Surgical or laser dermabrasion may induce long remissions.

■ Grover Disease

Acquired pruritic disease, generally of older men and affecting the trunk. Clinically, there are tiny extremely pruritic papules and dry skin. Histopathology shows acantholysis in a variety of patterns. It is generally self-limited and difficult to treat but may respond to UV or psoralen plus UVA (PUVA) irradiation and lubricants.

D. Follicular Keratoses

■ Keratosis Pilaris

Common disease affecting up to 50% of the population. Features rough follicular plugs, particularly over the triceps; they may have an erythematous rim; appearance compared to a kitchen grater. Lesions are not pruritic. It is often associated with atopic dermatitis, or ichthyosis vulgaris. It is treated with topical keratolytic agents.

Similar lesions may involve other areas:
• *ulerythema ophryogenes*—affects the lateral eyebrows and cheeks; heals with atrophic patulous follicles and loss of eyebrows

E. Porokeratoses

The unifying feature is histologic—a column of parakeratosis at the periphery of lesions, known as *cornoid lamella*.

■ Porokeratosis Mibelli

This is usually an acral annular lesion with a prominent rim and atrophic center. It is possibly viral in origin as it is more common in transplant patients. It is sometimes familial.

■ Superficial Disseminated Actinic Porokeratosis

Characterized by multiple annular lesions that are most common on sun-damaged skin of the forearms and legs. It tends to worsen in the summer.

F. Erythrokeratodermas

Erythrokeratoderma variablis is a rare disease caused by mutations in connexins, important proteins in cell communication. It features migratory erythematous patches and stable hyperkeratotic plaques. Therapy is retinoids and keratolytics.

Disorders of Keratinization

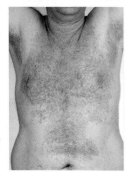

Darier disease

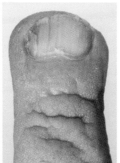

Nail streaks in Darier disease

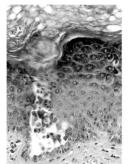

Histopathology: Darier disease with acantholysis and dyskeratosis

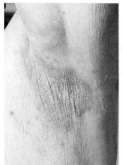

Hailey–Hailey disease

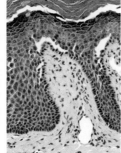

Histopathology: Hailey–Hailey disease with acantholysis

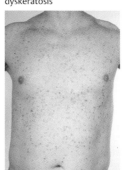

Grover disease

C. Dyskeratotic-acantholytic Disorders

Keratosis pilaris
D. Follicular Keratoses

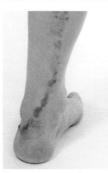

Porokeratosis of Mibelli
E. Porokeratoses

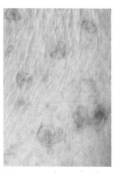

Disseminated superficial actinic porokeratosis

A. Mosaicism

Definition. A *mosaic* is an organism with genetically different populations of cells arising from a homogenous zygote. In contrast, a *chimera* results when two genetically different zygotes fuse.

Pathogenesis. While mosaicism can involve any organ, it is especially easy to see in the skin. When mutations occur in the 8–32-cell embryo, a somatic mosaic results. When such mutations involve genes that are important in skin differentiation, a mosaic pattern following Blaschko lines results. These lines reflect the distortions that occur as a round early embryo is converted into a human form. The best examples are epidermal nevi.

B. Epigenetic Mosaicism

Definition. All females are epigenetic mosaics because of the Lyon hypothesis and random inactivation of one X chromosome. Often, a mutation may be fatal in a male but, because of mosaicism, compatible with life in a female.

Clinical features. Several genodermatoses are characterized by marked female predominance, linear skin lesions, and other signs of mosaicism. None are amenable to therapy.

■ Incontinentia Pigmenti

This is caused by a mutation in the *NEMO* (nuclear factor κB essential modulator) gene which controls apoptosis. It presents at birth and goes through four stages:
- linear vesicles rich in eosinophils
- verrucous lesions, also subungual
- postinflammatory hyperpigmentation
- atrophic scars, especially on legs.

Patients may have dental, ocular, and central nervous system (CNS) problems.

■ Focal Dermal Hypoplasia (Goltz Syndrome)

This is caused by a mutation in the *PORCN* (porcupine homolog) signaling gene. Patients have linear atrophic steaks, herniation of fat, and periorificial papillomas, with associated oral, ocular, and skeletal changes. Histopathology shows almost complete absence of dermis.

C. Genomic Mosaicism

■ Lethal Mutations

Some mutations are so deleterious that they only exist in the mosaic state. Examples include:
- *pigmentary mosaicism of the Ito type*—hypopigmentation along Blaschko lines with a variety of systemic defects, depending on the nature of mosaic
- *McCune–Albright syndrome*—giant café-au-lait macules, with endocrine and skeletal defects. The activating mutation is in the *GNAS1* gene encoding the α-component of a G protein that regulates cAMP functions.

■ Nonlethal Mutations

Happle described two patterns of mosaicism that any autosomal dominant disorder can display:
- *type I*—a localized band of neurofibromas in an otherwise normal patient
- *type II*—a patient with full-blown neurofibromatosis but with a band that is even worse, with far more lesions.

D. Acquired Dermatoses in Blaschko Lines

Some acquired dermatoses are linear and appear to follow Blaschko lines. One explanation might be a silent mosaic, with a population of cells that are capable of reacting to a stimulus (infection, trauma) differently than the rest of the body.

■ Lichen Striatus

This usually occurs in children, with linear lichenoid papules usually running down the limb; it appears suddenly, and resolves spontaneously. It may be confused with epidermal nevus or linear lichen planus. Usually no therapy is needed; if pruritic, topical corticosteroids are used.

■ Others

Linear psoriasis, linear lichen planus, linear porokeratosis, and linear atrophoderma are all examples of possible mosaicism.

Mosaicism

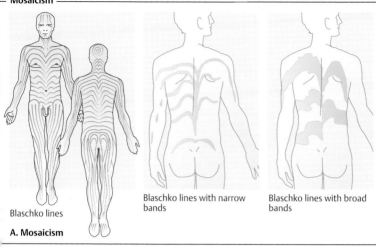

Blaschko lines

Blaschko lines with narrow bands

Blaschko lines with broad bands

A. Mosaicism

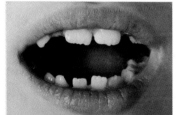

Dental anomalies
Focal dermal hypoplasia

B. Epigenetic Mosaicism

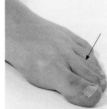

Syndactyly (arrow)

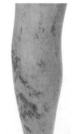

Linear atrophic streaks

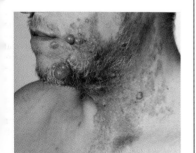

Segmental neurofibromatosis

C. Genomic Mosaicism

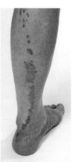

Linear porokeratosis

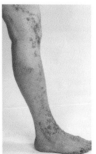

Linear lichen planus

D. Acquired Dermatoses in Blaschko Lines

A. Epidermal Nevi

Epidermal nevi are the prototype of cutaneous mosaicism. A mutation in early embryonic life leads to a localized area of abnormal skin. The umbrella term "epidermal nevus" has become accepted, although many skin components can be involved.

There are many different methods of classifying epidermal nevi:
- true epidermal nevi with only epidermal changes versus organoid nevi which also have dermal or adnexal involvement
- hard or verrucous nevi versus soft or papillomatous nevi
- histologic features—patterns such as epidermolytic hyperkeratosis, Darier disease, or Hailey–Hailey disease may be found.

B. Special Types

Some epidermal nevi can be identified clinically.

■ Nevus Sebaceus

Clinical features. These nevi usually occur on the scalp, with a bald patch at birth that becomes thicker and keratotic in puberty.
Histopathology. Microscopic features change with time. In childhood, there is papillomatous epidermal hyperplasia *without excess sebaceous glands.* Later it becomes organoid, with increased sebaceous and sweat glands, as well as epidermal proliferation. Adnexal tumors or, very rarely, basal cell carcinoma can develop within the lesion.
Therapy. Can be excised for cosmetic or functional reasons.

■ Becker Nevus

Clinical features. Initially, there is a slightly hyperpigmented area, typically on the shoulder; at puberty it becomes hairy; patients may have proliferation of the arrector pili muscles (smooth muscle nevus) with frequent goose bumps.
Histopathology. Basal layer hyperpigmentation, excess hairs, and often excess smooth muscles. Although frequently mistaken for a congenital hairy melanocytic nevus, no proliferation of melanocytes is found (Ch. 24.2)
Therapy. It is usually best not to treat. Lasers may help with epilation or depigmentation; but it is usually too large to excise.

■ Others

- *Nevus comedonicus*—many plugged follicular structures, resembling comedones of acne
- *Epidermolytic nevus*—verrucous nevus that is not clinically distinct but histopathology reveals epidermolytic hyperkeratosis. Patients with cutaneous and gonadal mosaicism can then have a child with congenital bullous ichthyosiform erythroderma (Ch. 20.1)
- *ILVEN (inflammatory linear verrucous epidermal nevus)*—verrucous nevus that appears permanently irritated or inflamed
- *Munro nevus*—a mutation in fibroblast growth factor leads to localized acne
- Eccrine, apocrine, and hair follicle nevi with overgrowth of respective adnexal structures

C. Epidermal Nevus Syndromes

Several epidermal nevi are associated with a variety of internal manifestations:
- *Becker nevus syndrome*—Becker nevus plus skeletal defects, ipsilateral breast hypoplasia
- *CHILD (congenital hemidysplasia with ichthyosiform nevus and limb defects) syndrome*—mutation in NAD(P)H steroid dehydrogenase-like protein, characterized by psoriasiform persistent patches that strikingly respect the midline and often favor the flexures (ptychotropism); there are also skeletal defects
- *Schimmelpenning syndrome*—nevus sebaceous, lid tumors, epilepsy
- *Proteus syndrome*—soft epidermal nevi in Blaschko lines, cerebriform connective-tissue nevi of the feet, macrodactyly.

D. Solitary Lesions

Occasionally, a banal papule or nodule will display the histologic features of epidermolytic hyperkeratosis, Darier disease, or Hailey–Hailey disease. One possible explanation is a late mutation involving only a single clone of cells. One distinct variant is *warty dyskeratoma*, which is typically a crusted papule on the head or neck of an adult, which has typical Darier-like changes confined to a single follicle or tiny cyst.

Epidermal Nevi

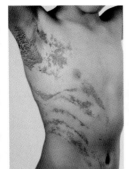

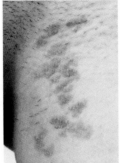

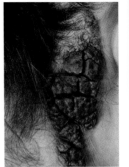

Epidermal nevus

Epidermal nevus

Verrucous epidermal nevus

A. Epidermal Nevi

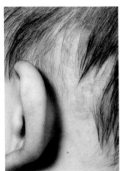

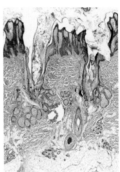

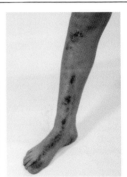

Nevus sebaceus

Histopathology: n. sebaceus w. papillomatosis + numerous sebaceous glands

ILVEN

B. Special Types

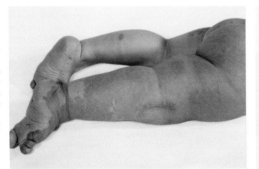

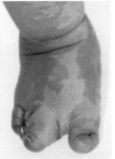

Proteus syndrome

C. Epidermal Nevus Syndromes

20 Genetic Diseases of the Epidermis

A. Seborrheic Keratosis

■ **Epidemiology**

This is the most common benign skin tumor; almost every elderly individual has several.

■ **Pathogenesis**

Some forms are associated with mutations in fibroblast growth factor (FGF) receptor 3. Sometimes it is clonal.

■ **Clinical Features**

Seborrheic keratoses are most common on the back, chest, and face. They start as well-circumscribed skin-colored or tan macules (erroneously known as senile or solar lentigo). They slowly become darker, thicker, and larger. Typically, they are described as resembling a "drop of dark wax" on the skin, as they are so superficial and delineated. The rough surface and plugs of keratin are diagnostically useful.
Clinical variants include:

- *irritated seborrheic keratosis*—tends to be smoother, erythematous, and sometimes pruritic; generally the result of rubbing from clothes
- *melanoacanthoma*—heavily pigmented seborrheic keratosis, often with dendritic melanocytes
- *stucco keratoses*—tiny white keratoses on the distal aspects of the legs, often with sun damage
- *eruptive seborrheic keratoses (Leser–Trélat syndrome)*—sudden eruption of many seborrheic keratoses is a rare paraneoplastic marker (Ch. 27.9)
- *dermatosis papulosa nigra*—tiny pigmented seborrheic keratoses seen on the cheeks of patients with colored skin.

■ **Histopathology**

Exophytic proliferation of basaloid tumor cells with a papillomatous or church-spire pattern, acanthosis, sometimes there is a reticulate pattern at the base, horn pseudocysts (keratin-filled invaginations, useful in dermatoscopy to identify seborrheic keratoses), and squamous eddies (retention eccrine ducts). Sometimes they are heavily pigmented.

■ **Differential Diagnosis**

There is no differential diagnosis for most lesions. Patients often suspect a melanocytic nevus or even melanoma. Dermatoscopy can identify the horn pseudocysts and confirm diagnosis if the lesion is irritated or otherwise hard to diagnose.

■ **Therapy**

No therapy is needed, but patients usually desire removal for cosmetic reasons. The simplest approach is curettage.

B. Acanthosis Nigricans

Acanthosis nigricans features velvety patches on the nape, as well as in the axillae and groin. Even though acanthosis nigricans and seborrheic keratosis share no clinical similarities, they are identical histologically. Acanthosis nigricans appears to be caused by excessive activity of insulin-like growth factor (IGF), explaining its association with insulin resistance and obesity, both in a variety of syndromes and in sporadic cases. In adults who are usually thin, it may be a paraneoplastic marker (Ch. 27.9).

C. Confluent and Reticulated Papillomatosis (Gougerot–Carteaud Disease)

This is a confusing disease, long considered a genetic disorder but apparently often triggered by *Malassezia* spp. Patients have hundreds of tiny <5 mm keratotic papules which are confluent and form a reticular (netlike) pattern on the trunk, below the breast, presternally, and on the nape. It is almost asymptomatic but unattractive. Under the microscope, it is identical to small seborrheic keratoses.

■ **Therapy**

Macrolides or tetracyclines for 4–8 weeks often bring marked improvement or clearing: if *Malassezia* spp. are identified, topical or systemic antifungal agents can be tried.

D. Clear Cell Acanthoma

This is an uncommon tumor that is almost never clinically recognized but has a striking microscopic picture. It presents as a slowly growing nodule usually on the shin of an older adult, generally with collarette scale and crust. Histology shows a psoriasiform pattern but the keratinocytes are swollen, clear, and on special staining rich in glycogen. The transition from clear cells to adjacent normal keratinocytes is extremely sharp. Treated by excision.

Benign Epidermal Tumors

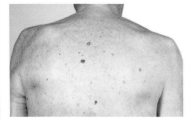

Multiple seborrheic keratoses

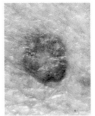

Different examples of seborrheic keratosis

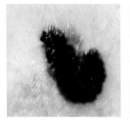

Melanoacanthoma

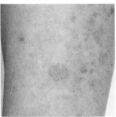

Flat seborrheic keratoses

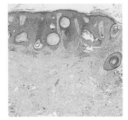

Histopathology: acanthosis with horn pseudocysts

A. Seborrheic Keratosis

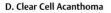

B. Acanthosis Nigricans

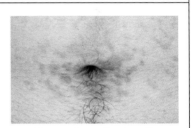

C. Confluent and Reticulated Papillomatosis (Gougerot–Carteaud Disease)

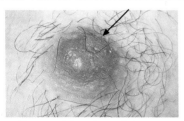

Red-brown nodule on the nipple (arrow)

D. Clear Cell Acanthoma

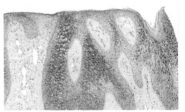

Histopathology: glycogen in the epidermis with periodic acid–Schiff stain

A. Cysts

Cysts are closed spaces surrounded by an epithelium and generally containing fluid or cellular secretions. Pseudocysts are clinically similar but do not have a true epithelial cover.

Epidermoid cyst. This is the most common cyst and one of the most common skin findings. It is usually a dome-shaped nodule with a central pore, being the hair follicle out of which the cyst develops. It may become inflamed from trauma or infection; if ruptured, it is generally painful. The cyst can usually be easily extracted through a small incision; if ruptured and scarred, it must be excised.

Trichilemmal cyst. This typically occurs on the scalp, and is often multiple. Larger cysts may have overlying pressure alopecia. It shells out like marble. Proliferating trichilemmal cyst is a rare variety that histologically looks like a squamous cell carcinoma (SCC) developing within the cyst.

Steatocystoma. These are yellow soft multiple broad-based cysts, usually on chest. The cyst wall contains sebaceous glands; the lumen has sebum and hairs. When multiple hairs are present, it is called a *vellus hair cyst*. Troublesome lesions can be excised, but the sternal area tends to scar so the results are not always pleasing. There is a temporary response to systemic retinoids.

Hidrocystoma. This is a cystic eccrine or apocrine tumor, typically located in the periorbital region. It is sometimes pigmented (*hidrocystome noir*) because eccrine sweat can contain pigment. Clinically, it is hard to separate from cystic basal cell carcinoma, which is common in the same location. Excision is curative.

Digital mucous cyst. This is a compressible 5–10 mm cyst on the back of a digit overlying the distal interphalangeal joint and approaching the nail fold. It is caused by outpouching of the synovium from a joint, or leakage of synovial fluid, which exudes as a tenacious gel when the pseudocyst is incised. The cyst usually recurs after drainage, so excision is preferred.

B. Adnexal Tumors

This is a large family of tumors with features of eccrine, apocrine, sebaceous, or hair follicle differentiation. Most present as red-brown nodules with few distinctive clinical features. All can be treated by excision.

Note: Multiple adnexal tumors usually suggest a syndrome with autosomal dominant inheritance.

Follicular tumors. The most common are epidermoid and trichilemmal cysts. Others include:

- *pilomatricoma*—common cystic childhood tumor, usually on the scalp or cheek, may drain chalky material; multiple tumors are a marker for myotonic dystrophy
- *trichoblastoma*—tumor of rudimentary hair follicles and papillae.

Eccrine tumors

- *poroma*—usually occurs on the scalp or soles of the feet; vascular and often missed as hemangiomas. Typically painful. Proliferation of sweat ducts. If purely epidermal, it is called *hidroacanthoma simplex*, if predominantly dermal, a *dermal duct tumor*.

Apocrine tumors

- *cylindroma*—usually on the scalp and multiple, described as "turban tumors." Often occur with trichoepitheliomas in Brooke–Spiegler syndrome.
- *hidradenoma papilliferum*—firm nodule in the anogenital region; proliferation of glandular and fibrous stroma with plasma cells.
- *mixed tumor of skin*—firm nodule with eccrine or apocrine ducts and a mesenchymal component that often resembles cartilage.
- *spiradenoma*—tender blue-red dermal nodule containing both secretory (clear) and dense eccrine cells.
- *syringoma*—multiple tiny skin-colored papules, usually periorbital; sometimes disseminated. Histology shows twisted eccrine ducts that have been compared with tadpoles.
- *syringocystadenoma papilliferum*—brown crusted tumor, often on the scalp and in association with nevus sebaceus.

Sebaceous tumors

- *sebaceous hyperplasia*—common yellow facial nodules consisting of a central pore and tiny surrounding sebaceous glands.
- *sebaceoma*—proliferation of basaloid cells with foci of sebaceous differentiation.

Note: When a patient has multiple or difficult-to-classify sebaceous tumors, always think of Muir–Torre syndrome and the risk of multiple underlying malignancies (Ch. 30.3).

Cysts and Adnexal Tumors

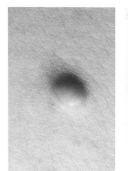

Epidermoid cyst

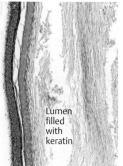

Histopathology: epidermoid cyst wall resembling normal epidermis

Lumen filled with keratin

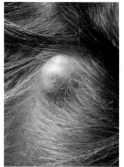

Trichilemmal cyst

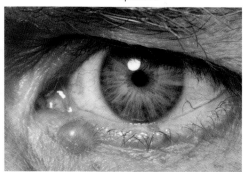

Hidrocystoma

A. Cysts

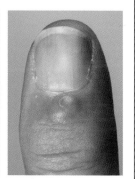

Digital mucous cyst

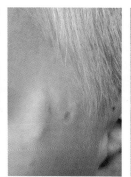

Pilomatricoma

B. Adnexal Tumors

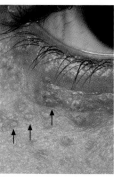

Syringomas (arrows)

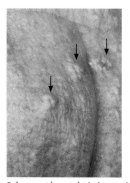

Sebaceous hyperplasia (arrows)

A. Malignant Adnexal Tumors

The only common malignant adnexal tumor is basal cell carcinoma (Ch.21.4), which is a trichoblastic carcinoma. The other adnexal tumors are sometimes malignant versions of benign tumors or entities without a benign parallel. All behave like a SCC, with local destructive growth and occasional lymphatic spread, but only rarely hematogenous dissemination. Therapy consists of complete excision with precise control of the margins. Micrographic surgery is often ideal. Chemotherapy is generally ineffective for widespread disease.

■ Porocarcinoma

This is the second most common adnexal tumor; it usually arises on the foot or shin of an elderly patient. There is histological overlap with poroma, but invasive growth, numerous mitoses and dedifferentiation, so it resembles a SCC. Recurrences and regional lymphatic spread with lymphedema are not uncommon; metastatic disease is treated with the same protocols as metastatic SCC.

■ Pilomatrical Carcinoma

This is a scalp tumor in the elderly, which is usually ulcerated; it sometimes appears to develop out of pilomatricoma.

■ Microcystic Adnexal Carcinoma

Firm nodule, usually in the mid-face. Histologic diagnosis is difficult; the superficial component may resemble syringoma or sclerosing basal cell carcinoma, while the deep (and often not sampled) component shows perineural invasive growth. Atypia and mitoses are uncommon. It is often much larger than clinically suggested and is best treated with micrographic surgery.

> **Caution:** When a deep mid-facial nodule is diagnosed histologically as syringoma or other adnexal tumor, always be suspicious and review the case with a dermatopathologist.

■ Papillary Adenocarcinoma

A destructive digital tumor with metastatic potential.

■ Sebaceous carcinoma

About 50% are on the eyelid and are often mistaken for chalazion, delaying correct therapy. Histologically, there is usually intraepidermal spread and thus it is misinterpreted as melanoma or Paget disease. Ocular lesions have 30% recurrence or metastasis rate; at other body sites, there is a better prognosis, presumably because lesions are more easily excised.

B. Paget Disease

Epidemiology. 0.5%–1% of breast carcinomas.
Pathogenesis. Spread of intraductal carcinoma cells into the skin.
Clinical features. Sharply bordered, often eroded scaly patch on one nipple; understandably misinterpreted as dermatitis.
Histopathology. Intraepidermal spread of large clear cells (Paget cells), which have no desmosomal contact to keratinocytes. The cells are periodic acid–Schiff (PAS) positive and express carcinoembryonic antigen (CEA), epithelial membrane antigen (EMA), and cytokeratins CK7 and CK19.
Differential diagnosis. Nipple dermatitis is usually bilateral. Nipple adenoma is a benign breast tumor which typically has draining crusted surface—the distinction is microscopic. Histologically, Bowen disease and melanoma must be excluded.
Therapy. Treatment of breast carcinoma with generous excision of involved skin.

C. Extramammary Paget Disease

Pathogenesis. Intraepidermal spread of an eccrine or apocrine duct carcinoma or, rarely, of an underlying adenocarcinoma (rectum, bladder, prostate, cervix).
Clinical features. Erythematous eroded scaly patch in the axillae or anogenital region.
Histopathology. Identical to Paget disease perhaps with slightly different markers, depending on the source.
Differential diagnosis. Dermatitis, tinea, and inverse psoriasis. It is often ignored or mistreated for years.
Therapy. Search for and treat the underlying tumor. If no tumor is found, as is usually the case, then generous local excision should be carried out, ideally with micrographic surgery. In addition, sonography should be used to evaluate the lymph nodes.

— Malignant Adnexal Tumors and Paget Disease —

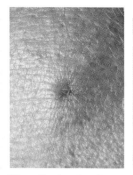
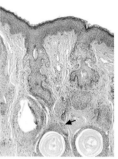
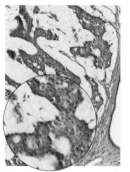

Microcytic adnexal carcinoma

A. Malignant Adnexal Tumors

Histopathology: microcystic adnexal carcinoma with small cysts extending to the depths of the tumor (arrow)

Histopathology: mucinous carcinoma with islands of malignant cells in lakes of mucin

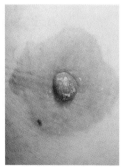
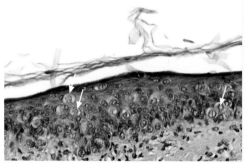

Erosive patch on the nipple

B. Paget Disease

Histopathology: intraepidermal spread of large pale malignant cells (arrows)

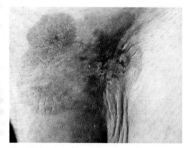
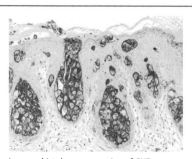

Sharply bordered erythematous plaques in inguinal fold

C. Extramammary Paget Disease

Immunohistology: expression of CK7

21 Tumors of the Epidermis

A. Basal Cell Carcinoma

■ Definition

Basal cell carcinoma (BCC) is the most common malignant tumor and by far the most common skin cancer. It grows slowly and may eventually become locally destructive, but almost never metastasizes. For this reason, some regard it as semi-malignant and use designations like basal cell epithelioma.

■ Epidemiology

BCC is often ultraviolet (UV) induced; individuals with skin types I and II are more affected. The age peak is 60–80 years. The incidence is increasing; in Northern Europe and USA, it is 200:100 000; in Australia, it is 10-fold higher. BCC is also roughly 10 times more common than SCC.

If BCC appears in childhood or young adult life, it suggests the presence of nevoid basal cell carcinoma syndrome (NBCCS).

■ Pathogenesis

It differentiates in the direction of hair follicle precursor cells (trichoblastic carcinoma). The key factor appears to be altered regulation of the sonic hedgehog pathway. The main etiologic factors are:

- *genetic factors*—skin type, *Patched (PTCH)* mutations in NBCCS; xeroderma pigmentosum
- Patched is a membrane-bound protein that blocks the stimulation of "smoothened by hedgehog" (SMOH). This in turn regulates Gli, TCF-β, and Bcl-2, important regulators of cell growth. Alterations in Patched lead to BCC by allowing unregulated cell growth.
- *UV irradiation*—UVB and UVA are both important cofactors
- *immunosuppression*—impaired T-cell response as in patients with iatrogenic immunosuppression following solid organ transplantation; SCC is more favored than BCC. Some immunosuppressive agents may also affect cell cycle control.
- *ionizing radiation*—after radiation therapy, the latency period for BCC is 10–20 years
- *carcinogens*—arsenic salts cause BCC with a considerable latent period. They were formerly used for psoriasis and asthma therapy, and are still present in ground water—especially in Bangladesh, where millions of people have chronic arsenic poisoning
- *chronic wounds and scars*—a risk factor, but not as great as for SCC.

■ Clinical Features

Some 80% of BCCs are on the face, usually nose, forehead, temples, or cheeks. On the trunk, superficial BCCs are most common. The backs of the hands are never affected, despite considerable sun exposure. Lesions on the shins tend to present as ulcers. BCCs grow slowly, may ulcerate, then seem to heal, and first come to clinical attention again months later. The main problem is relentless local infiltration, potentially involving vital structures such as the eye. There are three main clinical types (nodular, sclerosing, and superficial) and many different variants:

Nodular or solid BCC. This is the most common variant, a firm irregular nodule with tel angiectases and a border resembling a bead of pearls. It often presents with central ulceration or crust. Subtypes include:

- *cystic BCC*—translucent glassy pink tumor, sometimes fluctuant, rarely identified correctly clinically
- *pigmented BCC*—similar to nodular but brown to gray-black in color; more common in individuals with skin types IV–VI; rare in those with blue eyes.

Sclerosing (sclerodermiform or morpheaform) BCC. This presents as indurated scar, often on the face, such as in the nasal fold or near the ear. Clues such as telangiectases or a pearly border are often missing. All hair follicle tumors have a complex interplay between epithelium and stroma; here the stroma completely dominates. It is difficult to diagnose and to treat, as the tumor margins are very indistinct (iceberg phenomenon). It is best treated with micrographic surgery.

Superficial BCC. Also known as multicentric BCC, this variant mimics a patch of dermatitis. Typically, there are multiple flat red-brown macules and patches on the trunk, often with scale and a hint of pearly border. This is the most common type of BCC in arsenic toxicity and immunosuppression.

Fibroepithelioma (Pinkus tumor). This is a fleshy nodule usually on the flank, with unique histological appearance; lacy interconnecting basaloid tumor strands are dominated by mesenchymal proliferation.

Aggressive variants

- *ulcerated BCC*—sometimes BCCs reach considerable size before they are brought to medical attention, as they are usually painless and simply ignored. As they develop over years, central ulceration with hemorrhage and crusting occurs. The pearly border is often the only clue to the nature of the ulcer .

Basal Cell Carcinoma

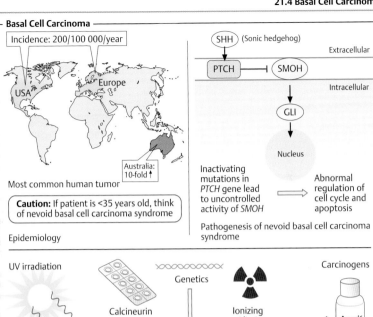

Incidence: 200/100 000/year

USA Europe

Australia: 10-fold ↑

Most common human tumor

Caution: If patient is <35 years old, think of nevoid basal cell carcinoma syndrome

Epidemiology

SHH (Sonic hedgehog)

Extracellular

PTCH ⊣ SMOH

Intracellular

GLI

Nucleus

Inactivating mutations in *PTCH* gene lead to uncontrolled activity of *SMOH*

⟹

Abnormal regulation of cell cycle and apoptosis

Pathogenesis of nevoid basal cell carcinoma syndrome

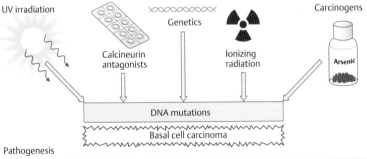

UV irradiation

Genetics

Calcineurin antagonists

Ionizing radiation

Carcinogens

Arsenic

DNA mutations

Basal cell carcinoma

Pathogenesis

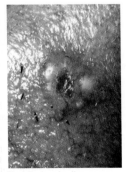

Nodular basal cell carcinoma

Sclerosing basal cell carcinoma

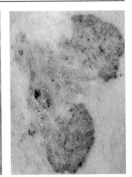

Superficial basal cell carcinoma

Clinical features

A. Basal Cell Carcinoma

21 Tumors of the Epidermis

- An old name for this type of BCC was *ulcus rodens* (rodent ulcer), as larger ignored lesions did often look as if they could have been caused by a gnawing mammal. Other BCCs become extremely aggressive, growing deeply and invading the skull, brain, or other structures; they are designated *ulcus terebrans*

■ Histopathology

The number of patterns is just as great as the clinical variants. The classic lesion is a basaloid tumor arising from the epidermis or hair follicle and featuring peripheral palisading (outer row of uniformly lined up basaloid cells) and clefting (separation between tumor and stroma). Superficial BCCs bud from the basal layer of the epidermis and resemble distorted hair germs. The stroma tends to dominate in the sclerosing and fibroepithelioma types. Pigmented BCCs have dendritic melanocytes and increased melanin.

■ Differential Diagnosis

The choices vary with the subtypes—nodular BCCs are confused with adnexal tumors and fibromas; superficial BCCs with Bowen disease, Paget disease, and dermatitis; sclerosing BCCs with a scar; and pigmented BCCs with melanoma.

■ Course

Recurrence rates depend on treatment; with micrographic surgery <1%; with routine surgery or radiation, 5%. Metastasis is very rare (0.003%) and occurs only with large often neglected tumors, or from secondary SCC.

■ Therapy

The decision on how to treat is based on the type of tumor, site, previous treatment, and age and health of the patient. Options include:
- *excision*—micrographic surgery with cosmetic repair (Ch. 22.3) is the quickest therapy and offers maximum margin control, fewest recurrences, and the best cosmetic results. It is the therapy of choice for facial BCC (especially around the nose, eyes, and ears), sclerosing BCC, and recurrences. Even ulcerated or deeply invasive tumors can usually be cured, so that there is no reason not to treat even advanced tumors in elderly patients with multiple comorbidities. Standard excision is also acceptable, but carries a higher recurrence rate because of the ten-

dency of BCC to have such an irregular border that cannot be clinically visualized. It should be reserved primarily for primary nodular tumors not on the face.
- *radiation therapy*—an option for older patients (total of 50–70 Gy, usually in 15–20 sessions
- *curettage*—usually combined with electrocautery. Unacceptable recurrences and poor cosmetic results; today it is reserved for superficial BCC. No histological control possible
- *laser ablation*—same disadvantages as curettage
- *cryotherapy*—superficial tumors can be frozen without monitoring; no histological control is possible; larger tumors in difficult sites (such as around eyes) are sometimes treated by deep cryotherapy with temperature probes
- *immunotherapy*—imiquimod is approved for treating superficial BCC. It stimulates toll-like receptor 7 and the resultant inflammatory response directs cytokines against the tumor cells. Not for problem areas (midface, around the eyes or ears), for sclerosing BCC, or for recurrences
- *photodynamic therapy*—useful for multiple superficial BCC on the trunk.

> **Caution:** Both imiquimod and photodynamic therapy, as well as occasional radiation therapy, may produce superficial clearing but leave residual tumor at the depths, leading to deep, destructive hidden recurrences.

> **Note:** The risk for a second unrelated BCC in a patient is around 30%; thus every patient with a BCC should be followed lifelong for new BCC.

B. Nevoid Basal Cell Carcinoma Syndrome (Gorlin syndrome)

Autosomal-dominant disorder with mutations in *PTCH* gene. Patients usually present in childhood with multiple, usually superficial, BCC, sometimes resembling nevi or skin tags (Ch. 30.3). The patients also have palmar pits, acral epidermoid cysts, jaw cysts (odontogenic keratocysts), frontal bossing, calcification of the falx cerebri, and skeletal defects. They are also at risk for medulloblastoma and benign ovarian fibromas. Patients can be treated with all the modalities mentioned above except radiation therapy, as their skin is radiation sensitive and they rapidly develop multiple new BCC in irradiated fields.

Basal Cell Carcinoma

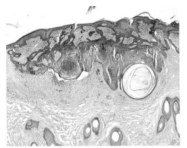

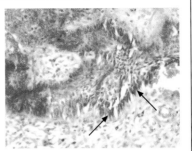

Overview showing basaloid tumor islands
Histopathology

Higher view showing peripheral palisading (arrows)

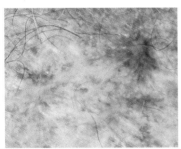

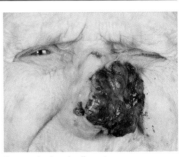

Recurrent basal cell carcinoma
Course

Destructive basal cell carcinoma

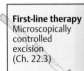
First-line therapy
Microscopically controlled excision (Ch. 22.3)

Nodular/sclerosing

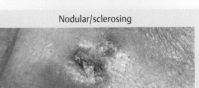

If inoperable; ionizing radiation 50–70 Gy

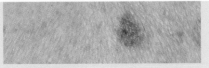

Superficial basal cell carcinoma

Curettage, shave excision, excision

Cryotherapy

Topical immuno-therapy

Photo-dynamic therapy   PDT

Therapy

A. Basal Cell Carcinoma

SCC arises from the epidermis or mucosal epithelium, often has an in situ phase, and then enters the dermis or lamina propria, becoming an invasive tumor with risk of metastasis.

A. Carcinomata In Situ

■ Actinic Keratosis

Pathogenesis. Actinic keratosis (AK) is an extremely common tumor, especially in skin types I and II; it is a SCC in situ induced by chronic exposure to UV irradiation.

Clinical features. AK occurs in the areas of heaviest sun exposure—the forehead, bald scalp, cheeks, nose, tips of the ears, and lower lip, as well as the backs of the hands and forearms. Early lesions are more likely to be felt than seen; they are tiny skin-colored or pale pink rough circumscribed macules and papules, which slowly become thicker and larger. When they are irritated or markedly hypertrophic, it is impossible clinically to distinguish them from a SCC. Some patients have a "field cancerization" effect with hundreds of AKs; it is most common on a bald scalp in elderly, immunosuppressed patients.

The natural history of AK is very variable ranging from self-healing to rare (0.5–3.0%) progression to SCC.

Therapy. Most lesions are best treated with superficial cryotherapy, which is quick, cheap, and effective. If there are many lesions, topical therapy is an option. Both 5-fluorouracil and imiquimod induce enough inflammation to destroy lesions; diclofenac in hyaluronic acid seems to promote regression of early AK.

Curettage, shave excision, or photodynamic therapy are other possibilities. Excision is reserved for thicker AKs when SCC cannot be clinically excluded. Since the time to develop an AK is 10–20 years, for almost all patients subsequent light protection will, over years, reduce the burden of new lesions.

■ Bowen Disease

This is a SCC in situ but not on sun-exposed skin; in the past, it was frequently caused by arsenic exposure; sometimes human papillomavirus (HPV) is identified in the tumor. An oval red-brown patch or plaque with variable scale can be confused with a patch of dermatitis or psoriasis.

> **Caution:** Always biopsy therapy-resistant patches of dermatitis or psoriasis to exclude Bowen disease, superficial BCC or lymphoma.

Histology reveals acanthosis with bulbous rete ridges, individual cell keratinization and numerous mitoses, When there is dermal invasion, it is Bowen carcinoma, identical to any other SCC. Therapy is excision.

■ Erythroplasia of Queyrat

Erythroplasia of Queyrat is SCC in situ on the transitional epithelium of the penis, female genitalia, or mouth. It presents as a harmless looking red velvety patch with a sharp border. Histology is SCC in situ. In the oral cavity, erythroplasia is more worrisome than leukoplakia. Therapy is excision.

■ Arsenical Keratoses

Exposure to inorganic arsenic (iatrogenic, industrial exposure, contained ground water) causes a variety of changes. The most dramatic is hypo- and hyperpigmentation, described as "rain drops on a dusty road." In addition, SCC in situ develops in the form of arsenical keratoses on the palms and soles, as well as more typical Bowen disease elsewhere. Superficial BCCs also occur. Similar lesions may develop with chronic exposure to pitch and tar, as well as ionizing radiation. Standard therapy suffices.

■ Special Variants

Cutaneous horn (cornu cutaneum). This clinical diagnosis describes a protuberant mass of compacted keratin (horn). The clue is at the base of the horn, where on histological examination one may find a verruca, seborrheic keratosis, or SCC (in situ or invasive). The lesion should be excised.

Leukoplakia. Leukoplakia is the generic name for white plaques on mucosa. Causes include:
- *candidiasis* which can be scraped off
- *trauma* (prosthesis, chewing) with reactive hyperplasia (mucosal callus)
- *genetic disorders* such as pachyonychia congenita, white sponge nevus
- *carcinoma in situ*—on the lower lip, SCC in situ is known as actinic cheilitis. It is usually scaly or crusted but sometimes white. In the mouth, danger areas are the side of the tongue and the gutter between the labial and gingival mucosa. Oral lichen planus is also a precancerous condition. Oral speckled leukoplakia (leukoplakia plus erythroplasia) is almost always SCC in situ. Risk factors include tobacco, heat, and HPV.

Therapy: address the suspected cause; if there is no response, biopsy, and excise if SCC in situ

Squamous Cell Carcinoma and Metastases

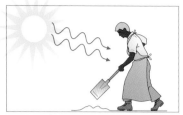

UV exposed areas

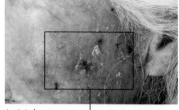

Actinic keratoses

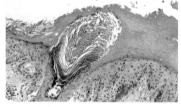

Histopathology: actinic keratosis with pink and blue hyperkeratosis with epidermal atypia

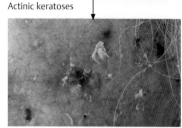

Actinic keratoses: close-up view

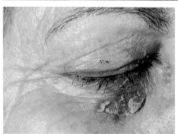

Bowen disease

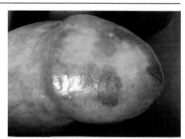

Erythroplasia of Queyrat

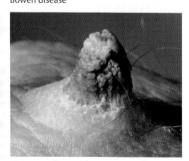

Cutaneous horn with squamous cell carcinoma at base

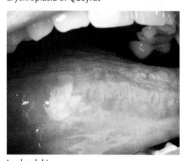

Leukoplakia

A. Carcinomata In Situ

B. Squamous Cell Carcinoma

■ Definition

SCC is the second most common malignant skin tumor (most common in black individuals and organ transplant patients) and most common mucosal malignancy. It is a destructive growth with a risk of lymphatic and hematogenous spread for tumors thicker than 5 mm.

■ Epidemiology

SCC affects the same group as AK. The incidence in Germany is 30:100 000, but much higher in Australia and Southwestern USA. 30-fold increased in immunosuppressed patients.

■ Pathogenesis

SCC arises from AKs or other SCC in situ. Risk factors include:
- *UV irradiation*—UVB is the most carcinogenic part of the spectrum
- *infection*—HPV is increasingly being implicated (usually HPV 16 and 18, but also others)
- *immunosuppression*—SCC is a major problem following solid organ transplantation through the combination of HPV, UV damage and calcineurin inhibitors; it also occurs in hematologic malignancies
- *genetic factors*—xeroderma pigmentosum and disorders with nucleic acid repair defects predispose to SCC
- *carcinogens*—arsenic, tobacco, tar soot
- *chronic inflammation and scars*—classic sites were draining tuberculosis or osteomyelitis sinuses; today burn scars, radiation dermatitis (>10 Gy; >10 years latency), acne inversa, and chronic leg ulcers are the biggest culprits. Chronic dermal inflammation is also a factor; both lichen planus (on oral mucosa) and lichen sclerosus et atrophicus (on genital mucosa) are rarely, but potentially, premalignant.

■ Clinical Features

SCC develops out of actinic keratoses, so they have the same distribution—sun-exposed skin of the face, forearms, and backs of the hands. Lesions that are larger, thicker, crusted, ulcerated, or resistant to therapy may be SCC. The risk of metastasis from a SCC arising from an AK is low. There are variants where the risk of metastasis is higher:
- *lower lip*—most common site on face; arises from actinic cheilitis or tobacco
- *border and tip of the tongue*—mostly in pipe smokers; high risk of metastases
- *penis*—usually on the glans; main factors are HPV infection and smegma, as SCC is much less common in circumcised men
- *vulva*—often related to HPV16 and 18; rarely associated with lichen sclerosus et atrophicus or even lichen planus.

■ Histopathology

Irregular pattern of epidermal maturation, individual cell keratinization, mitoses, and strands of atypical epithelium extend into the dermis. Well-differentiated tumors have swirls of keratinization (squamous eddies). The most important prognostic parameters are tumor depth and fibrotic stromal reaction (desmoplastic SCC).

■ Differential Diagnosis

Actinic keratosis, keratoacanthoma, Bowen disease, BCC, verruca, amelanotic melanoma, malignant adnexal tumors.

■ Course

The outlook depends primarily on tumor thickness. Tumors <2 mm in depth never metastasize; those of 2–6 mm, around 4% metastasize; and of those >6 mm, 20% metastasize. Tongue, penis, and vulvar carcinomas have relatively worse prognosis, as do sclerosing SCCs.

■ Therapy

Excision. Excision with adequate safety margins is the standard. In high-risk locations such as the face (eyes, ears, nose), and for sclerosing tumors, micrographic surgery is the best approach. A sentinel lymph node biopsy can be considered for patients with high-risk tumor who are good operative candidates.
Radiation therapy. Good option for inoperable SCC, although an operation is usually less demanding. Usually 50–70 Gy are given in 15–2 dosages. Other indications include consolidation therapy after an incomplete excision, recurrence, and metastases.
Systemic therapy. Polychemotherapy for metastatic SCC usually includes 5-fluorouracil, platins, and epidermal growth factor (EGF) receptor antagonists. While relatively high remission rates can be achieved, cure rates are very low.

— Squamous Cell Carcinoma and Metastases —

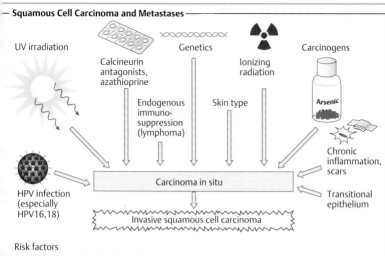

Risk factors

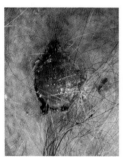

Squamous cell carcinoma

Extensive squamous cell carcinoma with metastases

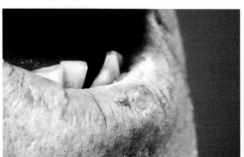

Squamous cell carcinoma of the lower lip

B. Squamous Cell Carcinoma

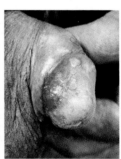

Squamous cell carcinoma of the penis

> **Note:** All patients with SCC >5mm or immunosuppression should be followed closely for three years for cutaneous and lymph node recurrence. They are also at risk for a second tumor. AKs should be treated aggressively. Most patients benefit from consequent light protection.

C. Variants of Squamous Cell Carcinoma

■ Keratoacanthoma

A rapidly growing skin-colored or pink nodule with a central keratin plug that arises from the hair follicle. It often regresses spontaneously within 6 months. About 2% progress and are then called SCC. Multiple keratoacanthomas suggest Muir–Torre syndrome with associated malignancies (Ch. 30.3). Histology overlaps with SCC; a key factor is the overall symmetrical pattern of keratoacanthoma. Treatment is excision.

■ Verrucous Carcinoma

A group of highly differentiated SCCs associated with HPV in most cases. They are clinically verrucous, and have histology with little atypia, and low risk of metastasis. All are treated by excision. Members of the group include:

- *oral florid papillomatosis (Ackerman tumor)*—oral verrucous tumor, presents as leukoplakia; HPV 6 and 11 and tobacco are cofactors
- *papillomatosis cutis carcinoides*—typically on the shins of elderly patients; perhaps associated with chronic venous insufficiency
- *Buschke–Löwenstein tumor (condyloma giganteum)*—a giant papillomatous genital tumor associated with HPV 6 and 11
- *epithelioma cuniculatum*—exophytic tumor on the sole; also HPV-related.

D. Skin Metastases

■ Pathogenesis

Tumors that commonly metastasize to the skin can be recalled with the acronym BLOCK (breast, lung, ovary, colon, kidney). Breast carcinoma accounts for 70% of all cutaneous metastases in women, followed by the lungs, kidney, and ovaries. In men, lung carcinoma is 25%, followed by colorectal and renal cancers.
- Cutaneous metastases can be the first sign of a malignancy or of its recurrence.

- Skin metastases mean stage IV disease and a poor prognosis.
- Carcinomas are much more likely to metastasize than sarcomas.
- Tumors tend to spread to nearby structures: breast → thoracic wall, lungs → thoracic wall, renal → lower back, colon → umbilicus.
- In 5% of patients presenting with a cutaneous metastasis, no primary is found.

> **Note:** Melanoma is responsible for 20%–30% of all cutaneous metastases.

■ Clinical Features

Suddenly appearing red-brown papules and nodules, usually multiple but occasionally solitary, are typical. Sometimes there are clues to the possible underlying tumor, although a final answer depends on the pathology of the primary and metastatic lesions.

- *Carcinoma en cuirasse* is metastatic breast carcinoma which is both erythematous, resembling erysipelas, and sclerotic. Metastases that block lymphatic drainage create obstruction and a *peau d'orange* effect. Breast carcinoma also commonly goes to the eyelids and scalp. Metastases can appear 10–15 years after the primary tumor.
- Renal cell carcinoma metastases are often very vascular and mistaken for a hemangioma; this is common on the scalp.
- Gastric and ovarian carcinomas may metastasize to the umbilicus (*Sister Mary Joseph nodule*).

■ Histopathology

Without a history and index of suspicion, mistakes are easy. Adenocarcinomas can be called sweat gland tumors, small cell lung tumor mistaken for Merkel cell carcinoma, epidermotropic metastatic melanomas called primary tumors, or sclerotic metastases interpreted as scars. Immunochemical stains are usually needed to confirm the diagnosis.

■ Therapy

Chemotherapy is based on the stage and other problems; individual lesions can be excised or irradiated.

21 Tumors of the Epidermis

Squamous Cell Carcinoma and Metastases

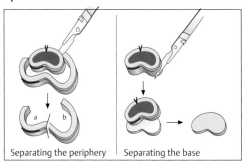
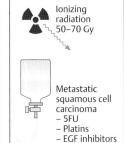

Separating the periphery | Separating the base

Ionizing radiation 50–70 Gy

Metastatic squamous cell carcinoma
– 5FU
– Platins
– EGF inhibitors

Therapy: microscopically controlled excision

B. Squamous Cell Carcinoma

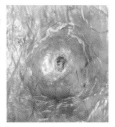
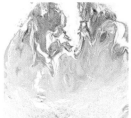
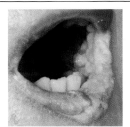

Keratoacanthoma | Histopathology: cup-shaped hyperkeratotic tumor | Verrucous carcinoma: oral florid papillomatosis

C. Variants of Squamous Cell Carcinoma

Common sources of skin metastases

 B Breast Breast carcinoma

 L Lung Lung carcinoma

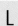 O Ovary Ovarian carcinoma

 C Colon Colon carcinoma

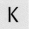 K Kidney Renal carcinoma (metastases often look like hemangiomas)

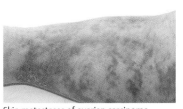
Skin metastases of ovarian carcinoma

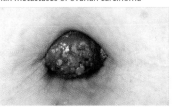
Sister Mary Joseph nodule

D. Skin Metastases

A. Benign Tumors of Fat

■ Lipoma

This is the most common human tumor and is occasionally multiple. It does not resolve with weight loss. Characterized as a discrete subcutaneous mass with pebbly surface, there are many clinical variants:

- *angiolipoma*—often tender because of vasospasms or thrombi in small vessels
- *spindle-cell lipoma*—usually on the nape of the neck in adults
- *subfascial lipoma*—forehead lesion.

All can be easily excised if they are functionally or cosmetically disturbing or painful. There is no malignant potential.

■ Nevus Lipomatosus

This is characterized by multiple grouped soft compressible papules and nodules, usually on the buttocks in girls; it results from herniations of fat through thinned dermis. They can be excised but are sometimes quite large, leading to marked scarring.

■ Benign Symmetrical Lipomatoses

This is a heterogenous group of disorders with multifocal or diffuse proliferation of fat. Most common in men (M:F = 10:1), with alcohol abuse being a major risk factor. Fat accumulation occurs independent of nutrition, and also can be triggered by human immunodeficiency virus (HIV) protease inhibitors. The classic type I pattern is a massive deposition about the neck; type II (pseudoathletic or Madelung disease) involves the shoulder girdle, giving a false image of muscular development; type III affects the hips. Treatment can be attempted with liposuction or lipolysis.

B. Benign Tumors of Connective Tissue

■ Scars and Keloids

Scars can be flat, atrophic, or hypertrophic. A hypertrophic scar is confined to the site of the tissue damage. A keloid results when the reparative process extends beyond the bounds of the original scar. Common sites are the midchest following cardiac surgery, in acne scars, and especially on ear lobes after piercing. Black individuals are more likely to develop keloids. Treatment is difficult; any manipulation may result in a worse keloid. The best results are obtained with shave excision, cryotherapy, laser ablation, intralesional corticosteroids, combined with compression.

■ Skin Tags

Tiny skin-colored or tan papules, typically on neck, axillae, or groin; they are also known as soft fibromas and more common in overweight and older individuals. Larger lesions can be confused with papillomatous melanocytic nevi. Shave or scissor excision is curative.

■ Dermatofibroma

Other names include histiocytoma and hard fibroma. This reactive process is usually secondary to arthropod assaults or folliculitis. It is most common on the legs and is characterized by a red-brown poorly circumscribed nodule which dimples when laterally compressed (*Fitzpatrick sign*). An atrophic form on the shoulder girdle clinically resembles BCC. Histopathology shows spindle-cell proliferation with peripheral entrapment of collagen and overlying epidermal hyperplasia. It can be excised but often heals with a poor scar.

■ Angiofibroma

This is a proliferation of small vessels with perivascular fibrosis. There are many variants:

- *fibrous papule of the nose*—a small solitary inconspicuous nasal papule
- *tuberous sclerosis*—facial papules mistakenly called adenoma sebaceum are angiofibromas (Ch. 30.1)
- *genital lesions*—*pearly penile papules* (tiny papules on the corona of glands) and *hirsuties vulvae* (similar lesions of introitus) are normal variants usually mistaken for warts

■ Nodular Fasciitis

This is a subcutaneous mass, usually on the forearm, with a history of rapid growth after trauma. Histologically, it is very worrying with myxoid stroma and many mitoses, but it is entirely harmless and easily excised.

■ Chondrodermatitis Nodularis Chronica Helicis

This is a tongue-twister but a common problem. It is a painful nodule on the helix (*sleeper's nodule*) and a result of microtrauma. Inflammation extends to underlying cartilage. Intralesional corticosteroids or cryotherapy can be tried, but excision is usually required.

Benign Tumors of Fat and Connective Tissue

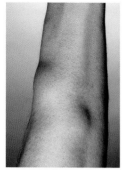

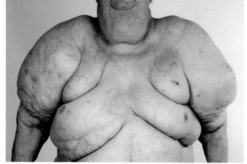

Lipomas

Benign symmetrical lipomatosis

A. Benign Tumors of Fat

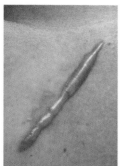

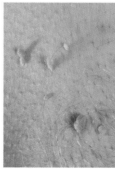

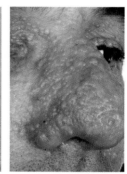

Keloid

Skin tags

Angiofibromas in tuberous sclerosis

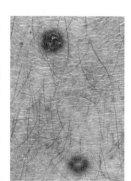

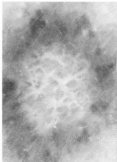

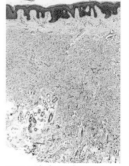

Dermatofibromas

Dermatoscopy of dermatofibroma

Histopathology: dermato-fibroma with overlying acanthosis

B. Benign Tumors of Connective Tissue

A. Leiomyoma

The different varieties of leiomyomas reflect the varying distribution of smooth muscle in the skin.

■ Piloleiomyoma

Develops from the arrector pili muscles and is characterized by soft red-brown nodules that are often multiple. It may be painful, especially when manipulated, which induces contraction. Multiple piloleiomyomas may be associated with both uterine leiomyomas and, rarely, with papillary renal carcinomas. Differential diagnostic considerations include Spitz nevus and mastocytoma for solitary red-brown lesions. Individual lesions may be excised; multiple lesions are sometimes treated with calcium-channel or α-adrenergic blockers to relax smooth muscle and diminish pain, but results are not dramatic.

Note: The acronym ANGEL is a useful way to remember the painful cutaneous tumors: *An*giolipoma, *N*eural tumors, *G*lomus tumor, *Ec*crine tumors, *L*eiomyoma (Ch. 13.1).

■ Angioleiomyoma

A solitary tender nodule on the leg; histology shows a prominent vessel with proliferation of peripheral vascular smooth muscle about it. It is often quite tender.

■ Other Leiomyomas

The smooth muscles of the dartos of the scrotum and nipple are other loci where smooth muscle tumors may develop.

■ Smooth Muscle Hamartoma

A solitary patch with increased smooth muscle; a clinical feature is prominent goose bumps (*cutis anserina*) when touched or otherwise stimulated. It often occurs beneath Becker nevus (Ch. 20.3) and follows Blaschko lines.

■ Accessory Nipple

This is a papillomatous nodule in the milk line from the axilla through the nipples to the groin; it is usually recognized clinically. Histologically, there is dermal accumulation of smooth muscles with easily overlooked epidermal hyperpigmentation, mammary glands, and ducts. Multiple accessory tumors may be a sign of Wilms' tumor (nephroblastoma).

B. Rhabdomyoma

Cutaneous tumors involving striated muscle are very uncommon. The muscles of facial expression are the only superficial striated muscles; occasionally skin-tag–like papules on the face will contain striated muscle and thus be capable of spontaneous motion. If striated muscle is identified in a lesion, be suspicious of associated malformations such as accessory tragus or branchial arch or cleft malformation.

C. Osteoma

Cutaneous bone formation is a rare but fascinating event. Most cutaneous ossification is secondary to trauma or fibrous proliferations and frequently associated with calcification. Two relatively common scenarios are multiple tiny facial or presternal osteomas in acne scars, and extrusion of ectopic bone on the digits of patients with CREST syndrome (Ch. 17.4). Rare causes of primary cutaneous ossification include:

- *idiopathic osteoma cutis*—subcutaneous bony mass with no obvious predisposing event
- *pseudohypoparathyroidism* with a defective G-protein pathway and inability to respond to parathormone. It is associated with a variety of metabolic problems and cutaneous osteomas
- *platelike cutaneous osteoma*—an embryologic throw-back to turtles or dinosaurs that have/had subcutaneous bones. Patients have disks or sheets of bone just below the dermis
- *subungual exostosis*—the most common osteoma seen in skin, but not cutaneous in origin. It arises from the bone of the distal digit of a toe, usually the great toe, and erodes through the skin, causing a friable subungual mass. Radiology confirms the diagnosis; excision is curative.

D. Chondroma

Cutaneous chondromas are exceptionally rare. If cartilage is found in a facial lesion, it almost certainly represents an accessory tragus or other embryologic rest. Occasional extraskeletal chondromas may be found on the soft tissue of the hands and feet. Subungual chondroma is invariably part of a subungual osteoma.

Other Benign Soft-tissue Tumors

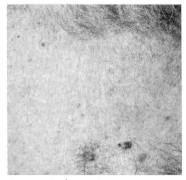

Accessory nipple: overview

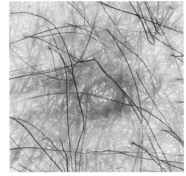

Accessory nipple: close-up

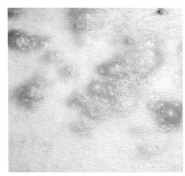

Piloleiomyomas

A. Leiomyoma

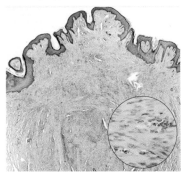

Histopathology: leiomyoma with bundles of spindle-shaped smooth muscle cells with cigar-shaped nuclei

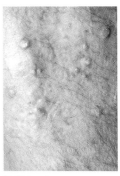

Multiple osteomas

C. Osteoma

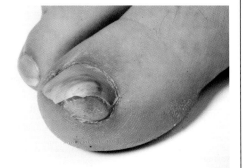

Subungual exostosis

Sarcomas are malignant tumors arising from mesenchymal structures. They present as irregular subcutaneous or deeper masses which are difficult to manage. Most cutaneous sarcomas can be completely excised and have a good prognosis. Advanced tumors may require radiation therapy or chemotherapy. Only a small number are relevant for dermatologists. The most common are dermatofibrosarcoma protuberans (DFSP) and Kaposi sarcoma (Ch. 22.6), a malignant vascular proliferation which is also a marker for HIV/AIDS.

A. Dermatofibrosarcoma Protuberans

■ Epidemiology

Even though it has a tongue-twister for a name, DFSP is the second most common cutaneous sarcoma with an incidence of 1 : 100 000; 10 %–15 % develop in children and adolescents.

■ Pathogenesis

DFSP is usually caused by a fusion gene involving platelet-derived growth factor-β (*PDGFB*) and collagen (*COL 1A1*). The collagen promoter stimulates the overproduction of functional PDGFB, which binds to the PDGF receptor on the DFSP cells and triggers their proliferation via tyrosinase kinase pathways.

■ Clinical Features

Irregular multilobular nodule or plaque. The typical site is the shoulder girdle. It is firm and not moveable and is usually mistaken for a scar. It is slow growing and may be pigmented (*Bednar tumor*). Giant cell fibroblastoma is a variant seen in infants.

■ Histopathology

Spindle-cell tumor with a storiform (irregularly whorled) pattern, irregular periphery, often infiltration of fat septae. Tumor cells are CD 34+.

■ Differential Diagnosis

The differential diagnostic considerations for a "scar" when there has not been an injury include, in addition to DFSP:
- sclerosing basal cell carcinoma (Ch. 21.4)
- scar sarcoidosis (Ch. 17.7)
- desmoplastic malignant melanoma (Ch. 24.3)
- acne keloidalis (Ch. 26.1)
- cutaneous metastases, especially from breast carcinoma (Ch. 21.5).

■ Therapy

Wide local excision is the standard, but micrographic surgery is ideal, as it can be combined with CD 34 staining. In larger or more aggressive tumors, postoperative radiation therapy is recommended when a complete excision cannot be guaranteed. The monoclonal antibody imatinib mesylate directly blocks several protein tyrosine kinases including the PDGF receptor, rendering the tumor less susceptible to overstimulation. It can be used for inoperable, recurrent, or metastatic DFSP.

B. Other Cutaneous Sarcomas

A distinction must be made between the rare lesions involving the dermis and top of subcutaneous fat from those arising in the deep soft tissues and secondarily impinging on the skin. The latter are both more common and much more aggressive.

■ Malignant Peripheral Nerve Sheath Tumor

Roughly 50 % develop in patients with neurofibromatosis, usually in association with a plexiform or deep neurofibroma. These tumors can occasionally start in the skin.

■ Atypical Fibroxanthoma

Crusted nodule in sun-damaged skin. Histology shows many bizarre cells; pattern seen in many tumors including squamous cell carcinoma, melanoma, and, rarely, primary mesenchymal tumor viewed as a superficial variant of malignant fibrous histiocytoma. Complete local excision is usually curative.

■ Leiomyosarcoma

These are locally aggressive tumors of smooth muscle that may recur but almost never metastasize. More common in HIV/AIDS patients.

■ Liposarcoma

This is the most common soft-tissue tumor, but almost never involves the skin until late in its course. Does not develop from lipoma. There are many histological variants.

■ Rhabdomyosarcoma

This is the most common sarcoma of children; it can occasionally present in the skin or female genitalia (botryoid tumor).

— Soft-tissue Sarcomas —

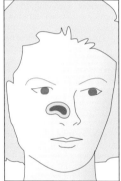

Dermatofibrosarcoma protuberans

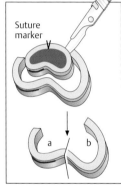

Histopathology: spindle-cell tumor usually extending into fat septa

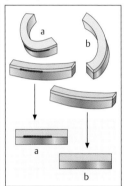

Immunohistopathology: tumor cells with CD34 positivity

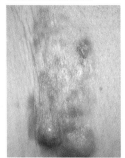

1. Excision "en bloc"

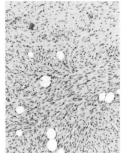

Suture marker

2. Separating the marked borders

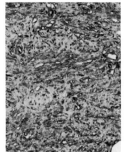

3. Embedding the tissue from the periphery

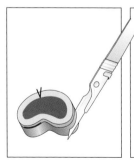

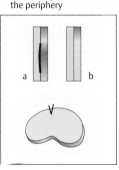

4. and **5.** Separating the base and embedding it

6. Examination of all borders, showing residual tumor in section a

Microscopically controlled surgery: 3D histology using the "Tübinger" torte method

A. Dermatofibrosarcoma Protuberans

One must carefully distinguish between:
- *malformation*—present at birth, often segmental, and permanent
- *hemangioma*—usually appear after birth, less often segmental, and many heal spontaneously.

Both can be associated with visceral involvement. Newer imaging procedures identify vascular structures more precisely and have shown many long-held concepts to be wrong.

A. Capillary Malformations

■ Telangiectases

These are small capillary malformations with dilated vessels; they can be congenital or acquired (pregnancy, collagen–vascular diseases, sun-damaged skin).

■ Stork Bite

Pink-red macule or patch on the nape or forehead tends to regress.

■ Port-wine Stain

Also known as nevus flammeus, circumscribed segmental pink or deep red-purple patch which grows with the patient and may thicken with nodules. About 15% are associated with syndromes:
- *Sturge–Weber syndrome*—association of port-wine stain involving 1st trigeminal distribution with ocular and CNS complications
- *Klippel-Trenaunay syndrome*—port-wine stain on an extremity with venous and lymphatic malformations, a tendency to thrombosis because of low flow, and overgrowth (both soft tissue and bones).

B. Venous Malformations

These are characterized by easily compressed blue-purple deep nodules. Patients often have recurrent episodes of clotting, presumably because of slow flow. On the face, they are associated with cerebral developmental venous anomalies. On the limbs, vascular nodules may involve the musculature causing pain and dysfunction.
Associated syndromes include:
- *blue rubber bleb nevus syndrome*—rubbery, often tender, venous malformations affecting the the skin and gastrointestinal tract.

C. Lymphatic Malformations

■ Lymphangioma Circumscriptum

Numerous translucent firm "pseudovesicles" resembling frog spawn. Distribution is segmental, on the skin or mucosa.

■ Cavernous Lymphangioma

This involves a deeper accumulation of the lymphatics, typically involving a limb or the head and neck region. *Cystic hygroma* of the neck is a variant. The tongue may be involved causing macroglossia. It is sometimes diffuse involving an entire limb.

D. Arteriovenous Malformations

Complex malformations involving the skin may initially resemble port-wine stain but are later distinguished because of pulsations, warmth, bruit, and pain. There is a risk of high-output cardiac failure because of arteriovenous shunting.
- *Parkes Weber syndrome*—vascular stain of limb with overgrowth in association with arteriovenous shunting.

E. Therapy

Capillary lesions can be treated with pulsed dye laser. Venous malformations can often be sclerosed or excised. Superficial lymphatic lesions can be easily excised, but often have deep feeder vessels. Deeper or more diffuse lesions are a problem. Arteriovenous lesions are the greatest challenge; they are generally approached with surgery and embolization. In some cases, amputation is necessary.

F. Acroangiodermatitis

Circumscribed livid to brown-black plaque and nodules. Clinically, mimics Kaposi sarcoma, secondary to chronic venous insufficiency or arteriovenous malformations. Histology clarifies the diagnosis. No treatment is needed.

G. Glomus Tumor

Glomus tumors or glomangiomas are firm tender subcutaneous nodules, most often acral, which may be solitary or multiple and are sometimes familial. When subungual, they are extremely painful and distort nail growth. Excision is curative.

– Vascular Malformations

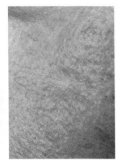

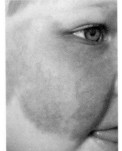

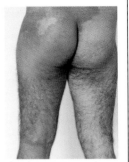

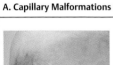

Telangiectases

Port-wine stain

Klippel–Trenaunay syndrome

A. Capillary Malformations

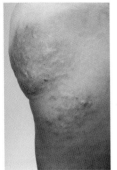

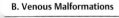

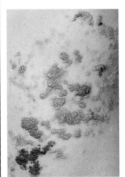

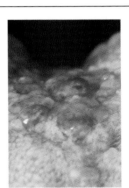

Lymphangioma circumscriptum

Lymphangioma on the tongue

B. Venous Malformations

C. Lymphatic Malformations

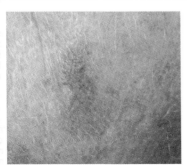

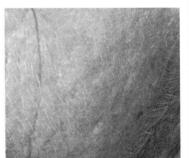

Capillary malformation on cheek before and after laser therapy

E. Therapy

A. Infantile Hemangioma

■ Epidemiology

This is the most common vascular lesion, also known as capillary hemangioma. It is present in 5%–10% of infants; F:M = 3:1; the greatest risk factor is low birth weight, which also predisposes to multiple tumors.

■ Pathogenesis

Infantile hemangiomas have a unique vascular phenotype and are composed of Glut-1 + endothelial cells similar to the placental microvasculature.

■ Clinical Features

Classic name of "strawberry hemangioma". The head and neck are common sites. Starts as a blanched macule with telangiectases, and evolves into a rubbery red tumor. During regression, it develops a gray sheen, flattens, and heals with scarring. High-risk hemangiomas are segmental, facial, or impinge on vital structures.

■ Variants

Variants include:
- *congenital*—fully developed at birth; lack Glut-1; divided into RICH (rapidly involuting congenital hemangioma) and NICH (noninvoluting)
- *multiple*—if there are more than five hemangiomas, look for liver involvement
- *periorificial*—around the mouth, nose, eyes, and anus; may interfere with vital functions and are more easily ulcerated
- *syndromal:* PHACE syndrome (*p*osterior fossa Dandy–Walker malformation, segmental *h*emangioma, *a*rterial anomalies, *c*ardiac anomalies [coarctation], *e*ye anomalies). F:M = 9:1.

■ Differential Diagnosis

Usually clear, but segmental forms can be confused with port-wine stains.

■ Course

In 80%, growth has stopped by 6 months and involution starts by 1 year; 50% have resolved by 5 years, and 70% by 7 years. Larger hemangiomas take longer to resolve and leave more cosmetic defects. Complications include:

- *ulceration*—usually uneventful; treated with antiseptic dressings
- *scarring*—facial lesions usually leave a scar
- *periorbital and periorificial*—risk of amblyopia, as well as disturbed maturation of the jaw or nose; sometimes interferes with eating or breathing
- *vascular problems*—risk of shunting and high-output cardiac failure. Rarely, *Kasabach–Merritt syndrome* develops with consumptive coagulopathy and risk of bleeding
- *aggressive growth*—tumors that grow aggressively after laser or cryotherapy may need systemic therapy.

■ Therapy

- Observation for low-risk lesions.
- Early cryotherapy may induce regression
- Tunable dye laser destruction very early in life.
- Other options include topical or intralesional corticosteroids and excision.

For high-risk lesions:
- systemic propranolol has become the treatment of choice
- systemic corticosteroids
- interferon (IFN)-α should not be used in the first year
- surgery or embolization of major arterial feeder vessels.

B. Pyogenic Granuloma

This is a reactive vascular proliferation in response to trauma, characterized by a red nodule that is usually friable with a bloody surface. Typical clinical settings are umbilicus of newborn, gingivae (especially in pregnancy), or the nail fold. Histology shows classic lobular proliferation of small vessels. Differential diagnosis: amelanotic melanoma. Therapy involves mild destructive measures, such as chemical or electrical cauterization, or laser destruction. Recurrence is common.

C. Eruptive Angioma

This is the most common vascular lesion; tiny ruby-colored papules occur most often on the trunk of older individuals. Some patients may have hundreds. No therapy is required. Lesions can be ablated with a laser.

Hemangiomas and Other Benign Vascular Tumors

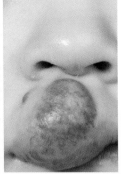
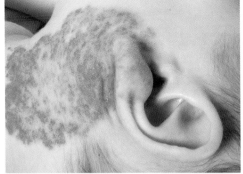

Hemangiomas of the lip and neck; the latter has extensive gray areas suggesting involution

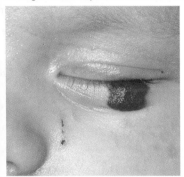
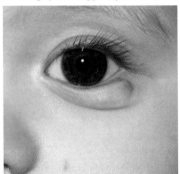

Hemangioma before and after cryotherapy
A. Infantile Hemangioma

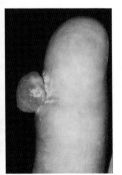
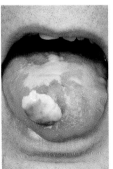
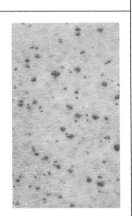

Typical eroded polypoid lesion on the finger and hyper-keratotic pedunculated papule on the tongue

B. Pyogenic Granuloma

C. Eruptive Angioma

A. Kaposi Sarcoma

■ Pathogenesis

The most important factors are infection with human herpes virus 8 and immunosuppression; the cell of origin is most likely lymphatic endothelial cells.

■ Clinical Features

There are four distinct clinical settings:
- *classic*—elderly men of Mediterranean, Jewish extraction; usually on the feet
- *African*—the most common tumor in equatorial Africa with expression ranging from a fulminant lymphadenopathic form to chronic skin lesions
- *iatrogenic*—complication of immunosuppression
- *HIV/AIDS*—first reliable marker for AIDS; more common in homosexual men.

Individual lesions are highly variable, ranging from pale brown macules in skin lines to red-brown nodules and plaques, to eroded tumors. Oral involvement is common in HIV/AIDS and indicates systemic diseases. Larger lesions may become ulcerated and bleed; systemic involvement may include gastrointestinal, pulmonary, and lymph node disease.

■ Histopathology

Early patch lesions have subtle vascular slits; later plaque lesions reveal spindle-cell proliferation with red blood cells in slits. Cells stain with lymphatic markers.

■ Differential Diagnosis

- *Acroangiodermatitis* (pseudo-Kaposi sarcoma) describes red-brown nodules arising in stasis dermatitis.
- Bacillary angiomatosis from *Bartonella henselae* in HIV/AIDS.

■ Therapy

Therapy must be adjusted to the clinical situation. In HIV/AIDS, highly active antiretroviral therapy (HAART) is clearly most important. In elderly asymptomatic individuals, no treatment, cryotherapy, or local radiation therapy (20–30 Gy) is best. In advanced KS, systemic IFN-α (3×10^6 IU thrice weekly) or liposomal anthracyclines are preferred.

B. Angiosarcoma

■ Clinical Features

The typical clinical setting is an erythematous tumor on the face or scalp of an elderly individual, usually a man. It may initially present an edematous patch or bruiselike change, and is thus often misdiagnosed. Variants include:
- *Stewart–Treves syndrome*—angiosarcoma developing in an area of chronic lymphedema, most often post-mastectomy
- *postirradiation*—once again, this is more common on the breast, years after radiation for carcinoma.

Note: Any vascular proliferation in irradiated skin should be suspected of being an angiosarcoma.

■ Histopathology

Vascular slits, atypical endothelial cells, and later clusters of malignant cells. Sometimes the only clue to the origin is special stains (factor VIII, *Ulex*) or cytoplasmic vacuole formation. Margins are indistinct and hard to delineate.

■ Therapy

Generous surgical excision with control margins and consolidation radiation therapy offer the only chance of cure, but the outlook dismal, with 5-year survival about 10%.

C. Other Vascular Tumors

There is a wide variety of other tumors; diagnosis is usually based on histology. Simple excision is curative.

■ Angiokeratoma

Dilated vessels extend to just under the epidermis with a hyperkeratotic reaction:
- common finding on the scrotum and labia of the elderly
- multiple tiny lesions are a marker for Fabry disease (Ch. 27.7).

■ Angiolymphoid Hyperplasia with Eosinophilia

This presents as red-brown nodules, usually on the head and neck, often about the ears. It features a combination of vessels with prominent endothelial cells, lymphocytic infiltrate, and usually abundant eosinophils.

Malignant and Other Vascular Tumors

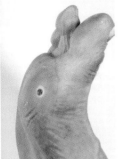

Polypoid lesion

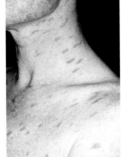

Multiple lesions following skin lines

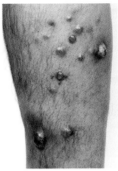

Nodules

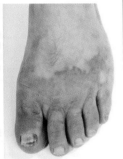

Discolored patch

A. Kaposi Sarcoma

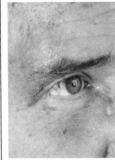

Typical angiosarcoma as subtle facial patch

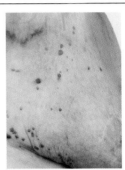

Metastotic angiosarcomas

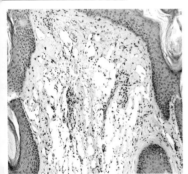

Histopathology: irregular vascular spaces insinuating between bundles of collagen

B. Angiosarcoma

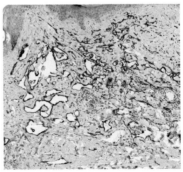

Immunohistopathology: expression of lymphatic marker D2-40

A. Benign Neural Tumors

The hallmark of neural tumors is that they are often painful. They may also be indicators of underlying disorders. Solitary lesions are treated with simple excision, which is curative.

■ Neurofibroma

Common solitary tumor presents as skin-colored nondescript papule, clinically confused with melanocytic nevus or skin tag. Histopathology reveals loosely arranged Schwann cells with mucinous stroma and mast cells. If multiple, always exclude neurofibromatosis 1—look for café-au-lait macules and axillary freckles (Ch. 30.1).

■ Plexiform Neurofibroma

Deep dermal/subcutaneous bundle of thickened nerve fibers, often described as a "bag of worms." It is pathognomonic for neurofibromatosis 1 and often covered by large café-au-lait macules. About 10% of plexiform neurofibromas undergo malignant transformation; this accounts for 50% of malignant peripheral nerve tumors.

■ Neurilemmoma

Also known as *schwannoma*, it is characterized by a subcutaneous encapsulated nodule histologically show an orderly arrangement of palisaded neural cells. Usually solitary, but if multiple consider neurofibromatosis 2 (Ch. 30.1). Psammomatous melanotic schwannoma is a feature of Carney syndrome (Ch. 30.3); it features dendritic melanocytes and psammoma bodies (lamellar calcified spheres).

■ Traumatic Neuroma

This usually occurs on the hands or feet (*Morton neuroma*) or following obvious trauma. It is also common in amputation stumps. Typically, it is painful. Histology shows neural elements entwined with scar tissue.

■ Mucosal Neuroma

This presents as glassy papules on the oral or ocular mucosa; it is a sign of multiple endocrine neoplasia (MEN) IIB (Ch. 30.3).

Caution: Be very skeptical of traumatic mucosal neuroma—almost unheard of! Think of MEN.

■ Granular Cell Tumor

Peculiar tumor whose etiology was long debated but appears to be neural; 40% occur on the tongue, others can be anywhere on skin. often has a verrucous surface. Congenital epulis is a variant in infancy. Typical reactive epidermal changes are easily mistaken for squamous cell carcinoma, especially on the tongue. Bundles of polygonal tumor cells occur more deeply, with eosinophilic periodic acid–Schiff (PAS)+ cytoplasmic granules. It is sometimes associated with nerves. S100, neuron-specific enolase, and other neuronal markers are positive. Excision is curative.

B. Merkel Cell Carcinoma

Epidemiology. This is an aggressive tumor of the elderly that is at least as common as cutaneous lymphoma. Merkel cell carcinoma (MCC) was first identified in the 1970s as a trabecular carcinoma. Previously, most were erroneously diagnosed as lymphomas or metastatic small cell tumors.

Pathogenesis. Merkel cells are neuroendocrine cells in the lower epidermis, intimately connected with sensory nerves. Merkel cell polyomavirus (MCV) infects 15%–25% of adults, but is found in >80% of MCC. Ultraviolet (UV) exposure and immunosuppression appear to play a role.

Clinical features. MCC occurs almost exclusively in sun-damaged skin of older patients. MCC are erythematous or blue-red nodules usually on the head and neck, which grow very rapidly.

Histopathology. "Murky cell" probably describes the cells best; they are small, often grouped (trabecula), poorly defined blue-gray cells which are positive for cytokeratin 20 (CK20) and some neural markers.

Differential diagnosis. Lymphoma, adnexal tumor, metastasis of pulmonary small cell carcinoma

Therapy. Excision with micrographic control employing CK20 as a marker and combined with sentinel lymph node biopsy. Consolidation radiation therapy with up to 50 Gy to the excision site and regional nodes. 30%–50% die of metastatic disease. Patients respond poorly to chemotherapy; regimens include carboplatin and etoposide.

Note: MCC is far more aggressive than any other cutaneous malignancy.

Neural Tumors

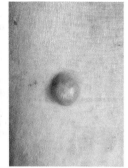

Neurofibroma

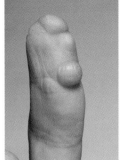

Neurofibroma

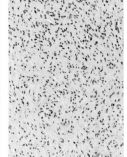

Histopathology: monotonous spindle-cell tumor

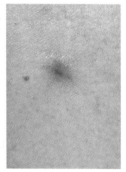

Neurilemmoma

A. Benign Neural Tumors

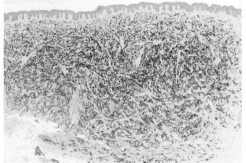

Immunohistopathology: granular cell tumor with S100 positivity

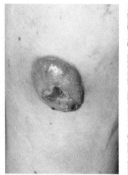

Clinical features

B. Merkel Cell Carcinoma

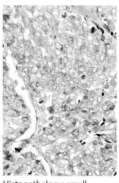

Histopathology: small murky blue-gray tumor cells

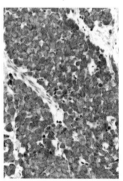

Immunohistopathology: tumor cells show CK20 positivity

22 Tumors of the Dermis and Subcutis

A. Definition and Classification

Lymphoma is a malignant proliferation of lymphocytes. Cutaneous lymphoma (CL) initially appears in the skin and remains confined there for at least 6 months. Divided into cutaneous T-cell lymphoma (CTCL) and cutaneous B-cell lymphoma (CBCL).

B. Epidemiology

The skin is the second most common extranodal site for lymphoma, after the gut. The incidence is around 0.5:100 000; 75% are CTCL.

C. Pathogenesis

Epstein–Barr virus plays an important role in Burkitt lymphoma in Africa and in several B-cell lymphomas in immunosuppressed individuals. The cause of most lymphomas is a mystery.

D. Parapsoriasis

This is a confusing concept, with no clear consensus on how the two types are related:
- *small-patch parapsoriasis*—multiple salmon-colored 1–2 cm macules with fine scale. Histopathology shows superficial mild dermatitis. It is asymptomatic but difficult to treat; PUVA or UVB 311 nm is most effective. There is no relationship to mycosis fungoides and the course is benign.
- *large-patch parapsoriasis*—large erythematous violet atrophic patches often on buttocks or trunk. Usually, < 10% surface area is involved. Histopathology usually just shows mild inflammation. Probably early mycosis fungoides but has a very slow course and little impact on the patient's life. It can usually be controlled with PUVA or UVB 311 nm.

E. Mycosis Fungoides

Epidemiology. Mycosis fungoides (MF) accounts for most cases of CTCL and is the most common CL, making up 40%–50% of most series. Incidence of 1–3:1 000 000.
Pathogenesis. Usually develops from large patch parapsoriasis.
Clinical Features. There are three classic stages:
- *patch*—oval patches with fine wrinkling (pseudoatrophy); most common on buttocks and trunk. It is asymptomatic and persists for years. We view *large-patch parapsoriasis* as a variant of patch-stage MF with a very low risk of progression

- *plaque*—the patches become thicker, as they are infiltrated by tumor cells. It lasts for 2–5 years. Patients usually have scale; pale and dark plaques often appear together
- *tumor*—large often ulcerated tumors admixed with patches and plaques. Poor prognosis.

Note: *MF d'emblée presenting with primarily tumors is quite uncommon.*

There are also several variants:
- *follicular*—lymphocytes infiltrate hair follicles and cause boggy mass with alopecia
- *hypopigmented*—more common in black individuals, often seen in younger patients
- *pagetoid reticulosis (Woringer–Kolopp disease)*—solitary patch with sharp border; usually acral; responds well to PUVA or low-dose radiation therapy (20–30 Gy)
- *leonine*—advanced disease may have marked facial infiltration (*leonine facies*)
- *granulomatous slack skin*—loose folds of damaged skin in the axillae and groin.

Histopathology. The histology also varies with stage; the sparse infiltrate in the patch stage is subtle, while the large tumor masses cannot be overlooked. The plaque stage features epidermotropic infiltrates of atypical T cells, usually CD4+, rarely CD8+. Tumor cells are usually monoclonal T lymphoblasts. There are no specific or sensitive staining patterns for MF.
Differential diagnosis. Early lesions are confused with dermatitis, psoriasis, lupus erythematosus, and dermatophyte infections.
Therapy. The therapy depends on the stage:
- *patch*—either observation, UVB 311 nm, or any of the other treatments for plaque stage
- *plaque*—UVB 311 nm, PUVA, topical (corticosteroids, retinoids [bexarotene], nitrogen mustard). The best method is likely PUVA plus systemic interferon (IFN)-α or retinoids (bexarotene). Electron beam therapy or 20–30 Gy radiation to selected plaques.
- *tumor*—PUVA plus systemic IFN-α or retinoids, spot radiation therapy to troublesome tumors. Some chemotherapy regimens produce only short-term improvement.

Prognosis. The 10-year survival data are patch, 97%; disseminated plaque, 83%; tumor 42%; lymph node involvement, 20%.

— Cutaneous Lymphomas —

Type of lymphoma	% of CL	5-year survival
Primary cutaneous T-cell lymphomas (CTCL)		
Mycosis fungoides	40–50%	88%
Patch		98%
Plaque		83%
Tumor		42%
Sézary syndrome	3%	24%
Lymphomatoid papulosis	12%	100%
Anaplastic large-cell lymphoma	8%	95%
Subcutaneous panniculitis-like lymphoma	1%	80%
Primary cutaneous B-cell lymphomas (CBCL)		
Marginal zone B-cell lymphoma	5–10%	>95%
Follicle center lymphoma	11%	95%
Diffuse large B-cell lymphoma, leg type	3–5%	55%

A. Definition and Classification

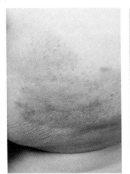

Patch stage

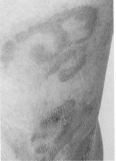

Plaque stage

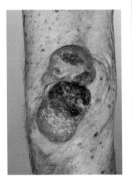

Tumor stage

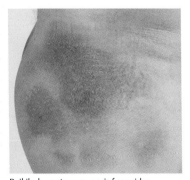

Poikilodermatous mycosis fungoides

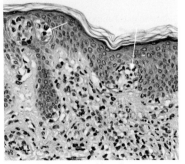

Histopathology: atypical lymphocytes
in the epidermis (Pautrier micro-abscess↑)

E. Mycosis Fungoides

F. Sézary Syndrome

A combination of erythroderma, marked lymphadenopathy, and >20% circulating atypical T cells with cerebriform nuclei, it usually involves older adults, with a poor prognosis. The differential diagnosis is that of erythroderma (Ch. 13.3). Treatment is as for tumor-stage MF except that extracorporeal photophoresis is often helpful.

G. Other Cutaneous T-cell Lymphomas

■ CD 30 + T-cell Lymphoproliferative Disorders

CD 30 is a cytokine receptor found on many activated T cells and 20% of CL. Variants include:
Lymphomatoid papulosis. Patients develop crops of erythematous papules and nodules, often hemorrhagic and crusted and occasionally ulcerated, which spontaneously regress and then generally recur at intervals. Histologic examination reveals wedge-shaped infiltrate of large atypical lymphocytes. Responds to antibiotics or low-dose methotrexate.
Primary cutaneous anaplastic large-cell lymphoma. Single or multiple red-brown nodules often grouped or limited to one body region. Nodal form, which has a different marker profile and worse prognosis. Therapy is excision or radiation therapy; 5-year survival >90%.
Hodgkin lymphoma. Rarely involves the skin, but tumor cells are generally CD 30+.

> **Note:** Patients with any CD 30 + disorder are at risk for the other disorders as well as for mycosis fungoides. The overall risk of developing lymphoma in lymphomatoid papulosis is <10%.

■ Subcutaneous Panniculitis-like T-cell Lymphoma

Malignant lymphocytes proliferate in subcutaneous fat, mimicking panniculitis. Phagocytosis may be seen, as well as rimming of fat cells by tumor cells. When associated with γ–δ T cells or hemophagocytosis, the outlook is worse.

H. Cutaneous B-cell Lymphomas

■ Marginal Zone B-cell Lymphoma

Presents as solitary or multiple nodules, usually on the trunk, most often in men aged >40–50 years. It accounts for 5%–10% of CL. The proliferative cell is the marginal-zone cell at the periphery of a lymphoid follicle. Histology shows CD 5–, CD 19+, CD 20+ with light chain restriction. Similar tumors in the gut are triggered by *Helicobacter pylori* and respond to antibiotic therapy, so a trial is worthwhile. Generally treated by excision or radiation therapy. Advanced disease responds to rituximab (anti-CD 20 antibody).

■ Follicle Center Lymphoma

The most common BCL (11% of CL). It is extremely low-grade, often diagnosed in the past as pseudolymphoma. Presents with red-brown nodules, favoring face, scalp, and upper back. Histology reveals a prominent follicular pattern with centrocytes and centroblasts; CD 5+, CD 19–, CD 20+ with light-chain restriction. Treatment as for marginal zone BCL.

■ Diffuse Large B-cell Lymphoma, Leg Type

The only other somewhat common BCL (3%–5% of CL) with a relatively poor prognosis, occurring most often, but not always, on the legs. There is a diffuse infiltrate of medium to large centroblast-like and immunoblast-like cells; histology shows CD 19+, CD 20+, Bcl-2+. It needs more aggressive therapy; excision and radiation therapy are often insufficient; rituximab or polychemotherapy is needed.

I. Pseudolymphoma

This term was formerly used to indicate benign cutaneous lymphocytic infiltrates. Modern studies show many are low-grade B-cell lymphomas, while others are:
- borrelial lymphocytoma (Ch. 33.4)
- lupus tumidus (Ch. 17.5)
- reactions to arthropod assault
- tumors with dense lymphocytic infiltrates
- drug reactions (rare cause)

Cutaneous Lymphomas

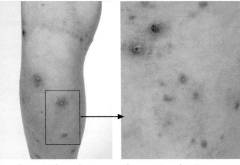

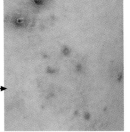

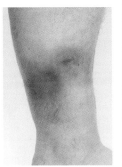

Lymphomatoid papulosis

Close-up view showing hemorrhagic necrotic papules

Subcutaneous panniculitis-like lymphoma

G. Other Cutaneous T-cell Lymphomas

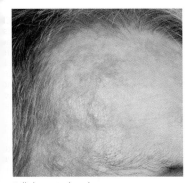

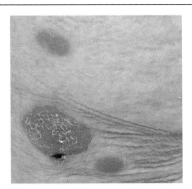

Follicle center lymphoma

Diffuse large B-cell lymphoma, leg type

H. Cutaneous B-cell Lymphomas

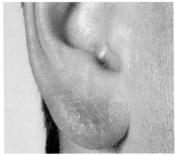

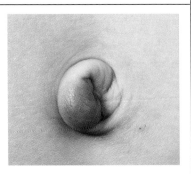

Earlobe and umbilicus: borrelial lymphocytoma

I. Pseudolymphoma

A. Introduction

Mast cells are derived from bone marrow and most common in a perivascular location in the barrier organs—the skin and mucosa. Their granules contain many mediators, which can be released upon mechanical, pharmacologic (aspirin, codeine), or immunologic stimulation.

Mastocytosis denotes a group of disorders characterized by the abnormal accumulation of mast cells in the skin and other tissues. In adults, mutations in the kit ligand are often found. About 80% of patients have only skin involvement, while 20% have systemic disease. The diagnosis is usually confirmed on biopsy. Mast cells contain granules identified with Giemsa or toluidine blue stain and are positive for CD117 (kit ligand). The childhood forms all tend to resolve spontaneously, while the adult forms are persistent. Some patients present with aspirin or codeine intolerance, as the clinical findings may be ignored until these agents cause mast cells to degranulate.

B. Mastocytoma

Clinical features. Mastocytoma usually presents as a solitary pruritic, red-brown nodule, most common in infants. Manipulation may cause erythema and wheal formation through release of mediator substances (*Darier sign*).
Histopathology. Accumulation of round or cuboidal cells, sometimes mistaken for melanocytic nevus or glomus tumor.
Differential diagnosis. Spitz nevus and xanthogranuloma are similar.
Therapy. Treatment is excision; some may resolve spontaneously.

C. Urticaria Pigmentosa

Clinical features. This usually affects children, with multiple red-brown macules that may be admixed with nodules or plaques. Because of the larger number of mast cells, patients more often develop urticaria and have more severe pruritus than with mastocytoma. Variants include:

- *bullous form*—the entire infant represents an exaggerated Darier sign. Surprisingly, this usually resolves spontaneously
- *hemorrhagic variant*—heals with hyperpigmentation

Systemic manifestations may include diarrhea and hypovolemia. Bone involvement may cause pain or osteoporosis.

Note: Always suspect mastocytosis in patients with severe or unexplained anaphylaxis.

Histopathology. Biopsy shows varying amounts of mast cells, usually around vessels with increased basal layer melanin.
Differential diagnosis. Syndromes with multiple melanocytic nevi or lentigines must be ruled out, but a history of Darier sign or severe urticaria helps.
Therapy. Antihistamines for pruritus; PUVA, IFN-γ-and topical corticosteroids can suppress mast cells.

D. Telangiectasia Macularis Eruptiva Perstans

This tongue-twister, usually called TMEP, is a form of diffuse mast cell disease in adults combining the tan macules of urticaria pigmentosa with multiple telangiectases. Treatment is as for urticaria pigmentosa.

E. Systemic Mastocytosis

Clinical findings. Many patients have both cutaneous and systemic findings. Most common is smoldering disease with skin, bone marrow and bone involvement. Rare forms include mast cell leukemia.

Any adult with cutaneous mastocytosis should be screened with serum tryptase level; a level of >15 ng/mL suggests systemic involvement. The next steps are bone marrow biopsy, bone density determination, and gastrointestinal examination. Bad prognostic signs are:

- >200 ng/mL serum tryptase
- ≥30% mast cells in bone marrow
- evidence of myelodysplastic or myeloproliferative disorder
- lymph node, spleen, liver, or gut involvement.

Therapy. Mainstays include systemic antihistamines, bisphosphonates, corticosteroids, and IFN-α. Kit kinase inhibitors only help in around 5% of cases. Patients should carry an emergency set for anaphylaxis.

Mast Cell Disorders

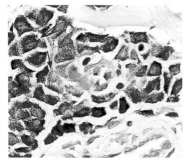

Histopathology: mast cell with granules (arrows) stained with toluidine blue stain

A. Introduction

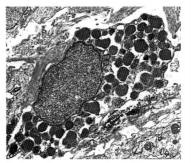

Electron microscopy: mast cell with granules

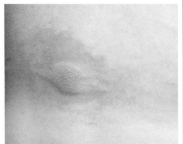

Solitary mastocytoma with Darier sign

B. Mastocytoma

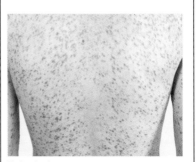

Urticaria pigmentosa

Urticaria pigmentosa: close-up view

C. Urticaria Pigmentosa

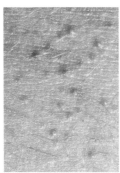

Urticaria pigmentosa: positive Darier sign

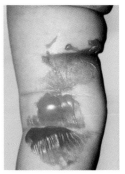

Bullous mastocytosis

Two types of disorders are included under this old name—disorders of Langerhans cells and of macrophages. They should be clearly distinguished, as they are clinically different and have different prognoses. The macrophage disorders include juvenile xanthogranuloma, sinus histiocytosis, and many rare entities.

A. Langerhans Cell Disease

■ Pathogenesis

Langerhans cell disease (LCD) is an uncommon monoclonal proliferation of Langerhans cells, but with a tendency to spontaneous regression.

■ Clinical Features

There are four variable pictures with frequent overlaps:
- *Letterer–Siwe disease*—usually occurs in infants, but also older children and adults. Purpuric papules favor the flexures, and are often widespread. Almost all have systemic involvement; 90% survive but frequently with residual defects
- *Hashimoto–Pritzker disease*—present at birth with multiple nodules that tend to regress in the first few days of life; rare transition to Letterer–Siwe disease
- *Hand–Schüller–Christian disease*—a triad of bony defects, diabetes insipidus, and exophthalmos; skin lesions tend to be yellow nodules in the flexures
- *eosinophilic granuloma*—usually occurs in adults; presents with focal destructive lesions in the mandible (*floating teeth*) and long bones; occasionally there are solitary skin nodules

■ Histopathology

Histiocytosis X was used to describe the entire group, unified by similar histologic features. There is an infiltrate of large kidney-shaped cells, which are often epidermotropic and stain positively for S 100, CD 1 a, and langerin (CD 207). Birbeck granules can be seen on electron microscopy, but this is no longer required for diagnosis.

■ Differential Diagnosis

At birth, the entire spectrum of TORCH (toxoplasmosis, other infections, rubella, cytomegalovirus, herpes simplex virus) infections with extramedullary hematopoiesis, congenital leukemia, mast cell disease. In infants, diaper der-

matitis. In older individuals, all forms of dermatitis and inverse psoriasis; nodules may suggest xanthogranuloma, mastocytoma, o Spitz nevus.

> **Note:** All infants with persistent, especially purpuric, flexural dermatitis should be biopsied to exclude LCD.

■ Complications

Prognosis is directly related to the degree o systemic involvement; patients should be staged using a standard scheme that weight clinical, laboratory, and radiological findings Between 50% and 70% of children have systemic disease. Lung, lymph node, spleen, an bone marrow involvement is unfavorable. Ir adults, solitary skin or bone disease are more common. Mastoid infiltrates suggest systemic involvement.

■ Therapy

Local lesions can be excised or curetted (bone) Topical corticosteroids or nitrogen mustard (ir adults only) are also helpful. Those with exten sive disease should be treated according to protocol; vincristine and prednisolone with 6-mercaptopurine added for maintenance i standard; options include thalidomide, metho trexate, and cladribine.

B. Sinus Histiocytosis with Massive Lymphadenopathy

Sinus histiocytosis with massive lymphade nopathy (SHML) is also known as Rosai–Dorf man disease. Usually presents in children, with massive cervical lymphadenopathy that tend to resolve spontaneously. About 15% presen with primary skin lesions, usually red-brow or skin-colored deep nodules. Under the mi croscope, there are lymphocytes and clear cell that resemble sinus histiocytes of lymph nodes. They stain with S-100 and macrophag markers but lack CD 1 a and langerin. Gian cells containing multiple lymphocytes (*em peripolesis*) are pathognomonic.

■ Therapy

Lesions can be excised if desired.

Histiocytoses and Leukemia

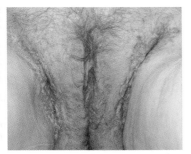

Hemorrhagic eroded flexural papules; in the adult here, but a classic finding in infants

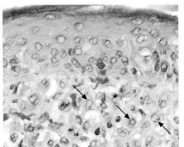

Histopathology: kidney-shaped dermal macrophages (arrows)

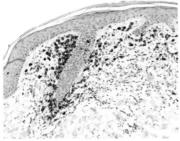

Immunohistopathology: tumor cells with langerin (CD207) positivity

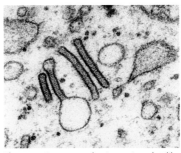

Electron microscopy: classic tennis-racket-like Birbeck granules

Variant	Systemic involvement	Affected organs
Letterer–Siwe	Very common	Lymph nodes, liver, spleen , bone marrow
Hashimoto–Pritzker	Rare	
Hand-Schüller–Christian	Common	Pituitary, bones
Eosinophilic granuloma	Uncommon	Bone, rarely skin

Disorder	S100	CD1a	CD68	Birbeck granules	Langerin (CD207)
Langerhans cell disease	+	+	−	+	+
Sinus histiocytosis with lymphadenopathy	+		+/−	−	−
Xanthogranuloma	−	−	−	−	−

A. Langerhans Cell Disease

C. Juvenile Xanthogranuloma

■ Clinical Features

Juvenile xanthogranuloma (JXG) is a common lesion in children. Yellow-red nodules are usually on the scalp or flexures.

> **Note:** There is a slight risk of eye involvement. Ophthalmologic examination should be obtained if the child is aged <2 years and has multiple lesions of recent onset.

■ Histopathology

Biopsies show an infiltrate of CD68+ macrophages with Touton (wreathed) multinucleated giant cells.

■ Differential Diagnosis

Mast cell tumor and Spitz nevus.

■ Therapy

In children, JXG almost always regresses spontaneously; in adults, it is persistent and often excised.

D. Other Macrophage Disorders

All these diseases are variants on JXG with yellow to red-brown papules and nodules. There is little tendency to regression. Solitary lesions can be excised or otherwise ablated. No effective systemic therapy is available.

- *Benign cephalic histiocytosis*—most common variant: tiny papules on the cheeks of small children, which resolve spontaneously.
- *Multicentric reticulohistiocytosis*—acral nodules are associated with destructive arthritis (almost all), autoimmune diseases (15%), and associated malignancies (15%). Histology shows multinuclear macrophages with ground-glass cytoplasm.
- *Xanthoma disseminatum*—grouped yellow to red-brown papules in the flexures and around eyes. Disease is persistent and associated with diabetes insipidus. The lesions are xanthomas, full of foamy macrophages, but lipid values are normal.
- *Eruptive histiocytosis*—multiple small red-brown papules, which wax and wane. Occasionally a paraneoplastic marker.
- *Progressive nodular histiocytosis*—many red-brown papules (xanthomas) and deep nodules (spindle-cell xanthogranuloma).

- *Erdheim–Chester disease*—systemic xantho granulomas, usually involving bone but also retroperitoneal fibrosis, CNS, heart, and kidneys; sometimes with cutaneous lesions. Usually fatal in 3–5 years.

E. Leukemia

Leukemia may involve the skin in two basic ways:
- specific infiltrates where leukemic cell spread to the skin via blood
- nonspecific changes as a result of immuno suppression or bleeding disorders.

■ Leukemia Cutis

Specific infiltrates indicate advanced disease. Most common are widespread livid or bruise like papules and nodules which appear rapidly, often overnight. Unusual features include:
- rarely, the cutaneous infiltrate may preced the systemic disease. About 7% of acute my eloid leukemias present in the skin. The most exceptional variant is the granulocyti sarcoma (*chloroma*).
- adult T-cell leukemia has the highest inci dence of cutaneous involvement, over 50%
- leukemic infiltrates may concentrate i scars (zoster, indwelling catheters)
- extensive gingival infiltrates are seen in 50% of myelomonocytic leukemia
- leonine facies occasionally result from di fuse infiltrates
- Sweet syndrome (Ch. 17.2) is sometimes th first sign of acute myeloid leukemia.

■ Nonspecific Changes

Typical infections include persistent herpe simplex, atypical zoster, and severe staphylo coccal pyodermas, especially perioral. Reduce platelets or leukemia-related disturbances i coagulation lead to purpura and bruising, es pecially on the legs. Hemorrhagic panniculiti is another clue to leukemia.

■ Therapy

Treat the leukemia, not the skin. Disturbing le sions can be palliated with 20–30 Gy ionizing radiations, which melts them but does not af fect the prognosis.

— Histiocytoses and Leukemia —

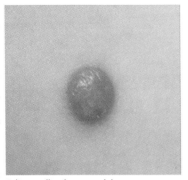 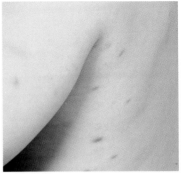

Solitary yellow-brown nodule   Multiple small papules

C. Juvenile Xanthogranuloma

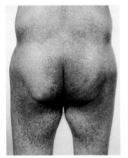  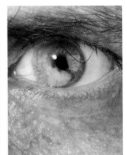

Xanthoma disseminatum   Xanthoma disseminatum: close-up view of confluent red-brown papules   Xanthoma disseminatum: periorbital papules with infiltration of cornea

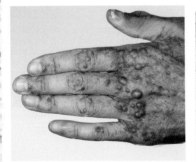 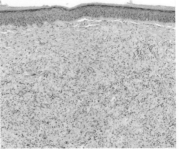

Xanthoma disseminatum

D. Other Macrophage Disorders

Histopathology: xanthoma disseminatum with dermal infiltrate of foamy macrophages with occasional giant cells

A. Vitiligo

Definition. Acquired depigmentation of skin secondary to loss of melanocytes; harmless but very disturbing to patients.

Epidemiology. Prevalence 1%, peak onset in young adult life; 30%–40% have family history.

Pathogenesis. Neural, traumatic, and autoimmune factors are postulated to damage melanocytes. Cytotoxic T cells may administer the final blow to melanocytes. It is associated with autoimmune thyroid disease (up to 30% in adults), alopecia areata, uveitis, and pernicious anemia, also as part of the polyglandular autoimmune disease or aberrant IL-1 signaling.

Clinical features. Vitiligo presents with sharply circumscribed, white macules and patches of varying sizes and shapes. Initially these have an erythematous border, reflecting inflammation. The most common pattern is an acrofacial type, with periorbital, perioral, hand, foot, and genital involvement. Other patients may have segmental disease, scattered, or diffuse patches. The hairs in vitiligo patches are usually white, but can retain their pigment.

Histopathology. Special stains (melanin, S-100) show loss of melanocytes; this is hard to appreciate on routine sections.

Differential diagnosis. Chemical depigmentation through paraphenolic compounds is identical. Piebaldism has larger midline patches at birth. Many other disorders are similar but hypopigmented—not depigmented—lichen sclerosus et atrophicus and systemic sclerosis (confetti pattern in blacks) are atrophic-sclerotic; pityriasis alba and pityriasis versicolor have marked scale; postinflammatory hypopigmentation occurs especially in psoriasis and syphilis; leprosy has anesthetic patches. *Nevus anemicus* also appears at birth; pallor is caused by catecholamine hypersensitivity with permanent vasoconstriction.

Therapy. In perhaps 30% of patients, a satisfactory repigmentation can be achieved; in another 30%, there is some degree of color change, which often does not matter to the patient. This leaves at least 40% of treated patients unhappy and distressed. Usual agents include:

- topical corticosteroids or calcineurin inhibitors, with little evidence
- phototherapy with ultraviolet (UV)B 311 nm or psoralen plus UVA (PUVA)
- maximum UVB and UVA protection to protect white areas and avoid tanning the surrounding skin
- camouflage with special makeup.

Skin grafting or other ways to transplant melanocytes to depigmented areas are possible, but must be combined with subsequent UVB therapy. It is unclear if this approach increases the risk of melanoma.

B. Albinism

Definition. Diffuse hypo- or depigmentation caused by genetic defects in melanin production or transfer; the number of melanocytes is normal. In oculocutaneous albinism (OCA, autosomal recessive), melanin is missing in the skin, hair, and eyes. In ocular albinism, the defects are primarily in the eye.

Clinical features. Pale to white skin and hair, with subtle variations between types:

Tyrosinase-negative OCA1. No activity of tyrosinase, the most important enzyme in melanin production; white skin, hair, blue eyes with red reflex; impaired vision, nystagmus and photophobia. No pigmented nevi.

Tyrosinase-positive OCA2. OCA2 is the most common form, with a prevalence in USA of 1:15 000 in black individuals and 1:36 000 in white individuals. Mutation in protein P blocks formation of eumelanin, but other forms are still produced. Patients have white skin at birth, but later develop a pale tan with freckles and slightly pigmented nevi. OCA2 has fewer ocular problems than OCA1.

Albinoid Disorders. Membrane protein defects lead to impaired melanin transfer, associated with defects in other cells. *Chediak–Higashi syndrome* and *Griscelli syndrome* feature pigmentary dilution with a gray sheen and macrophage defects with severe infections. *Hermansky–Pudlak syndrome* has tyrosinase-positive albinism plus platelet defects.

C. Piebaldism

Mutations in *c-Kit* and other melanocyte trafficking genes lead to altered migration of melanocytes from the neural crest to the skin during embryogenesis. Patients are born with sharply defined areas of depigmentation usually involving the anterior scalp (poliosis, white forelock), face, chest, knees, and elbows. Typically, patients have pigmented islands within white patches.

Vitiligo and Albinism

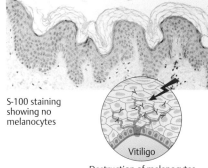

S-100 staining
showing no
melanocytes

Vitiligo

Destruction of melanocytes

Pathogenesis

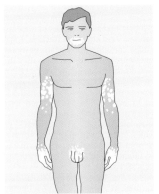

Pattern of distribution

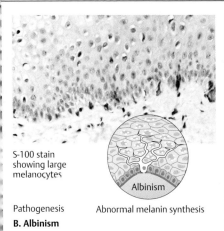

A. Vitiligo

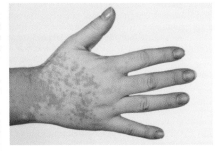

S-100 stain
showing large
melanocytes

Albinism

Abnormal melanin synthesis

Pathogenesis

B. Albinism

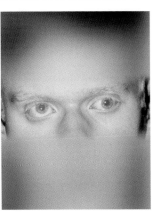

Red eye reflex

A. Melanotic Spots

Melanotic spots have an increase in melanin but not an increased number of melanocytes.

Ephelides. Also known as freckles, epiphelides are most common in redheads or blonds with type 1 Celtic skin; they are typically tan to red-brown on the forehead and across the cheeks, as well as on the forearms and shoulders; they darken with sun exposure and regress somewhat in winter. Other pigmented lesions do not vary in color with the seasons.

Café-au-lait macule. Homogenous light tan macules or patches typically 2–10 cm in size. Present in 15 % of individuals, but five or more in an infant or child suggests neurofibromatosis (Ch. 30.1).

Becker nevus. Hamartoma with increased pigment present at birth; often overlooked until puberty when hairs appear, making it more noticeable. (Ch. 20.3).

Melanotic mucosal macule. Irregular brown-black macules on the lips, buccal mucosa, glans, or labia minora. Sometimes biopsy is needed to exclude melanoma.

B. Melanocytic Nevi

■ 1. Lentigo Simplex and Multiple Lentigines

Lentigo simplex presents with a dark brown small macule with increased melanocytes in the basal layer without nests. It overlaps with junctional nevus but is not related to solar or senile lentigo, which is a flat seborrheic keratosis. Multiple lentigines are markers for several syndromes:

Peutz–Jeghers syndrome. Lentigenes on the lips, perioral area, and backs of the hands are a marker for hamartomatous small intestinal polyps (which often cause intussusception) and increased risk of ovarian and testicular carcinomas.

Carney complex. Lentigines, blue nevi, cardiac and cutaneous myxoma, pigmented nodular adrenal hyperplasia (Cushing syndrome), testicular tumors.

LEOPARD syndrome. Acronym for *l*entigines, *E*CG (electrocardiographic) changes, *o*cular hypertelorism, *p*ulmonary stenosis, *a*bnormal genitalia, *r*etarded growth, and *d*eafness.

■ 2. Dermal Melanocytosis

Blue-gray usually congenital lesions contain dermal melanocytes. The deeper location of the melanin is responsible for the blue-gray-black tones.

Mongolian spot. A blue-gray patch over the sacrum, which is present in 90 % of Asian infants but uncommon in white babies; it tends to regress.

Nevus of Ota. Unilateral blue-gray discoloration in 1st and 2nd branches of the trigeminal nerve, with discolored temple, cheek, and sclera. It is usually seen in Asians.

Nevus of Ito. Unilateral blue-gray patch on the shoulder and scapular region; also occurs most frequently in Asians.

Blue nevus. Localized collection of pigmented melanocytes in the dermis; usually present at birth or noticed in early childhood. Most lesions are blue-gray dome-shaped nodules. Blue nevi that appear in adult life should be suspected of being melanoma and excised.

■ 3. Common Melanocytic Nevi

Melanocytic nevi are benign proliferations of melanocytes and the most common human tumor. In this section, nevus is used to mean melanocytic nevus. They may be congenital or acquired. Most appear at puberty or in young adulthood. They may flare during pregnancy. An average individual has 10–50 nevi, some of which regress. These nevi are symmetrical and regular, tan, brown or black macules or papules, usually less than 5 mm in diameter.

Nevi are traditionally classified on their histological pattern:
- *junctional nevu*—melanocytes at the dermal–epidermal junction (DEJ)
- *dermal nevus*—melanocytes in the dermis
- *compound nevus*—melanocytes in both sites.

There are several clinical types of nevi:
- *Clark nevus*—flat or slightly elevated, sometimes mammillated nevus, often with shades of brown and red
- *Miescher nevus*—a dome-shaped smooth facial nodule, often with little pigment
- *Unna nevus*—papillomatous usually heavily pigmented nevus, generally on the trunk; easily irritated.

Histologic features of benign nevi include symmetry, uniform nests of melanocytes at the DEJ and/or in the upper dermis, and maturation of deeper melanocytes.

■ Dysplastic Nevi

Occasional patients have multiple large atypical nevi that continue to develop throughout life; they have an increased risk of melanoma and sometimes have affected family members. They have been designated as having dysplastic nevus syndrome or familial atypical multiple mole melanoma syndrome.

Melanotic Spots and Melanocytic Nevi

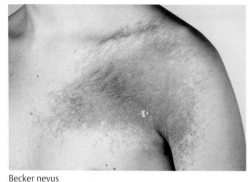

Becker nevus

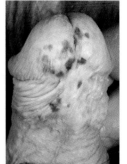

Melanotic mucosal macules

A. Melanotic Spots

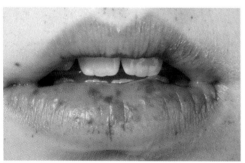

Peutz–Jeghers syndrome

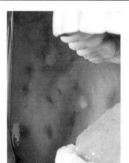

Peutz–Jeghers syndrome

1. Lentigo simplex and multiple lentigines

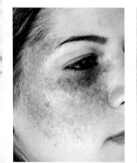

Nevus of Ota
2. Dermal melanocytosis
B. Melanocytic Nevi

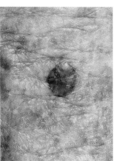

Blue nevus

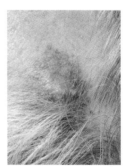

Blue nevus

However, there are no repeatable clinical or histological criteria to diagnose an individual lesion as a dysplastic nevus, or to separate it with certainty from melanoma.

> **Note:** The clinical ABCD rule is helpful for separating unequivocally benign nevi from dysplastic or atypical nevi and melanomas. It is not helpful for separating the latter two groups. The following features help to identify atypical nevi:
> - asymmetry
> - border (irregular, leakage of pigment)
> - color (multiple colors)
> - diameter (>5 mm).
>
> Another way to identify atypical nevi is the "ugly duckling sign"—looking for the one nevus that a person has that is quite different from all the others.

■ Halo Nevus

Also known as *Sutton nevus*, this lesion is surrounded by a halo of depigmentation. The nevus may become pale or even disappear. The histologic correlate is lymphocytic infiltrates at the DEJ, perhaps reflecting autoimmune destruction of melanocytes. A solidary halo nevus is harmless. Adults with multiple halo nevi should be checked for a melanoma, which may trigger an antimelanocyte immune response.

■ Spitz Nevus

This common childhood nevus presents as a red-brown papule, often on the face. Under the microscope, a combination of spindle and epithelioid melanocytes is seen, sometimes with mitoses in the upper reaches. Distinguishing between a Spitz nevus and melanoma is perhaps the hardest task in dermatopathology. Spitz nevi should always be completely excised. Reed nevus is a superficial variant of Spitz nevus.

■ Nevus Spilus

This variant of café-au-lait macule is spotted with multiple small nevi and is often segmental. It often alarms the patient but is harmless.

■ Congenital Nevus

These lesions are present at birth; they are designated as small (<1.5 cm in diameter), medium (1.5–20 cm), or large (>20 cm). Often they contain hairs. Congenital nevi are melanoma precursors. The risk is very small for small lesions (<1 %) but increases to around 5 % for larger lesions. Giant lesions covering a large portion of the body (bathing trunk nevus) including the dorsal midline are at risk for neurocutaneous melanosis. All but the smallest congenital nevi should thus be excised as soon as possible.

■ Differential Diagnosis

The main question is melanoma; other considerations are seborrheic keratosis, Becker nevus, angiokeratoma, dermatofibroma, and adnexal tumors.

> **Note:** The most useful tool in distinguishing between nevi and melanomas, helping to decide which lesions should be examined histologically, is dermatoscopy (Ch. 9.1).

■ Therapy

Ordinary melanocytic nevi require no therapy. If they are cosmetically disturbing or frequently irritated, they can be excised. If a nevus cannot be unequivocally identified as benign by clinical and dermatoscopic criteria, it should be excised and examined histologically. Tangential excisions are best reserved for exophytic nevi; complete removal of the base of the lesion should be aimed for.

> **Caution:** Never treat nevi with destructive measures such as by laser ablation. If a nevus is removed, it must be examined microscopically.

Patients with multiple atypical nevi require monitoring every 6–12 months. Computerized image analysis systems may be useful for those with large numbers of lesions.

Medium and large congenital nevi should be excised as soon as possible. Usually staged excisions are used. Smaller lesions can be watched or excised in adulthood.

Melanotic Spots and Melanocytic Nevi

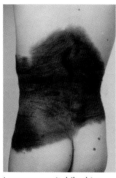

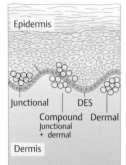
Location of nests of melanocytes

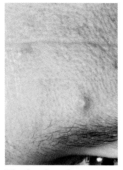
Miescher dermal nevus

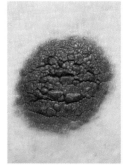
Unna papillomatous nevus

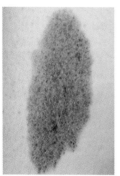
Small congential nevus

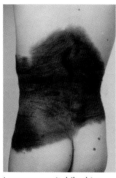
Large congenital (bathing trunk) nevus

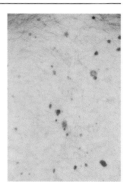
Multiple dysplastic nevi

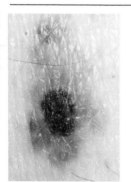
Close-up of dysplastic nevus

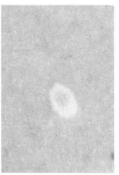
Halo nevus

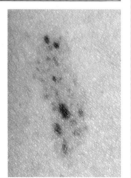
Nevus spilus

B. Melanocytic Nevi

A. Definition

Melanoma is a malignant tumor of epidermal melanocytes with metastatic potential, which causes the majority of skin-cancer-related deaths. It is also called malignant melanoma, but we will use melanoma—as all melanomas are malignant

B. Epidemiology

Melanoma is the tumor with the most rapidly increasing incidence worldwide. Its incidence is 15–20:100 000 in Northern Europe and USA; this is a lifetime risk of developing melanoma of 2%. The risk is inversely related to skin color. The peak age is around 60 years but varies with the type of melanoma; superficial spreading melanoma appears much sooner than lentigo maligna melanoma. Acrolentiginous melanoma is equally common in all races, and thus the most common melanoma of darker individuals. As the incidence has increased, the tumors have been identified at an earlier stage with a better prognosis. Over half of all melanomas are ≤0.75 mm thick, so that >95% of patients never develop metastases.

C. Pathogenesis

■ UV irradiation

Both UVB and UVA increase the risk of melanoma. Intermittent excessive exposure—such as bad sunburns during childhood—correlates better with superficial spreading and nodular melanoma, while chronic long-term exposure fits with lentigo maligna melanoma. Inflammatory cytokines and growth factors may combine with UV to increase risk.

■ Inherited Factors

The genetic contributions are usually complex. For example, pale-skinned individuals with mutations in the MCR1 gene have a 17-fold increased risk of developing a melanoma with BRAF mutation. Other inherited factors include:
- hair color (red 5-fold higher risk than black)
- freckling
- number of nevi (>50 carries 5-fold higher risk than <10)
- >5 dysplastic nevi
- personal or family history of melanoma.

■ Melanoma Genes

A series of gene mutations have been associated with melanoma.
- Mutations involve either signal transduction of a tyrosine kinase receptor (c-Kit, EGFR, FGFR, ErbB-2), the proliferation and differentiation cascade which is triggered by this signal (N-RAS, BRAF, ERK, $p15_{INK4b}$, $p16_{INK4a}$, $p19^{ARF}$, and genes associated with Rb or p53 like MITF), or the survival and differentiation cascade (PI3K- and AKT cascade with PTEN and GNAC).
- Different types of melanoma are associated with different cascades; GNAC is involved in almost 50% of ocular melanomas.
- Abnormal signal cascades may serve as a point of attack for therapy of metastatic melanoma, such as using imatinib for c-Kit mutations.

■ Other Risk Factors

Congenital nevi develop into melanomas in 5%–10% of cases, but make up a small portion of the number. About 30%–40% of superficial spreading melanomas are histologically associated with a preexisting nevus; in the other types, precursor lesions are not seen.

D. Clinical Features

Melanoma can arise anywhere on the skin or mucosa; the clinical spectrum is very broad. The following types are identified, but there are frequent overlaps:
- superficial spreading melanoma (SSM)—the "red, white, and blue" tumor; accounts for 55% of all melanomas, with mean age of occurrence of 53 years. It has a radial growth phase but this is shorter than for lentigo maligna melanoma (LMM). It starts as a brown or brown-black macule which, over months, spreads laterally developing an irregular border and areas of regression. It may also develop a nodular component, suggesting vertical or invasive growth. The back is the most common site in men, and the legs in women
- nodular melanoma (NM)—brown-black tumor with rapid onset of vertical growth phase over months, so that the precursor lesion is not appreciated. Often crusted or ulcerated. It makes up 30% of melanomas; the mean age of onset is 56 years and it has a poor outlook, as it is rarely thin at diagnosis
- lentigo maligna—(LM) is a melanoma in situ in sun-damaged skin, most commonly the

Melanoma

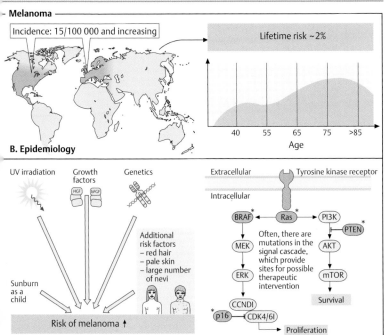

Incidence: 15/100 000 and increasing

Lifetime risk ~2%

Age

B. Epidemiology

UV irradiation

Growth factors

HGF   bFGF

Genetics

Additional risk factors
– red hair
– pale skin
– large number of nevi

Sunburn as a child

Risk of melanoma ↑

C. Pathogenesis

Extracellular — Tyrosine kinase receptor
Intracellular

BRAF* ← Ras* → PI3K
                        PTEN*
MEK   AKT
ERK   mTOR
CCNDI   Survival
p16* — CDK4/6I
            Proliferation

Often, there are mutations in the signal cascade, which provide sites for possible therapeutic intervention

Pink–commonly mutated molecules

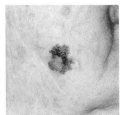

Lentigo maligna melanoma

Superficial spreading melanoma

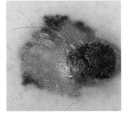

Nodular melanoma

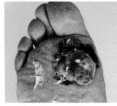

Acrolentiginous melanoma

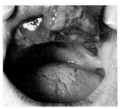

Amelanotic mucosal melanoma

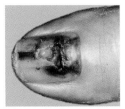

Subungual melanoma

D. Clinical Features

face of women. The irregularly shaped and variably pigmented gray, brown, and black patch spreads for many years. The invasive growth phase occurs as a nodule in the midst of the patch; the tumor is then known as lentigo maligna melanoma (LMM) and accounts for 9% of melanomas

- *acrolentiginous melanoma (ALM)*—located on the hands or feet, often sub- or periungual, or mucosal. It accounts for 4% of melanomas; average age of onset is 63 years. It is equally common in white and dark skin and thus the most common melanoma in black individuals. Histologically and genetically, it resembles LMM. Subungual lesions often have pigmentation of the nailfold (*Hutchinson sign*). Amelanotic subungual lesions are usually missed as pyogenic granuloma.

There are several other clinical variants:
- *amelanotic melanoma*—skin-colored to pink (lacks melanin); thus often overlooked. Usually NM or ALM
- *desmoplastic melanoma*—superficial component is LMM, but the deep portion elicits a desmoplastic stromal response and may infiltrate nerves (neurotropic); often missed as LM and scar
- *ocular melanoma*—usually arises on the chorioid or iris, but can involve the retina. It has a tendency to liver metastases

Note: If a melanoma is suspected during pregnancy, the lesion should be excised—there is no reason to wait!

E. Histopathology

Most tumors can be identified with certainty, as they feature irregular proliferations of atypical melanocytes in both the epidermis and dermis. Melanocytes can spread within the epidermis (horizontal growth phase with pagetoid pattern) as well as invading the dermis (vertical growth phase). They may follow nerves or adnexal structures, as well as invading vessels. Many melanomas are diagnosed in situ with only epidermal involvement.

A great deal of useful information can be obtained by histologic study of a melanoma:
- *adequacy of excision*—the lateral and deep margins must be checked carefully, paying special attention to nerves, adnexal structures, and vessels
- *tumor thickness*—the Breslow thickness or tumor depth (TD) in mm is measured from the granular layer to the deepest part of tu-

mor. It is the most important independent prognostic variable
- *Clark level*—the depth of penetration is based on which tissue level in invaded; scored I–V; this is not as useful as thickness
- *ulceration*—an independent prognostic factor whose presence or absence should always be stated
- mitoses in thin melanomas
- *special stains*—markers for melanocytes such as S-100, HMB-45, or Melan-A are not always helpful in deciding the question of nevus or melanoma, but are extremely useful in identifying the extent of the tumor. Molecular analysis or comparative genomic hybridization may help identify difficult tumors as benign or malignant.

F. Differential Diagnosis

The key question is nevus versus melanoma. Other possibilities include seborrheic keratosis, pigmented basal cell carcinoma, hemangioma, angiokeratoma, pyogenic granuloma, dermatofibroma, and adnexal tumors.

G. Diagnostic Approach

The clinical ABCD rule (Ch. 24.2) helps separate harmless nevi from atypical nevi. Dermatoscopy helps identify suspicious melanocytic lesions that require excision or close follow-up (Ch. 9.1). The patient's entire integument should be examined, searching for other melanomas.

The usual approach is to excise a suspicious lesion, get a histological diagnosis with TD, and then plan the definitive surgery. A partial biopsy does also not help the tumor spread—the patient's usual fear—but is so prone to sampling errors that it is rarely used. Sometimes the clinical and dermatoscopic findings are so definite that only a single surgical procedure is needed.

Preoperative 20 MHz sonography can assess TD, helping in operative planning. The patient should be examined for lymph node involvement, both clinically and with sonography. Baseline chest X-ray, abdominal sonography, and serum S100 levels should be determined; they are useful in monitoring for recurrence.

H. Prognosis

The TD is the most crucial prognostic factor; it correlates in almost linear fashion with 10-year survival. With a TD ≤0.75 mm, the 10-year survival is ≥97%; for >4.0 mm, it is only 43%. Put another way, patients with TD

— Melanoma —

Clark
level

I — Epidermis

II — Basement
membrane zone

Stratum papillare

III

Stratum reticulare

IV

V — Subcutis

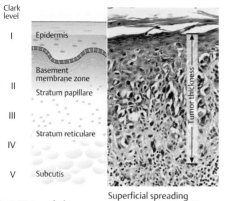

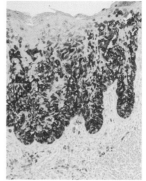

Superficial spreading
melanoma, Clark level II

Melanoma in situ with MelanA stain

E. Histopathology

For high-risk tumors: CT, MRI, PET

Serum S-100 levels for monitoring

Chest X-ray and abdominal sonography

Lymph node sonography and perhaps 20 MHz sonography to estimate tumor thickness

Whole body examination and palpation of lymph nodes

ABCDE rule with dermatoscopy

G. Diagnostic Approach

Most important prognostic factor: tumor thickness in mm

Positive sentinel lymph node

Other poor prognostic signs

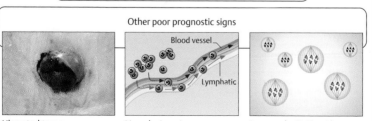

Blood vessel

Lymphatic

Ulcerated tumor

Vascular invasion

Increased mitotic rate

H. Prognosis

<1.5 mm have a very good outlook, although occasional metastases occur. Earlier diagnosis has ensured that melanoma mortality has increased much less than its incidence. Other adverse prognostic factors include:
• ulceration
• mitoses in thin melanomas
• invasion of lymphatics or blood vessels by tumor cells
• positive sentinel lymph node biopsy.

If regional and distant metastases develop, then the prognosis is dismal. Micrometastases have a better prognosis than those identified clinically or with sonography.

Follow-up with clinical examination, sonography and serum S100 is recommended for monitoring therapy, early diagnosis of progression and identification of second melanoma.

■ Metastasis

The risk of and time interval to metastasis correlate with TD. With TD < 1.50 mm, 50% of metastases appear within 26 months; if the TD is > 4 mm, then the interval is 10 months. In 70%, the regional lymph nodes are affected, emphasizing why sonographic control is crucial. Skin metastases < 2 cm from the primary are *satellite metastases*; those between the tumor and regional lymph nodes are *in-transit metastases*. Multiple cutaneous and subcutaneous metastases are not uncommon in advanced disease. Sites of *disseminated metastases* favor the liver, lungs, brain, and bones, as well as distant lymph nodes. The outlook for metastatic disease is dismal; long-term survival is < 3%.

■ Unknown Primary

About 5% of patients with metastatic melanoma have no history of melanoma and no primary tumor can be found. The suspicion is that some cases develop out of a melanoma that metastasized before completely regressing.

I. Therapy

■ 1. Excision of primary tumor

Complete excision of a melanoma prior to metastasis is the only cure. The recommended safety margin for the excision is shown opposite. If there are uncertainties, then the melanoma should be excised in toto and the margins of re-excision based on the histological diagnosis.

■ 2. Sentinel lymph node biopsy

Elective lymph node dissection reduces the risk of local metastases but does not improve survival.

Sentinel lymph node biopsy (SLNB) is widely used for melanomas with TD >1 mm. Using dyes and technetium-99, which are injected around the melanoma or the excision site, the first draining lymph node can be removed. About 20% of patients with TD >1 mm have histologic micrometastasis. These patients then often have lymph node dissection; they are less likely to develop additional nodal disease, but the overall survival benefit is the subject of study. SLNB is clearly of prognostic value; its therapeutic benefit remains controversial.

If a patient has clinical or sonographic evidence of lymph node involvement, then lymph dissection is undertaken without SLNB.

■ 3. Adjuvant Immunotherapy

Interferon (IFN)-α 3 × 10^6 IU 3 × weekly for 18 months improves the 5-year survival in patients with ulcerated or ≥ 2.0 mm TD melanomas and no sign of metastasis.

■ 4. Treatment of Metastases

Surgery of solitary metastases provides about 30% long-term survival. Multiple or nonoperable metastases require chemotherapy; for decades, dacarbazine (DTIC) has been the mainstay, but monotherapy produces up to 10% 4-year survival. With polychemotherapy (carboplatin and taxol), another 5% get long-term survival.

New therapies based on immune activation or targeted intervention with altered signaling molecules have greatly changed the systemic therapy of metastatic melanoma. Broad immune activation with anti-CTLA4 antibodies (tremelimumab and ipilimumab) and DTIC produce 15% 4-year survival. Interleukin 2 combined with peptide vaccine achieves similar results. Imatinib causes regression in the 1–2% of melanomas with appropriate kit mutations, while BRAF inhibitors (vemurafenib) can produce rapid regression but do not markedly improve survival. Solitary brain metastases can be give isolated sterotactic radiation, while multiple ones require whole-brain irradiation as well as chemotherapeutic agent (temozolomide/fotemustine) that cross the blood–brain barrier.

Melanoma

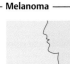

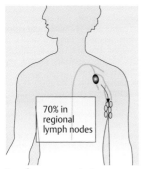

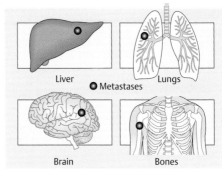

70% in regional lymph nodes

Lymphogenous metastases

Liver · Metastases · Lungs · Brain · Bones

Hematogenous metastases

Stage	10-year survival (%)
TD ≤ 0.75 mm	97
TD ≤ 1.5 mm	90
TD ≤ 4.0 mm	67
TD > 4.0 mm	43
Satellite/in-transit metastases	28
Regional lymph node metastases	19
Distant metastases	3

Survival based on tumor depth and metastatic disease

H. Prognosis

Tumor depth (Breslow)	Safety margin
in situ	0.5 cm
< 2 mm	1 cm
> 2 mm	2 cm

1. Excision of primary tumor

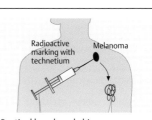

Radioactive marking with technetium · Melanoma

2. Sentinel lymph node biopsy

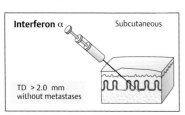

Interferon α · Subcutaneous

TD > 2.0 mm without metastases

3. Adjuvant immunotherapy

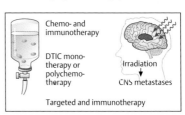

Chemo- and immunotherapy

DTIC mono-therapy or polychemo-therapy

Irradiation

CNS metastases

Targeted and immunotherapy

4. Treatment of metastases

I. Therapy

A. Definition

Vasculitis is an inflammatory condition with damage to blood vessels. It may be primary or associated with underlying disorder (autoimmune disease, drug reaction, infection, malignancy, serum sickness).

B. Classification

The most widely used scheme is the Chapel Hill classification, which is based on the size of the vessels affected.

C. Large-vessel Vasculitis

Temporal arteritis. Patients present with headache, visual disturbances, and a tender temporal artery; it is more common in women. Tongue pain may be an early sign; sometimes there is necrosis in an area served by the vessel. Diagnosis is made on vessel biopsy, showing granulomatous giant cell inflammation destroying internal elastic lamina. Markedly elevated erythrocyte sedimentation rate (ESR) and association with polymyalgia rheumatica.

Takayasu arteritis. This occurs primarily in young Asian women, with aortic involvement, occlusion of the arteries of the arm (pulseless disease), and claudication. Renal disease and hypertension are common.

D. Mid-sized-vessel Vasculitis

Polyarteritis nodosa. This typically presents with painful subcutaneous nodules, ulcers, livedo racemosa, but also leukocytoclastic vasculitis. It commonly occurs with renal disease and hypertension, gastrointestinal problems (ischemic colitis, ulcers), fever, myalgias, and neuropathy; the lungs are generally spared. Laboratory is normal except for rare pANCA. Usually requires prompt aggressive therapy with corticosteroids and azathioprine or cyclophosphamide.

Cutaneous polyarteritis nodosa. This is a pure cutaneous variant with painful nodules along the arteries.

Nodular vasculitis. Variant of panniculitis (Ch. 18.1) with vasculitis, and nodular lesions on the calves. It is sometimes associated with tuberculosis (*erythema induratum*)

E. Small-vessel Vasculitis

Several forms are associated with ANCA (antineutrophilic cytoplasmic antibodies) and usually do not show immunoglobulins (Igs) (pauci-immune vasculitis). All of the ANCA-associated vasculitides may present with leukocytoclastic vasculitis.

Wegener granulomatosis. The main target organs are the upper airways, lungs, and kidneys. Cutaneous involvement includes oral ulcers, pathergy (minor trauma induces diseases), and leukocytoclastic vasculitis. cANCA (cytoplasmic ANCA) is positive.

Microscopic polyangiitis. This form is associated with pulmonary and renal disease but never with eosinophilia or granuloma formation. Cutaneous involvement may occur; pANCA (perinuclear ANCA) is positive.

Churg–Strauss disease. Also known as allergic granulomatosis, this features asthma, rhinosinusitis, and eosinophilia, as well as granulomatous vasculitis. Chronic granulomatous pulmonary infiltrates are found.

Cryoglobulinemia. This is a combination of immune complex damage and intravascular gels of cryoprotein, often secondary to hepatitis C. Acral superficial ulcers are triggered by exposure to a sudden change in temperature.

Urticarial vasculitis. This is characterized by chronic recurrent urticaria with individual lesions persisting >24 hours, and fever, arthralgias, lymphadenopathy, and hypocomplementemia; may be part of SLE.

F. Leukocytoclastic Vasculitis

■ Epidemiology

This is the most common type of cutaneous vasculitis

■ Pathogenesis

Inflammation of postcapillary venules, which results from deposition of immune complexes in most instances.

■ Clinical Features

The prototypical finding is *palpable purpura*, usually on the legs. The spectrum is broad, including blisters, pustules, superficial ulcers and urticarial lesions. In many instances, it is limited to the skin.

> **Note:** All patients with vasculitis should be investigated for systemic disease (especially renal and pulmonary involvement) as well as for possible drug reaction, infection, or autoimmune disorder. If the disease persists or is atypical, an underlying malignancy should be excluded.

– Vasculitis and Purpura

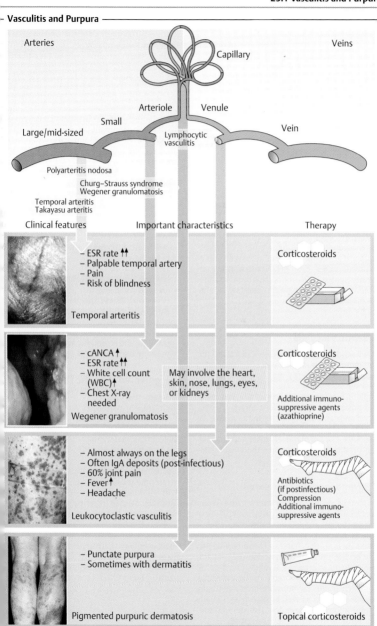

Arteries

Capillary

Veins

Arteriole   Venule

Small

Large/mid-sized   Lymphocytic
vasculitis

Vein

Polyarteritis nodosa

Churg–Strauss syndrome
Wegener granulomatosis

Temporal arteritis
Takayasu arteritis

Clinical features   Important characteristics   Therapy

– ESR rate ↑↑
– Palpable temporal artery
– Pain
– Risk of blindness

Corticosteroids

Temporal arteritis

– cANCA ↑
– ESR rate ↑↑
– White cell count
  (WBC)↑
– Chest X-ray
  needed

May involve the heart,
skin, nose, lungs, eyes,
or kidneys

Corticosteroids

Additional immuno-
suppressive agents
(azathioprine)

Wegener granulomatosis

– Almost always on the legs
– Often IgA deposits (post-infectious)
– 60% joint pain
– Fever ↑
– Headache

Corticosteroids

Antibiotics
(if postinfectious)
Compression
Additional immuno-
suppressive agents

Leukocytoclastic vasculitis

– Punctate purpura
– Sometimes with dermatitis

Pigmented purpuric dermatosis   Topical corticosteroids

A. to K. Vasculitis and Purpura–Clinical Features and Therapy

IV Dermatologic Diseases

■ Histopathology

The vessel wall is damaged with fibrin deposition. There is exocytosis of neutrophils into the dermis with nuclear debris (*leukocytoclasia*), and extravasation of erythrocytes. Direct immunofluorescence reveals deposits of IgG and complement in the vessel wall.

Henoch–Schönlein purpura is a variant, more common in children with gastrointestinal and renal disease, which features deposition of IgA in the vessel walls and kidneys.

G. Therapy

After eliminating possible triggers, the usual approach for persistent disease, especially with ulcerations or arthritis, is immunosuppressive therapy. Most respond to monotherapy with prednisolone 0.5–1.0 mg/kg daily, which is tapered after improvement. Combination with azathioprine is useful for resistant or recurrent cases. The ANCA vasculitides are usually treated with prednisolone and azathioprine or cyclophosphamide. Limited cutaneous disease sometimes responds to dapsone or colchicine.

H. Septic Vasculitis

Small acral petechiae, pustules, and more diffuse hemorrhage suggest vasculitis secondary to septicemia. Patients are ill with fever and systemic complaints. The most extreme example is meningococcal septicemia, but localized pustular vasculitis is a hallmark of gonococcal and candidal sepsis. Disseminated intravascular coagulation (DIC) is a form of septic vasculitis, but the massively distorted coagulation problems dominate, not the vessel damage.

I. Thromboangiitis Obliterans

Epidemiology. Also called Buerger disease, affects 25–45-year-old male smokers. Anti-nicotine antibodies are perhaps causative.
Clinical features. Typically, the legs are affected before the hands. Thrombophlebitis may be the presenting sign. The toes (or fingers) may initially be red, swollen, and painful; then they evolve into bizarre configurate macules with livedo racemosa, which eventually become necrotic, as well as petechiae. Usually chronic and progressive, the disorder is sometimes fulminant with severe gangrene.

Therapy. Treatment depends on the patient ability to stop smoking. Prostaglandins brin some relief. Amputation is often the sad resul

J. Purpura

Purpura is a general term for bleeding into th skin. Small lesions are designated petechiae while larger ones are bruises or ecchymose Small lesions generally suggest a problem wit platelets or vessel wall integrity, while hemo philia or thrombotic disorders usually hav larger areas of bleeding.

There are three general causes:

- *quantitative or qualitative platelet defects* the platelets may be destroyed by autoant bodies (idiopathic thrombocytopenic pu pura), medications, or bone marrow diseas (leukemia), or they may be abnormal (man inherited and some acquired disorders). He matological consultation is usually require to evaluate this aspect
- *vessel wall integrity*—biopsy looking fo lymphocytic vasculitis. Scurvy, Ehlers–Dar los syndrome, and amyloid can all weaken vessel wall. Minor trauma can produce larg patches of senile purpura in sun-damage skin of the arms
- *increased intravascular pressure*—prolonge standing and strenuous activity may eleva pressure and cause leakage.

K. Pigmented Purpuric Dermatoses

Pathogenesis. Increased hydrostatic presenc often coupled with mild venous insufficienc is the main factor. Drugs are an overrate cause.
Clinical features. Primary lesions are 2–3 m red-brown macules on the feet or shins. Var ants include:

- *Schamberg purpura*—most common for multiple red-brown macules
- *lichen aureus*—solitary yellow-brown patc usually over an incompetent vein
- other forms that may be annular, lichenoi or eczematoid; sometimes the lesions c alesce.

Histopathology. Perivascular lymphocytic i filtrates (lymphocytic vasculitis).
Therapy. Topical corticosteroids are used fo pruritus. Support hose may slow progressio

Vasculitis and Purpura

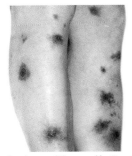

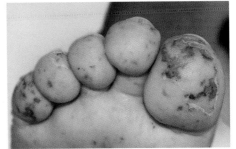

Septic vasculitis caused by *Fusaria* in an immunosuppressed patient

Distal septic vasculitis

H. Septic Vasculitis

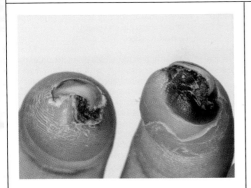

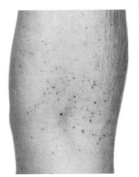

Idiopathic thrombocyto-penic Purpura

I. Thromboangiitis Obliterans

J. Purpura

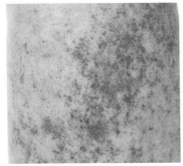

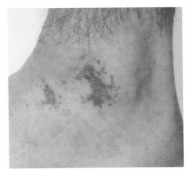

Schamberg purpura

Lichen aureus

K. Pigmented Purpuric Dermatoses

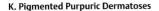

L. Antiphospholipid Syndrome

Epidemiology. Uncommon disorder of young women features:
- venous or arterial thromboses
- pregnancy events (fetal deaths, spontaneous abortions, premature births)
- antiphospholipid (APL) antibodies.

It may be primary or associated with other diseases (usually lupus erythematosus).

Pathogenesis. APL antibodies fall into two groups:
- anticardiolipin antibodies (IgG, IgM)
- "lupus anticoagulants" detected by functional tests.

Lupus anticoagulant is a confusing term, as the factors are not limited to lupus erythematosus and the patients experience thromboses, not bleeding. The battery of antibodies activates clotting factors in vitro and predisposes patients to thromboses (especially anti-$\beta2$ glycoprotein antibodies), even though 30% have thrombocytopenia.

Clinical features. The hallmark is livedo racemosa, a mottled or lightning figurelike vascular pattern due to hypoperfusion from vessel occlusion.

> **Note:** Livedo reticularis or cutis marmorata is normal mottled skin occurring as a vasoconstrictive response to cold. Livedo racemosa is always abnormal and reflects vascular obstruction.

Patients also present with Raynaud syndrome, ulcerations, and peripheral gangrene. Systemic problems include central nervous system (transient ischemic attacks and strokes), pulmonary (emboli and secondary hypertension), and placental thromboses. Two variants are:
- *catastrophic APL syndrome*—sudden onset with small-vessel occlusion in >3 organs; gloomy outlook
- *Sneddon syndrome*—livedo racemosa and CNS problems; not all have APL antibodies.

Histopathology. Vascular damage is hard to see in the skin; biopsy only in the pale area of occlusion, not the blue area of delayed flow. If lucky, a mid-sized vessel with endothelial damage and thrombus will be seen.

Therapy. Over 10% of the population has APL antibodies. Only those with thromboses require treatment—lifelong anticoagulation with coumarin derivatives. Pregnancy management is tricky and involves aspirin and/or heparin.

M. Livedo Vasculitis

This is an uncommon vasculitis, with livedo racemosa and superficial or starburst ulcerations, more common in spring and summer. It heals with white fibrotic scars (*atrophie blanche*) and is only occasionally associated with APL antibodies. Biopsy shows hyaline thickening of the vessel wall. Low-dose heparin is usual therapy; the role of aspirin and platelet inhibitors is unclear.

N. Pyoderma Gangrenosum

Despite the name, pyoderma gangrenosum (PG) is neither an infection nor a vasculitis, but instead a neutrophilic vasculopathy.

Epidemiology. The incidence is <1:100 000; it is often associated with chronic inflammatory diseases (Crohn disease, ulcerative colitis, rheumatoid arthritis) and IgA gammopathy (which it usually precedes).

Clinical features. This dramatic disease is diagnosed clinically by a sudden onset of a red papule or pustule, which dramatically expands into a large flat ulcer with a necrotic base and livid undermined border. The patient is always ill and the lesions are painful. They often have pathergy, developing new lesions at sites of minor trauma like needle sticks. Variants include:
- postoperative PG in surgical scars
- bullous PG, often on the hands and associated with hematologic malignancies.

Histopathology. It is not helpful; there is no vasculitis and only necrosis. Perivascular immunoglobulins are secondary.

Differential diagnosis. Exclude infections and factitial disease.

Therapy. Systemic corticosteroids are essential. Either use prednisolone 1 g daily for 5 days and then drop to 1–2 mg/kg daily, or start with prednisolone 1–2 mg/kg daily combined with steroid-sparing agents (ciclosporin or azathioprine); in either case, the dose should be tapered rapidly as improvement occurs. While wound care is important, it should be gentle; avoid surgical débridement which worsens lesions. Treat underlying disease aggressively.

O. Behçet Disease

Type of vasculitis with oral and genital ulcers, ocular inflammation (iritis, hypopyon), arthritis, and CNS problems. Skin features are thrombophlebitis, erythema nodosum, and pathergy.

Vasculitis and Purpura

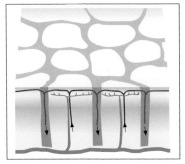

Livedo reticularis: netlike pattern, blanch with pressure

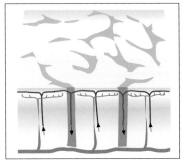

Livedo racemosa: lightening figures, do not blanch with pressure

Livedo reticularis

Livedo racemosa

L. Antiphospholipid Syndrome

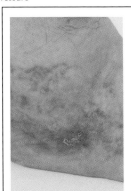

M. Livedo Vasculitis

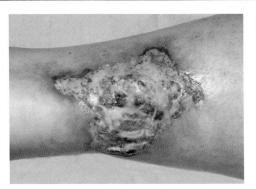

N. Pyoderma Gangrenosum

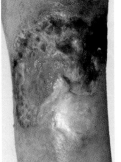

Phlebology is the study of diseases of veins. Almost all venous problems occur on the legs—the price we pay for being biped. Since every second individual has venous problems at some point in their life, the specialty is of great medical and economic importance.

A. Anatomy and Physiology

The venous flow from the legs to the heart goes through the superficial *epifascial veins* (great and small saphenous veins) and deep *subfascial veins* (popliteal and superficial femoral veins). These are connected by the transfascial *perforating veins*.

B. Chronic Venous Insufficiency

■ Pathogenesis

Varicose veins are dilated convoluted epifascial veins. Primary varicosities develop through wall defects, vessel dilation and incompetent valves. Predisposing factors are familial predisposition, advanced age, female sex, pregnancy, hormonal changes, overweight, and lack of activity. The most common cause of secondary varicosities is a deep vein thrombosis with resultant *post-thrombotic syndrome*. The muscle–joint pump fails to adequately drive blood centrally, leading to chronic edema and a cascade of events in the skin and underlying tissues, resulting from chronic hypoxia.

■ Clinical Features

Veins affected by varicosities include:
- *truncal*—involve greater and small saphenous veins; usually the incompetence is at the site of termination
- *accessory truncal*—branches of both saphenous veins are affected by reflux from the main vein
- *perforating*—when incompetent, blood refluxes from the deep to superficial veins; typical sites are just above the ankle or below the knee
- *reticular*—convoluted small subcutaneous veins, often on the lateral shin or in the popliteal fossa. Asymptomatic
- *starburst*—netlike dermal veins; only of cosmetic significance
- *pudendal*—incompetent ovarian plexus; lower abdominal pain (pelvic congestion syndrome)
- *varicosities of pregnancy*—more than 50% of women develop varicosities during pregnancy; in addition to the legs, vaginal, vulvar, and suprapubic lesions are common. Some improve after pregnancy.

If the venous flow is obstructed, the pressure increases with reflux. This leads to *chronic venous insufficiency* (CVI), which is divided into three stages:
- *grade I*—edema, corona phlebectatica (perimalleolar telangiectases)
- *grade II*—edema, stasis dermatitis, dermite ocre (yellow-brown hemosiderin deposits after vessel leakage), dermatosclerosis (reactive dermal and subcutaneous fibrosis) atrophie blanche (white pale scars)
- *grade III*—venous ulcers (usually medial and distal; never on feet or toes).

Symptoms include pruritus or feelings of pressure or heaviness in the legs; these initially improve when the leg is elevated. Later stasis dermatitis and allergic contact dermatitis secondary to numerous topical treatments may develop. Over 70% of leg ulcers are venous in origin, lateral and surprisingly asymptomatic initially. Severe pain suggests an infection or allergic contact dermatitis. Ulcers may spread to encompass the entire circumference (spat ulcers). Atrophie blanche is frequently ulcerated, very painful, and slow to heal.

■ Differential Diagnosis

Other causes for edema (heart failure, renal disease, lymphatic obstruction) should be excluded. Allergic contact dermatitis should be ruled out with patch testing. If an ulcer is lateral, more painful when the leg is elevated or affects the feet, suspect an arterial component.

> **Caution:** When a leg ulcer fails to respond to therapy, always biopsy the edge to exclude an ulcerated tumor.

■ Therapy

Initial steps include physical activity, weight loss, and compression therapy with stockings or elastic wraps.

Starburst and reticular varicosities, as well as the "finger-pointing veins" that often surround an ulcer, all benefit from *sclerotherapy*. Foam sclerotherapy is more effective for larger vessels. The sclerosing material is manipulated to make it foamy; this ensures more prolonged contact with the vessel wall but at lower concentrations, improving efficacy and reducing irritation. *Endoluminal* therapy causes thermal damage with radio waves or a diode laser, which is threaded into a vein.

IV Dermatologic Diseases

Diseases of Veins

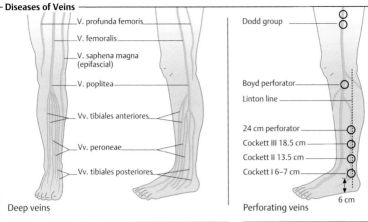

V. profunda femoris

V. femoralis

V. saphena magna (epifascial)

V. poplitea

Vv. tibiales anteriores

Vv. peroneae

Vv. tibiales posteriores

Deep veins

Dodd group

Boyd perforator

Linton line

24 cm perforator

Cockett III 18.5 cm

Cockett II 13.5 cm

Cockett I 6–7 cm

6 cm

Perforating veins

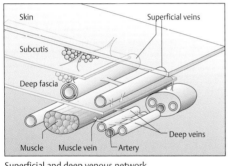

Skin

Superficial veins

Subcutis

Deep fascia

Deep veins

Muscle   Muscle vein   Artery

Superficial and deep venous network

A. Anatomy and Physiology

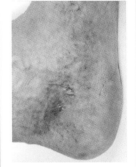

Corona phlebectatica
CVI Grade I

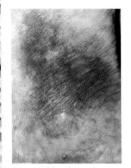

Atrophie blanche and
purpura jaune d'ocre
CVI Grade II

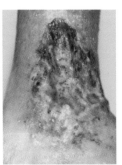

Stasis ulcer CVI Grade III

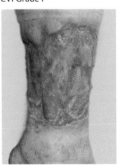

Circumferential (spat) ulcer

B. Chronic Venous Insufficiency

The standard procedure for truncal varicosities is crossectomy, addressing the high-level incompetence by ligating the vein near its end and its secondary branches, followed by *vein stripping*. Accessory truncal and reticular varicosities can be excised through tiny incisions (phlebectomy). Perforating veins can be closed with epifascial or endoscopic subfascial ligations.

In addition to addressing the CVI, the leg ulcer requires specific therapy. It must be débrided, either surgically or with proteolytic enzyme creams. Secondary infections should be controlled with disinfectants, and granulation tissue and wound healing encouraged with special dressings, such as hydrocolloid plasters. For chronic refractory ulcers, a variety of surgical procedures such as shave excision, fibrosectomy, or fasciotomy are available. Adjacent stasis dermatitis should be treated with topical corticosteroids.

C. Thrombophlebitis

The three main factors predisposing to thrombi are known as the *Virchow triad*:
- endothelial cell damage
- reduced blood flow
- increased blood coagulability.

Thrombophlebitis is inflammation of a superficial vein with partial or complete thrombotic closure of the lumen. The area is erythematous and warm, while the vein is palpable as a deep cord. *Varicophlebitis* is an inflamed thrombus in a varicosity.

Clinical features. The affected vein is firm and tender; the adjacent skin is erythematous, edematous, and painful. One-third of patients with thrombophlebitis have deep vein thrombosis at the same time. Duplex sonography should be performed to rule out deep thrombosis or an ascending phlebitis in a varicosity, which can also cause a pulmonary embolus, if it reaches the junction of the great saphenous vein and femoral vein.

Therapy. Mobilization and compression are the mainstays. Often, low-molecular-weight heparin in either prophylactic or a weight-adjusted dosages is used. A thrombectomy via a tiny incision brings quick pain relief. Systemic nonsteroidal anti-inflammatory drugs (NSAIDs) are sufficient for pain. A thrombus near the junction may require an emergency crossectomy.

D. Deep Vein Thrombosis

A deep vein thrombosis is a blood clot closing the lumen of a vein of the deep venous system. It carries the risk of breaking apart, giving rise to a life-threatening pulmonary embolus.

Pathogenesis. The most common causes are prolonged bed rest after surgery and long periods of sitting, as on cramped overseas flights. Risk factors include obesity, pregnancy, estrogens, advanced age, dehydration, and associated illnesses like infections and tumors. Patients with factor V Leiden mutation, protein C or S deficiency or antithrombin II deficiency are at increased risk.

Clinical features. Deep vein thrombosis presents with acute pain and cyanosis and swelling of the affected leg, often accompanied by fever, chills, and tachycardia. The greatest acute risk is pulmonary embolus. A long-term problem is the post-thrombotic syndrome with chronic venous insufficiency.

> **Caution:** In bedridden patients, the signs and symptoms are often less dramatic. Sometimes acute pulmonary embolus is the presenting sign.

Therapy. Immediate anticoagulation is the most important step; low-molecular-weight heparin given subcutaneously and oral coumarin should be started. The platelet count (risk of heparin-induced thrombocytopenia) and prothrombin time or international normalized ratio (INR) should be monitored. When an INR of 2–3 has been reached for 3 days, heparin therapy can be stopped. The oral anticoagulants should be continued for 3–6 months. Patients with a genetic predisposition and recurrent disease are often anticoagulated for life.

Compression therapy should also be instituted immediately; once it is in place, the patient should be ambulatory unless iliofemoral thrombosis is extensive, compliance poor, or home support lacking.

Prophylaxis. Early mobilization, compression stockings, adequate fluids, and breathing and leg exercises should be used. Subcutaneous low-molecular-weight heparin should be used for high-risk situations.

Diseases of Veins

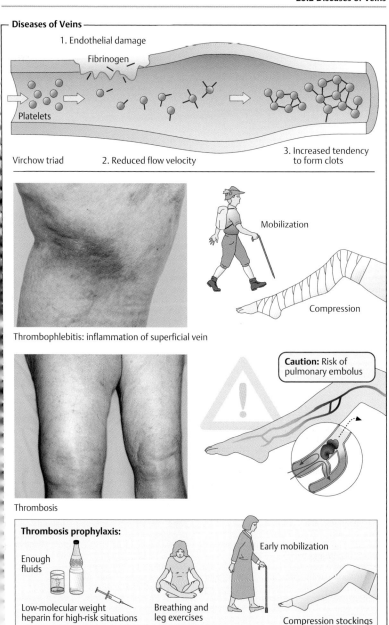

1. Endothelial damage

Fibrinogen

Platelets

Virchow triad   2. Reduced flow velocity   3. Increased tendency to form clots

Mobilization

Compression

Thrombophlebitis: inflammation of superficial vein

Caution: Risk of pulmonary embolus

Thrombosis

Thrombosis prophylaxis:

Enough fluids

Low-molecular weight heparin for high-risk situations

Breathing and leg exercises

Early mobilization

Compression stockings

C. and D. Thrombophlebitis and Deep Vein Thrombosis

A. Epidemiology and Pathogenesis

Acne affects almost every teenager, sometimes with resolution after puberty but often persisting into adult life. The pathogenesis is multifactorial—hormone mediated increase in sebum, disturbed follicular keratinization, and microbial interactions. Increased *fibroblast growth factor receptor*-2 *(FGFR2)* signaling and IL-1/TNF-driven inflammation play major roles.

B. Clinical Features

The primary lesion is a comedo or plugged follicle; it may be pale and closed (whitehead) or dark and open (blackhead). Migration of neutrophils through damaged follicular epithelium leads to papules and pustules. Invariably there is scarring; sometimes punched-out out circular (ice pick) scars; also keloids, mainly on the chest and back. There are many overlapping types of acne:

Acne comedonica. Usually mid-face and temples; this is the earliest stage with comedones.

Acne papulopustulosa. Inflammatory acne affecting the face, as well as the chest and back.

Acne conglobata. Repeated rupture of comedones and papules leads to painful nodular abscesses, which can persist and scar bad.

Acne neonatorum. Comedones and papules in pustules in newborn because of adrenal activity and androgen transfer from the mother; this resolves spontaneously.

Acne infantum. True acne in infants; it starts at 3–6 months, usually in boys, and persists. Parents often give a history of acne and children are at risk for severe acne later.

Acne fulminans. Acute severe acne conglobata in boys; with hemorrhagic jelly-like necrosis, joint pains, sterile osteomyelitis (often of the clavicle), and fever. **Caution:** Acne fulminans rarely is triggered when high-dose systemic retinoids are initiated.

Acne excoriée. Minimal acne with maximal picking. Psychological problems lead to excessive manipulation.

Acne venenata. Acne comedonica caused by cosmetics, oils, and other occlusive substances.

Acne mechanica. Repeated traumas (football helmet, headband, backpack straps) damage follicles and predispose to acne. Comedones in scars or secondary to pressure are often quite large.

Acneiform eruptions. Monomorphic follicular papules and pustules without comedones; these are usually triggered by corticosteroids, psychotropic agents, vitamins, halogenated compounds, or tetracycline. Anabolic steroids can also trigger or worsen typical acne (*body-builder's acne*).

Acne inversa. Nodules, abscesses, and foul-smelling draining sinuses in the axillae, groin, and buttocks; also known as *hidradenitis suppurativa*. It is usually mistreated as furuncles until advanced. It severely impairs quality of life. Late risks include squamous cell carcinoma and amyloidosis.

Gram-negative folliculitis. Monomorphic follicular pustules secondary to selection of Gram-negative organisms through long-term antibiotic therapy (Ch. 33.3).

C. Therapy

Be a friend to the patient. The psychological burden of acne in teenagers can scarcely be overestimated. No special cleansing rituals or stringent diets are needed. Avoid occlusive cosmetics.

Acne comedonica. Topical retinoids initially every other day, advancing to b.i.d. as tolerated; can be combined with benzoyl peroxide.

Acne papulopustulosa. Topical retinoids plus benzoyl peroxide and/or doxycycline. Systemic doxycycline for 6–9 months should be combined with topical retinoids or benzoyl peroxide. Refractory cases, especially if scarring, require systemic isotretinoin 10–20 mg p.o. daily for 6–9 months.

> **Caution:**
> - 1. Isotretinoin in women of child-bearing age is allowed only with effective contraception, because of the risk of severe teratogenic effects (Ch. 10–13).
> - 2. Do not combine isotretinoin and tetracycline; increased risk of pseudotumor cerebri.

Acne conglobata/fulminans. Systemic isotretinoin 10–20 mg daily, initially in combination with prednisolone 0.5–1.0 mg/kg daily.

Acne infantum. Benzoyl peroxide; if stubborn, topical retinoids.

Acne excoriée. Counseling; patients often need psychological support.

Contact acne, acneiform eruption. Avoid triggers; if severe, systemic retinoids.

Acne inversa. Early and extensive surgical excision, perhaps combined with isotretinoin and/or dapsone.

Gram-negative folliculitis. Systemic retinoids and culture-adjusted antibiotics.

— Acne —————————

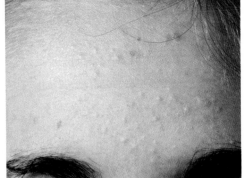

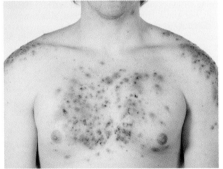

Acne comedonica

Acne papulopustulosa

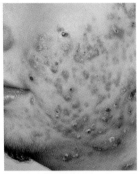

Acne papulopustulosa overlap with
acne conglobata

Acne conglobata from anabolic steroids

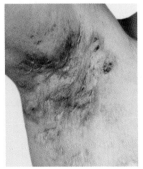

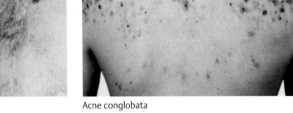

Acne inversa

Acne conglobata

B. Clinical Features

A. Epidemiology and Pathogenesis

Rosacea is a disease of middle-aged adults, with a peak age of 40–50 years. It is equally common in both sexes, but more severe in men. Causative factors include dysregulation of facial blood flow, skin type I–II (fair skin: "curse of the Celts"), chronic ultraviolet (UV) exposure, *Demodex* colonization, and induction of innate antimicrobial peptides. An older connection to gastrointestinal disease has not been substantiated.

B. Clinical Features

Rosacea is predominantly mid-facial (chin, cheeks, nose, and forehead); it may cause burning or stinging. Clinical types include:

Rosacea erythematoteleangiectatica. Transient, then persistent erythema because of dilated vessels, sometimes accompanied by burning. Triggers may include alcohol, warm drinks, hot spices, changing temperatures, and emotional stress.

Rosacea papulopustulosa. Additional edema and nonfollicular papules and pustules; there are no comedones. Occasionally there is extra-facial disease on the upper trunk, and a bald scalp.

Glandular-hyperplastic rosacea. Diffuse sebaceous gland hyperplasia with increase sebum production, lymphedema. A combination of sebaceous gland hyperplasia and dermal fibrosis leads to formation of *phyma*. Rhinophyma is most common, with an initially prominent erythematous nose that can become markedly distorted. Others include gnatophyma (chin) and metophyma (forehead).

■ Special Variants

Lupoid rosacea. Disseminated small red-brown granulomatous papules around the eyes and mouth.

Rosacea fulminans. An acute maximal variant that frequently affects young women, often during pregnancy. Confluent, fluctuant pustules and nodules on the forehead, chin, and cheeks. There are rarely systemic features but there is a severe emotional burden.

Ocular rosacea. Thirty percent of patients have eye involvement with blepharitis, conjunctivitis, iridocyclitis, and even ulcerated cornea. Some patients have eye disease with minimal or no skin findings. This must be managed with an ophthalmologist because of the risk of blinding.

■ Rosacea-like Dermatoses

Steroid rosacea. Chronic topical corticosteroid use on the face may help resolve underlying dermatitis but eventually causes erythema, telangiectases, and pustules. Burns and flares occur when corticosteroids are discontinued.

Perioral dermatitis. Grouped papules about the mouth (with pale spared zone adjacent to vermilion) or around eye. The trigger may be moisturizers, but the main factor is treatment with topical corticosteroids.

Demodicosis. Older adults may develop often unilateral grouped papules and pustules with fine scale, typically involving the cheek, nose, or forehead. Occasionally there are deep inflamed nodules. Lesions are full of *Demodex* mites, which can be seen under the microscope (Ch. 35.3).

Drug-induced rosacea. Antibodies against the epidermal growth factor (EGF) receptor and inhibitors of the EGF receptor tyrosine kinase used for targeted cancer therapy can cause a rosacea-like dermatosis; the worse the rash, the better the systemic response.

C. Therapy

All patients should avoid sunlight and irritating substances. Older preparations with sulfur and resorcin are no longer appropriate.

Mild rosacea. Long-term topical metronidazole 0.75% gel or cream; azelaic acid 15% cream.

Rosacea papulopustulosa. Systemic doxycycline 40–100 mg daily or isotretinoin 10–20 g daily for 6–9 months. Numerous precautions are required (Ch. 10.13).

Rosacea fulminans. Isotretinoin 10–20 mg plus prednisolone 0.5 mg/kg daily for weeks to months, with gradual taper.

Phyma and ectatic vessels. Surgical measures (dermabrasion, shaving) always combined with standard therapy.

Ocular rosacea. Doxycycline 40–100 mg daily for 6–9 months; an alternative is isotretinoin 10 mg daily.

Perioral dermatitis, steroid rosacea. Stop corticosteroids! Doxycycline 40–100 mg daily; consider topical calcineurin inhibitors to control steroid-withdrawal flare and burning.

Rosacea

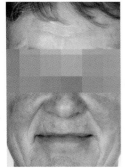

Rosacea erythemato-
teleangiectatica

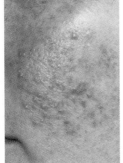

Rosacea
papulopustulosa

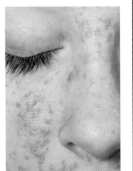

Lupoid rosacea

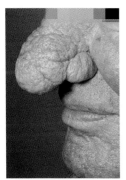

Rhinophyma

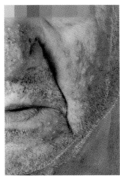

Rosacea-like dermatosis
secondary to anti-EGF therapy

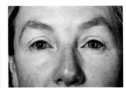

Ocular rosacea

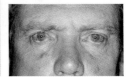

Ocular rosacea with
erythematous papules

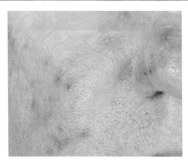

Demodicosis

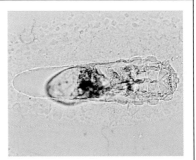

Demodex mite

B. Clinical Features

A. Primary Hyperhidrosis

■ Epidemiology and Pathogenesis

Primary hyperhidrosis is a common disorder, especially in younger individuals; there is up to 100-fold increased parasympathetic stimulation of eccrine sweat.

■ Clinical Features

Attacks of uncontrollable severe sweating on the hands, feet or axillae, sometimes stimulated by stress or heat, but often spontaneous. Patients suffer social and occupational stigmatization because of "sweaty hands" or "stinky feet," as well as increased problems with warts, erythrasma, keratoma sulcatum, and fungal infections.

■ Therapy

Aluminum chloride hexahydrate in 10%–20% gel administered via deodorant roller for axillary hyperhidrosis. Apply in the evening (time of least sympathetic activity) every night or every other night.

Tap-water iontophoresis is best for palmoplantar hyperhidrosis, initially daily until improvement, then several times weekly; commercial units deliver weak direct current in tap water. Home therapy is possible.

Botulinum toxin injections are an effective and safe option for localized hyperhidrosis. Toxin blocks the innervation of eccrine glands. It is costly and must be repeated every 6–12 months for the axillae and every 3–6 months for the palms of the hands and soles of the feet.

For generalized hyperhidrosis, *anticholinergic agents* can be tried, but their side effects (dry eyes and mouth, urinary retention) make use difficult.

Axillary sweat glands can be completely removed by excision or subcutaneous curettage. The ultimate step for hands is endoscopic sympathetectomy; there is risk of compensatory hyperhidrosis at other sites.

B. Secondary Hyperhidrosis

Increased sweating, especially at night, is a type B symptom, raising suspicion of chronic infections, autoimmune diseases, or malignancies. Sweating is an instrinsic part of hot flashes during menopause, along with erythema and warmth. Localized hyperhidrosis may be secondary to nerve damage (carpal tunnel syndrome, cervical rib, neurological disease).

Gustatory hyperhidrosis. Also known as *Frey syndrome* or auriculotemporal syndrome. Following facial nerve injury with misdirected regrowth of fibers, chewing stimulates not only parotid gland secretion but also sweating in the distribution of one or more facial nerve branches.

Eccrine angiomatous hamartoma. Nevoid increase of vessels and eccrine glands that presents with focal sweating.

Granulosis rubra nasi. Nasal erythema with drops of sweat, blisters, and pustules. Only seen in prepubertal children.

Ross syndrome. Unilateral segmental hypohidrosis of the trunk with compensatory contralateral hyperhidrosis. Unilateral lack of pupil and tendon reflexes.

C. Hypohidrosis and Anhidrosis

Reduced sweating with heat intolerance in systemic disorders (renal failure, hypothyroidism, Addison disease, diabetes insipidus) and neurological diseases (leprosy) and with marked dehydration. Anhidrotic and hypohidrotic ectodermal dysplasia are rare syndromes with reduced to absent sweat glands. A side effect of anticholinergic agents is reduced sweating.

D. Chromhidrosis and Bromhidrosis

Chromhidrosis. Exogenous discoloration of sweat, usually by drugs or dyes; there are many different colors (blue, green, red, gray-black).

Bromhidrosis. Penetrating, rancid, axillary odor secondary to hyperhidrosis, poor hygiene, and overgrowth of *Corynebacteria* causing trichomycosis axillaris.

E. Inflammatory Diseases

Miliaria. This results from occlusion of eccrine ducts. When the blockage is within the stratum corneum, *miliaria crystallina* results with tiny clear vesicles. *Miliaria rubra* and *miliaria profunda* have deeper obstruction with inflammation producing red papules.

Fox–Fordyce disease. Skin-colored axillary papules; occluded inflamed apocrine ducts (apocrine miliaria).

Neutrophilic eccrine hidradenitis. Painful erythematous papules on the palms of the hands and soles of the feet, usually following chemotherapy. Toxic agents are presumably accumulated in eccrine sweat, also causing *squamous metaplasia* of the duct wall. It resolves spontaneously.

Diseases of the Sweat Glands

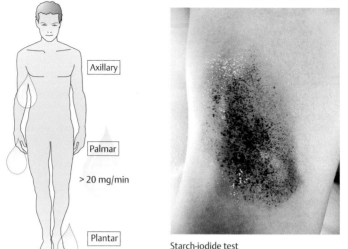

Axillary

Palmar

> 20 mg/min

Plantar

Starch-iodide test

1. Clinical features

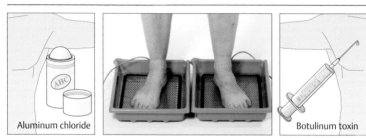

Aluminum chloride

Tap-water iontophoresis

Botulinum toxin

2. Therapy

A. Primary Hyperhidrosis

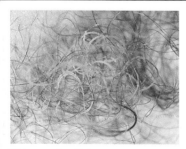

Trichomycosis axillaris

D. Chromhidrosis and Bromhidrosis

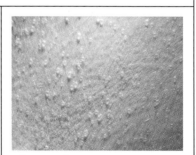

Miliaria crystallina

E. Inflammatory Diseases

26 Diseases of Adnexal Structures

A. Alopecia

Alopecia is loss of hair—usually divided into nonscarring and scarring variants.

Androgenetic alopecia. This develops in 50% of man via genetic sensitivity of the hair follicle to androgens. It usually starts in the 3rd decade, on either the temples or top of the scalp; it then spreads over years; 30%–50% of women develop diffuse thinning with a "widened part" after menopause. It is usually diagnosed by the patient or clinically; 2%–5% minoxidil solution applied 1–2× daily is effective, but must be used lifelong. In men, finasteride, a systemic 5α-reductase inhibitor, is more effective but expensive and also needed lifelong.

Telogen effluvium. Increased loss of telogen hairs months after stress, pregnancy, stopping oral contraceptives, or major illness. It results from alterations in the hair cycle rather than toxic damage, and rarely causes visible alopecia. It resolves spontaneously but causes much worry.

Catagen effluvium. Rapid loss over days of damaged bayonet hairs after chemotherapy or poisoning. Hairs are directly damaged.

Alopecia areata. Oval patches of complete hair loss; patients typically have "exclamation point" hairs at the periphery. It is nonscarring and usually resolves spontaneously but with a high recurrence rate. Hair may regrow with light or dark hairs. The alopecia can become more widespread and even lead to complete scalp hair loss (*alopecia totalis*) or total body hair loss (*alopecia universalis*). There is a poor prognosis with onset in childhood, family history, or associated nail dystrophy. Always check for thyroid disease.

Treatment is with topical or intralesional corticosteroids; larger areas or persistent disease are treated with topical diphencyprone immunotherapy (artificially induced contact dermatitis stimulates hairs). A short burst of systemic corticosteroids may arrest early severe cases.

Scarring alopecia. The most common causes are lupus erythematosus (LE) and lichen planus (LP). *Frontal fibrosing alopecia* is a variant of LP. The two are hard to separate unless there are findings elsewhere. Both are hard to treat. Pseudopelade of Brocq is a controversial form of noninflamed scarring alopecia; we consider it the end stage of LE or LP but others consider it a primary process.

Folliculitis et perifolliculitis capitis abscedens et suffodiens. Often associated with acne conglobata, acne inversa, and pilonidal cysts (*acne triad*), this is most common in black men. Follicular blockage leads to dilated ruptured follicles, which trigger a neutrophilic and granulomatous response. Bacteria are a secondary feature. Surgical removal is often the best approach.

Folliculitis decalvans. Pustules and crusts induced by *Staphylococcus aureus* progress to scarring with "paint brush" hairs. Responds well to rifampicin 300 mg daily, together with clindamycin 300 mg daily for 3–6 months.

Folliculitis nuchae. Keloids on the nape of the neck are far more common in black individuals; ingrown hairs trigger inflammation and secondary fibrosis with alopecia and keloid formation.

B. Hair Shaft Anomalies

Abnormal hair shafts tend to be fragile and break off. No treatment is possible, other than minimizing trauma.

- *Monilethrix*—multiple nodules make hairs more fragile. They break off at 5–25 mm, sometimes inflamed with follicular keratoses. This is most common on the occiput.
- *Trichorrhexis invaginata*—bamboolike junctions lead to breakage after just a few centimeters. Part of Comèl–Netherton syndrome (a rare ichthyosis).
- *Pili annulati*—intermittent pockets of air give hair a blond shimmer. It is not fragile.
- *Trichorrhexis nodosa*—this trauma-induced damage resembles interdigitating paint brushes; once again, hairs break off.
- *Uncombable hairs*—congenital malformation with triangular hairs that defy grooming.
- *Wool hairs*—curly or kinky hairs with axial turn and oval cross-section. This is normal hair for black individuals, but it is occasionally seen in others.

C. Hypo- and Hypertrichosis

These are seen in many genodermatoses—frontotemporal hypotrichosis in alopecia triangularis congenital; focal hypertrichosis is usually nevoid. Medications (ciclosporin, minoxidil) can cause diffuse acquired hypertrichosis. Acquired diffuse fine downy hairs are a paraneoplastic marker.

D. Hirsutism

Hirsutism is male-pattern hair growth in women. Virilism is a combination of hirsutism and altered secondary sexual characteristics. It is often a normal variant, but endocrine evaluation is required to exclude polycystic ovary syndrome and adrenal hyperplasia.

Diseases of the Hair

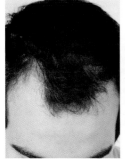

Androgenetic alopecia

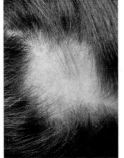

Alopecia areata

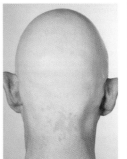

Alopecia totalis

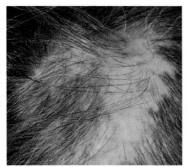

Lichen planus with scarring alopecia

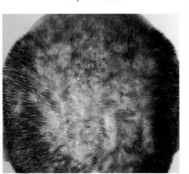

Folliculitis et perifolliculitis capitis abscedens et suffodiens

A. Alopecia

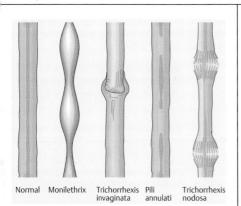

Normal Monilethrix Trichorrhexis invaginata Pili annulati Trichorrhexis nodosa

B. Hair Shaft Anomalies

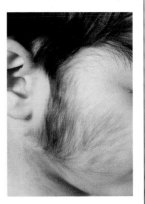

C. Hypertrichosis

A. Changes in the Nail Plate

Onychoschizia. Horizontal splitting of the nail plate, usually caused by a combination of drying and trauma; also seen with lichen planus and systemic retinoids.
Onychorrhexis. Notching and longitudinal splitting of the nail plate; once again, repeated drying is the main factor; others include iron and vitamin deficiencies.
Onycholysis. Partial separation of the nail plate from the nail bed. It occurs when wet work is combined with trauma, lifting up the nail; it can also be drug-related (photo-onycholysis from tetracyclines). Common in psoriasis.
Mees lines. White transverse streaks across the nail following severe illnesses or poisoning (like rings of a tree marking weather). When toxic damage to the nail matrix is greater, furrows may develop known as *Beau–Reil furrows*.
Trachyonychia. Thin fragile nails with a rough surface; seen in alopecia areata and lichen planus; when all the nails affected—*20-nail dystrophy*.
Koilonychia. Spoonlike nail deformation that is sometimes a marker for iron deficiency.
Watch-glass nails. Usually associated with clubbing as a sign of chronic pulmonary disease, the nails are curved and the angle between the nail plate and digit is lost.
Onychogryposis. Claw like deformity of the nail, usually related to prolonged pressure from shoes.
Tube nails. An almost cylindrical or rolled nail, associated with hallux valgus in older women.
Median canal dystrophy. A longitudinal canal in the middle of the nail from the matrix to the tip. The main causes are persistent trauma, as well as nail bed cysts and tumors. It may resolve spontaneously, or if the underlying cyst or tumor is excised.
Ingrown nail. Growth of nail into the nail fold, usually in young men on the medial side of the great toe, caused by tight shoes and incorrect trimming.

B. Changes in Nail Color

Terry nails. Vascular changes in the nail bed in cirrhosis, cardiac failure, and diabetes mellitus cause "milk glass" nails with loss of the lunula.
Half and half nails. Pale proximal and red-brown distal zone in renal disease.
Melanonychia striata or longitudinalis. Brown streaks, common in individuals with colored skin; can be induced by medication. Melanocytic lesions frequently involve the nail bed

and paronychium. A single uniform streak suggests a melanocytic nevus, while an irregular streak or nail fold discoloration (Hutchinson sign) suggests melanoma. Dermatoscopy may help. In case of doubt, then careful follow-up or deep nail bed biopsy, clearly informing the dermatopathologist of the clinical situation.
Yellow nail syndrome. A rare triad of yellow nails, pleural effusions. and lymphedema. The nails are thickened and slow growing; chronic pulmonary disease is common (bronchiectasis, bronchitis, rhinosinusitis).
Green nails. Caused by subungual colonization by *Pseudomonas aeruginosa*, producing green-black pyocyanin. Treat with antibacterial solutions or acetic acid.

C. Genetic Nail Anomalies

In *Darier disease*, nails have multiple longitudinal red and white stripes with distal notches. *Hailey–Hailey disease* has more discrete white stripes. Patients with *ectodermal dysplasia syndromes* have combinations of nail, hair tooth, and sweat gland changes. Painful subungual tumors develop in *incontinentia pigmenti* while in *pachyonychia congenital*, the nails are thickened. *Racquet nails* are short and widened, affecting one or both thumbs. *Tuberous sclerosis* features subungual angiofibromas *(Koenen tumors)*.

D. Tumors of the Nail Region

Verrucae vulgares are the most common subungual and periungual tumors. Bowen disease and squamous cell carcinoma of the digits are often caused by HPV. They are most common on the thumb, tend to be eroded and damage the nail bed and plate. About 3 % of melanomas arise in the nail bed, usually of the thumb or great toe (Ch. 24.3).

> **Caution:** Be suspicious of poorly healing nail injuries; think of melanoma (especially amleanotiuc melanoma) and squamous cell carcinoma.

Subungual exostosis or *subungual chondroma* is a slowly growing spur of bone or cartilage from the distal phalanx, which pushes up and damages the nail plate. *Glomus tumors* can present as blue subungual masses that are tender to touch or temperature change.

– Diseases of the Nails

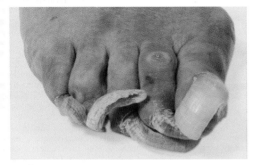

Onychogrypose

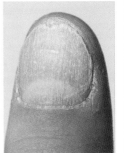

Trachyonychia

A. Changes in the Nail Plate

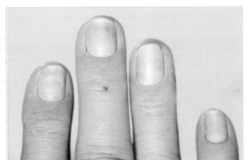

Yellow-nail syndrome

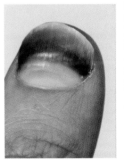

Green discoloration from *Pseudomonas*

B. Changes in Nail Color

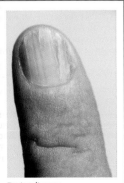

Darier disease

C. Genetic Nail Anomalies

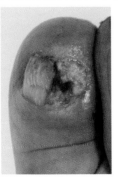

Bowen carcinoma

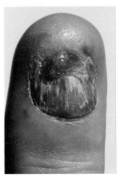

Subungual melanoma

D. Tumors of the Nail Region

A. Pathogenesis

Basic features. Amyloid is an extracellular protein, consisting of small straight fibrils made up of polypeptide chains arranged in β-pleated sheets. It is very resistant to degradation.
Types of amyloid. There are many different sources of amyloid. Examples include:
- immunoglobulin light chains (AL)
- acute phase reaction protein (serum amyloid A protein) (AA)
- keratin (AK)
- transthyretin (ATTR).

Identification in tissue. Amyloid is an amorphous protein that stains positively with Congo red and fluoresces with thioflavine T.

B. Systemic Amyloidosis

■ Plasma Cell-associated Amyloidosis

Pathogenesis. Associated with multiple myeloma and other monoclonal B-cell proliferations and characterized by deposits of AL. It sometimes precedes myeloma, when it is called *primary amyloidosis.*
Clinical features. Vessel fragility; pinch purpura, squint purpura; unexplained hemorrhage. Also infiltrates in the tongue (macroglossia). Deposits in many organs lead to a broad spectrum of changes including carpal tunnel syndrome, cardiac arrhythmias, renal failure, peripheral neuropathies, and gastrointestinal (GI) disturbances.
Histopathology. Amyloid in the vessel wall.

> **Note:** Biopsy the area of purpura. If no skin lesions are present, then carry out blind biopsy of the oral mucosa, rectum, or aspiration of abdominal fat.

Differential diagnosis. Other forms of purpura (Ch. 25.1).
Therapy. Search for and treat underlying disease.

■ Reactive Amyloidosis

Pathogenesis. "Wear and tear" or secondary amyloid, associated with systemic tumors, chronic disease (rheumatoid arthritis, leprosy), as well as familial Mediterranean fever.
Clinical features. Skin deposits are uncommon; renal disease is more likely. There are deposits of AA.
Therapy. Treat underlying disease.

■ Hereditary Amyloidosis

Numerous syndromes usually with cardiac and neurological findings; ATTR is derived from transthyretin, a transport protein.

C. Cutaneous Amyloidosis

■ Nodular Amyloidosis

Large, usually solitary, red-brown plaques or nodules, generally on the legs or trunk; infiltrates contain AK or AA; the latter is associated with myeloma. This is the only cutaneous form that has possible systemic involvement.

■ Lichen Amyloidosus

Pathogenesis. Occurs in response to marked rubbing, which presumably damages keratinocytes releasing keratin into the dermis.
Clinical features. Pruritic lichenoid papules usually on the shins.
Histopathology. Deposits of AK amyloid expanding dermal papillae.
Differential diagnosis. Lichen simplex chronicus or planus; perhaps thyroid dermopathy.
Therapy. Topical antipruritic agents and corticosteroids under occlusion; sometimes systemic retinoids.

■ Macular Amyloidosis

Pathogenesis. Even more dramatically associated with rubbing; also known as "bath brush" or "back scratcher" amyloidosis.
Clinical features. Hyperpigmented pruritic macules on the mid-back in areas that can be reached by the patient. Some individuals have *notalgia paresthetica* (Ch. 14.10).
Histopathology. Sparse deposits of AK amyloid, along with incontinence of pigment (melanin in dermal macrophages).
Differential diagnosis. Postinflammatory hyperpigmentation.
Therapy. Topical antipruritic agents.

D. Hyalinosis

Hyalin means glassy or translucent and refers to proteins that stain in an amorphous pattern. Sometimes such deposits are found in the skin.
- *Lipoid proteinosis*—rare autosomal dominant disorder with abnormal extracellular matrix protein 1. Tiny glassy nodules along the eyelids (*string of pearls*), lips, and hands also in the vocal chords, causing hoarseness

Amyloidosis and Hyalinosis

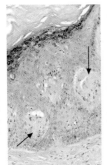

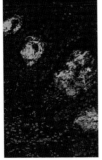

Histopathology: amyloid globules in dermal papillae

Immunohistopathology: amyloid deposits stain with thioflavine T stain

Systemic manifestations of amyloidosis

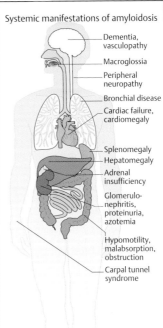

- Dementia, vasculopathy
- Macroglossia
- Peripheral neuropathy
- Bronchial disease
- Cardiac failure, cardiomegaly
- Splenomegaly
- Hepatomegaly
- Adrenal insufficiency
- Glomerulo-nephritis, proteinuria, azotemia
- Hypomotility, malabsorption, obstruction
- Carpal tunnel syndrome

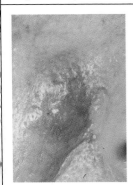

Periocular purpura

B. Systemic Amyloidosis

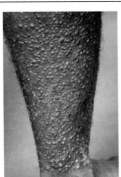

Nodular amyloidosis

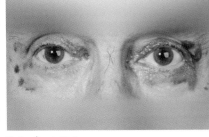

Lichen amyloidosus

Macular amyloidosis

C. Cutaneous Amyloidosis

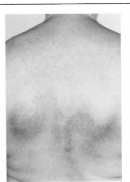

283

A. Overview

Diabetes mellitus (DM) is one of the most common metabolic disorders, with a prevalence of over 5% in western lands; 5%–10% have type I early-onset DM with pancreatic islet cell failure and the rest have type II adult-onset DM with insulin resistance and metabolic syndrome. Psoriasis patients often fall into the latter group.

B. Cutaneous Infections

The incidence of skin infections in patients with diabetes correlates to the blood sugar level and matches the general population in well-controlled patients. *Mucocutaneous candidiasis* sometimes heralds the onset of DM and often indicates poor control. Patients also have more tinea pedis, a particular problem because of their peripheral vascular disease. Therapy is needed to eliminate a potential portal for erysipelas. Staphylococci cause folliculitis and furuncles, often recurrent; streptococci cause impetigo and ecthyma but also necrotizing fasciitis and gangrene. Individuals with DM are at special risk for the latter. Erythrasma is common in the groin in overweight patients. Those with ketosis are at risk for *mucormycosis*, a life-threatening subcutaneous fungal infection of the mid-face.

C. Diabetes-associated Dermatoses

There are many uncommon cutaneous findings that can be associated with DM.
Acanthosis nigricans. Acanthosis nigricans is a sensitive marker for insulin resistance in a variety of syndromes, especially when associated with lipodystrophy. It is also common in overweight individuals with type II DM.
Aurantiasis. About 10% have yellow discoloration of thickened skin of the palms of the hands and soles of the feet caused by abnormal hepatic metabolism of carotenoids.
Bullous disease of diabetes. This rare form of subepidermal blisters is separated from more common autoimmune bullous diseases by negative immunofluorescence studies. It is associated with retinal disease.
Diabetic dermopathy. Small atrophic hyperpigmented patches on the shins are seen in 25%–30% and reflect vessel damage and leakage (*Binkley spots*).
Disseminated granuloma annulare. An association between widespread granuloma annulare and DM has been long postulated but is poorly supported by data,

Eruptive xanthomas. Patients with poorly controlled DM and secondary increase in triglyceride levels may have sudden onset of small yellow papules.
Necrobiosis lipoidica. This presents as yellow telangiectatic scar-like plaques on the shins. About 50% of patients have DM, but less than 1% of those with diabetes have necrobiosis.
Perforating disease. DM patients with renal disease often have marked pruritus, scratch and rub their skin, and develop a severe form of prurigo nodularis, which has been called perforating folliculitis or perforating disease of DM.
Pruritus. DM is one of the common systemic causes of pruritus, often associated with unexplained dermatitis or prurigo.
Rubeosis. Persistent facial flushing may be seen in adults with poorly controlled DM.
Sclerotic disorders. Adults with scleredema present with firm hard skin, usually of the back. There is an increase in both collagen fibers and mucin. *Diabetic stiff skin* typically involves the fingers.
Vitiligo. Patients with DM of either type are more likely to have vitiligo. Those with early-onset disease may have anti-insulin antibodies; both are linked to IL-1.

D. Diabetic Neurovascular Disease

Although there is increased large-vessel disease in DM, small-vessel disease (eyes and kidneys) and peripheral neuropathy are the major players. Both may be reflected in the skin, especially of the foot. Muscle atrophy, bone damage, and abnormal biomechanics combined with lack of sensation (neuropathy) and poor vascular supply lead to infarcts and painless ulcers. Patients must be taught foot care so they or their family members examine the feet daily, alert to early injuries or infections.

Note: Every patient with a painless or slow-to-heal foot ulcer (malum perforans) requires an investigation for DM.

E. Complications of Therapy

Injections of insulin may cause urticaria, although this is much less common with humanized insulin. After long use, lipoatrophy may occur in injection sites; paradoxically sometimes lipomas develop.

Diabetes Mellitus

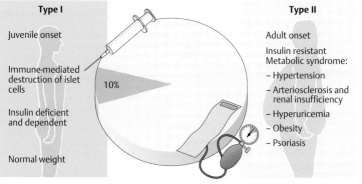

Type I

Juvenile onset

Immune-mediated destruction of islet cells

Insulin deficient and dependent

Normal weight

10%

Type II

Adult onset

Insulin resistant Metabolic syndrome:

– Hypertension

– Arteriosclerosis and renal insufficiency

– Hyperuricemia

– Obesity

– Psoriasis

A. Overview

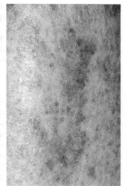

Diabetic dermopathy

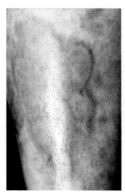

Necrobiosis lipoidica diabeticorum

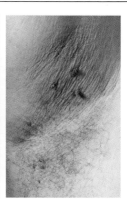

Pseudoacanthosis nigricans

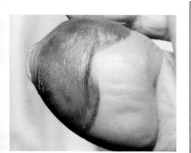

Bullous disease of diabetes

C. Diabetes-associated Dermatoses

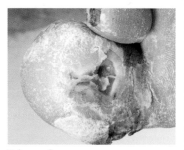

Malum perforans

D. Diabetic Neurovascular Disease

A. Pituitary Gland

The pituitary gland has few direct effects on the skin. Melanocyte-stimulating hormone influences pigmentation, so patients with panhypopituitarism tend to be pale. Acromegaly results from excessive production of growth hormone usually by pituitary adenoma; this results in coarse features, enlarged hands and feet, macroglossia, and acanthosis nigricans.

B. Thyroid Gland

Hyperthyroidism. This presents with warm, moist skin, sweaty palms, onycholysis (Plummer nail), and diffuse alopecia. The most common cause is *Graves disease*, which features orbital disease with exophthalmos, acropachy, and *pretibial myxedema*. The latter shows sharply demarcated plaques on the shins, often with "orange-peel" surface. Biopsy shows massive deposits of mucin.

Hypothyroidism. The most common cause in adults is autoimmune or Hashimoto thyroiditis. Symptoms are dry puffy skin, alopecia, and loss of the lateral one-third of the eyebrows (*Hertoghe sign*). The skin is yellow from carotinemia, but the sclerae are unaffected. Biopsy reveals discrete mucin deposits.

> **Note:** Assess thyroid function in all patients with cutaneous mucinosis.

Thyroid tumors. Multiple mucosal neuromas are a marker for medullary thyroid carcinoma in multiple endocrine neoplasia (MEN)2B syndrome.

C. Parathyroid Glands

Most cutaneous findings occur with secondary hyperparathyroidism in chronic renal disease (Ch. 27.5) with altered calcium metabolism. Pseudohypoparathyroidism is associated with end-organ resistance to parathyroid hormone and cutaneous bone formation.

D. Adrenal Glands

Cushing syndrome. Characterized by hyperadrenalism, this is commonly seen with dramatic skin findings but is almost always iatrogenic following systemic and, rarely, topical corticosteroids. It is rarely caused by pituitary tumors (*true Cushing disease*), adrenal adenomas, or carcinomas. Features include moon facies, lipodystrophy with truncal obesity and buffalo hump, hirsutism, acne and excessive striae.

Addison disease. Characterized by hypoadrenalism, Addison disease is usually caused by autoimmune adrenal damage or tuberculosis. The main cutaneous feature is diffuse hyperpigmentation of sun-exposed skin, the nipples, scars, palmoplantar creases, and mucosal surfaces. Sudden withdrawal of systemic corticosteroids after weeks of therapy leads to systemic features of hypoadrenalism (hypotension, hypothermia) but not cutaneous findings.

Hyperandrogenism. This is primarily a problem in women. After the testes, the adrenal glands are the second major source of androgens. Excessive production leads to acne, hirsutism, and even virilization (Ch. 26.4). Congenital adrenal hyperplasia should be excluded in adults with therapy-resistant acne.

Pheochromocytoma. The adrenal medulla is the most common site for these epinephrine-secreting tumors, which are an overrated cause of flushing but often lead to hypertension, palpitations, and panic attacks. It is associated with neurofibromatosis (Ch. 30.1) and MEN syndromes causing hypertension in both these. About 10% are malignant.

E. Pancreas

Most changes are secondary to DM (Ch. 27.2). *Necrolytic migratory erythema* consists of scaling plaques and crusted erosions at acral, perioral, and anogenital sites that are a sensitive marker for a glucagonoma. Pancreatic disease (both inflammation and tumors) is a cause of liquefying panniculitis, often with elevated lipase levels and saponification (Ch. 18.1).

F. Polyendocrine Diseases

Polyendocrine deficiency diseases. Often autoimmune, with defects in several endocrine glands as well as candidiasis, vitiligo, or alopecia areata.

- *MEN1*—parathyroid, islet cell and pituitary tumors; connective tissue nevi and angiofibromas just as in tuberous sclerosis but otherwise unrelated
- *MEN2A*—medullary thyroid carcinoma, pheochromocytomas, and parathyroid tumors; sometimes macular amyloidosis
- *MEN2B*—medullary thyroid carcinoma, pheochromocytomas, and multiple mucosal neuromas.

Endocrine Disorders

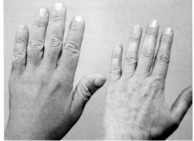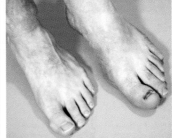

Acromegalic hand and foot in comparison to normal

A. Pituitary Gland

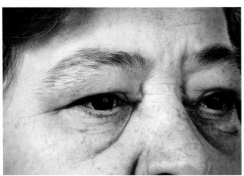

Thyroid orbital disease

Histopathology: mucin deposits

B. Thyroid Gland

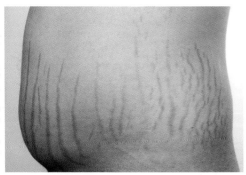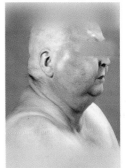

Striae in Cushing syndrome

Moon facies and buffalo hump

D. Adrenal Glands

A. Gammopathy

A gammopathy or paraproteinemia is an increase in the amount of plasma proteins, usually with an alternation of the electrophoretic pattern. There are two types:

- *polyclonal gammopathy*—response of multiple B-cell clones to antigen stimulation in chronic infections and a variety of diseases.
- *monoclonal gammopathy*—plasma cell clone that secretes *M protein*, producing a γ-electrophoretic spike.

Bence–Jones proteins are increased numbers of monoclonal light chains spilling into the urine.

B. Clinical Disorders

Multiple myeloma. This is the most common gammopathy, characterized by monoclonal proliferation of plasma cells with a light-chain spike and depression of other proteins. It appears primarily in patients aged >60 years with M protein and monoclonal overproduction of immunoglobulin (Ig)G, IgA, IgD, or light chains. Bone involvement is the most common clinical finding. Cutaneous findings are rare but can include purpura, pyoderma gangrenosum, and occasionally infiltrates of abnormal plasma cells.

> **Note:** Some patients have a monoclonal gammopathy of undetermined significance (MGUS) and go for long periods without other signs of systemic disease.

Plasmacytoma. Involvement of the skin with infiltrates of plasma cells occurs seldom and late in multiple myeloma. Rarely, *primary cutaneous plasmacytoma* may appear as a red-brown nodule. Because the lesion is small, little M protein is produced and a spike may not be seen, but if monoclonal, progression to B-cell lymphoma may occur.

Amyloidosis. Light-chain gammopathy with frequent deposits in cutaneous vessels, so it may present with purpura, as well as nodules or plaques (Ch. 27.1).

Waldenström Macroglobulinemia. This is a monoclonal proliferation of IgM-secreting plasma cells with diffuse involvement, also known as lymphoplasmacytic lymphoma. The typical cutaneous manifestation is *hyperviscosity syndrome* with impaired blood flow to skin, central nervous system (CNS), and kidneys, as well as bleeding disorder. It occasionally presents with IgM deposits in the skin, known as *cutaneous macroglobulinosis*.

Cryoglobulinemia. Cryoglobulins are monoclonal or mixed immunoglobulins that undergo reversible precipitation at low temperatures. Type I (20%) form is a monoclonal gammopathy usually IgM but occasionally IgG, IgA, or light chains, associated with lymphoproliferative disorders. Types II and III (80%) are mixed cryoglobulinemias containing rheumatoid factor or antibodies (monoclonal in II, polyclonal in III), which complex with the Fc portion of polyclonal IgG. It is caused by hepatitis C or autoimmune diseases such as lupus erythematous and Sjögren syndrome. Patients develop Raynaud phenomenon, vasculitis, and necrosis leading to coalescent ulcers on the shins and ankles. Purpura is more common in type II, often associated with arthralgias and weakness. Cold urticaria also occurs. Kidneys lungs, muscles, and peripheral nerves may be affected.

Cold agglutinin disease. Antibody cause sludging and hemolysis of erythrocytes when the patient is exposed to cold. It clinically mimics Raynaud syndrome.

C. Gammopathy-associated Diseases

Necrobiotic xanthogranuloma. Yellow plaques which almost invariably affect the periorbital region but may appear anywhere; over 90% of patients have gammopathy. Histology shows an admixture of necrobiosis, foam cells, and accumulations of lymphocytes.

Diffuse normolipemic plane xanthomas Widespread xanthomas with normal serum lipid values.

Scleromyxedema. Thickened skin with acral tightening. Patients may also have tiny papules (*lichen myxedematosus*). Unifying features are abundant mucin on biopsy and an association with gammopathy.

POEMS syndrome. The many facets of this rare syndrome are shown opposite. The skin findings include glomeruloid hemangiomas and sclerosis.

Waldenström purpura. Polyclonal gammopathy with purpura of extremities; a small number evolve into multiple myeloma or lymphoma; others have Sjögren syndrome or lupus erythematosus.

Follicular spicules. Crystals of paraproteinemia can be deposited in hair follicles, causing tiny spines. Crystals can also affect the cornea

> **Caution:** Patients with any of these findings should be monitored for development of a gammopathy with underlying B-cell lymphoma.

Gammopathies and Cryoglobulinemia

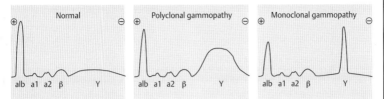

Serum protein electrophoresis

A. Gammopathy

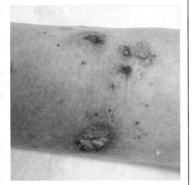

Vasculitis 2° to cryoglobulinemia

B. Clinical Disorders

P	Poly-neuro-pathy		Peripheral neuropathy
O	Organo-megaly		Hepato-megaly
E	Endo-crine disorders		Thyroid disease Diabetes mellitus
M	Mono-clonal gammo-pathy		Monoclonal gammopathy
S	Skin	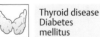	Sclerosis Glomeruloid hemangiomas

C. Gammopathy-associated Diseases

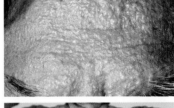

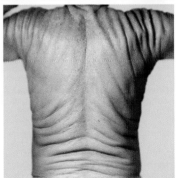

Scleromyxedema

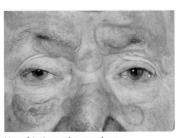

Necrobiotic xanthogranuloma

A. Cutaneous Signs of Hepatic Malfunction

Jaundice. Also known as icterus, patients have a yellow skin color caused by hyperbilirubinemia, due to either hepatic dysfunction or obstruction. The sclerae are also yellow, useful for differential diagnosis because in carotenemia and hemochromatosis they remain white.

Pruritus. Hepatic function should be evaluated in any patient with persistent pruritus.

B. Cutaneous Signs of Specific Liver Diseases

Hepatitis. Hepatitis C virus, and to a lesser extent hepatitis B virus, are associated with a variety of cutaneous problems including porphyria cutanea tarda, cryoglobulinemia, Gianotti–Crosti syndrome, urticaria, and in some populations lichen planus, especially mucosal variants.

Cirrhosis. Presents with telangiectases (spider nevi), palmar erythema, and prominent abdominal veins (caput medusae). There is also gynecomastia, loss of body hair, ascites with secondary leg edema, and easy bruising.

Primary biliary cirrhosis. A combination of pruritus, jaundice, and xanthomas; often associated with other autoimmune diseases.

Hemochromatosis. This is the most common genetic disorder, with abnormal iron absorption and hepatic deposition causing cirrhosis, arthritis, DM, and skin discoloration (Ch. 27.7).

Wilson disease. Autosomal recessive defect with mutations in the gene for ATP7B, an ATPase copper transport protein, leading to deposits of copper in the liver (cirrhosis, jaundice), brain, and eyes (*Kayser–Fleischer ring*—a pigmented band around the iris). The skin is gray-brown. Penicillamine therapy is likely to cause *elastosis perforans serpiginosa* (warty grouped papules reflecting extrusion of damaged elastin fibers through the epidermis).

C. Cutaneous Signs of Renal Failure/ Dialysis

Pruritus. The only cutaneous symptom reliably associated with renal disease is pruritus. Prior to the introduction of renal dialysis and renal transplantation, prurigo nodularis was considered a marker for chronic renal failure.

> **Note:** Nephrogenic pruritus responds well to broad-spectrum ultraviolet (UV)B, but not to UVB 311 nm. Some dialysis filter systems induce excruciating pruritus in rare patients; the only solution is to switch systems.

Perforating disease. Patients undergoing dialysis, especially because of renal failure from DM, are particularly likely to develop prurigo nodularis-like lesions. Histologically, the lesions are centered on hair follicles and may show epidermal perforation with discharge of dermal components.

Calciphylaxis. Patients in renal failure with secondary hyperparathyroidism may develop sudden vessel calcification. Selye called this calciphylaxis as an analog to anaphylaxis but the exact cause is unknown. Typically, there is irregular erythema, necrosis with black eschar and painful ulcerations. Precipitated calcium salts are sometimes found in the skin. It may also occur with massive hypercalcemia in sarcoidosis, tuberculosis of bone, osteogenic tumors, and as a paraneoplastic sign with lymphomas.

Nephrogenic systemic fibrosis. Cutaneous and systemic (often retroperitoneal) fibrosis in dialysis patients, caused by exposure to contrast material containing gadolinium. It may improve with transplantation. Cutaneous findings resemble the edematous phase of eosinophilic fasciitis or scleromyxedema.

Pseudoporphyria. Subepidermal blisters may develop, resembling porphyria cutanea tarda (but with normal porphyrins) or bullous pemphigoid (negative immunofluorescence) sometimes this is drug induced (furosemide, tetracyclines, nonsteroidal anti-inflammatory drugs [NSAIDs]); other cases are idiopathic.

D. Cutaneous Diseases with Renal Involvement

Several diseases seen or managed by dermatologists have a significant risk of renal disease. They include:

- *systemic lupus erythematosus (LE)*—assessment of renal status is crucial in all LE patients; it usually determines the course of therapy
- *systemic sclerosis*—scleroderma renal crisis is potentially fatal; renal disease is a major challenge in managing this disorder. It frequently starts with severe hypertension which must be rapidly controlled, starting with ACE inhibitors.
- *diabetes mellitus*—the most common cause of renal failure and the need for transplant
- many forms of cutaneous vasculitis, especially Henoch–Schönlein purpura, Wegener granulomatosis, and polyarteritis nodosa
- Behçet disease
- genodermatoses, including Fabry syndrome and nail-patella syndrome.

Hepatic and Renal Diseases

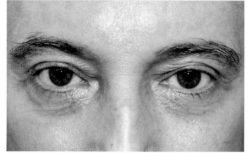
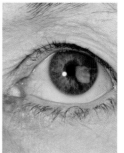

Jaundice of the skin and sclerae

A. Cutaneous Signs of Hepatic Disease

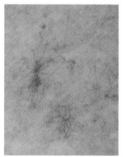
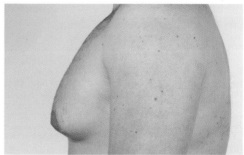

Spider nevi in a patient with cirrhosis

Gynecomastia

B. Cutaneous Signs of Specific Liver Diseases

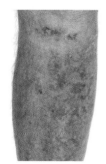
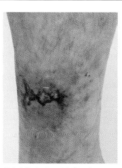
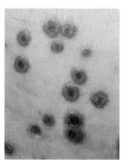

Renal pruritus with excoriations

Calciphylaxis with livedo

Perforating disease of dialysis

C. Cutaneous Signs of Renal Failure/Dialysis

A. Cutaneous Signs of Gastrointestinal Disease

Esophagus
- *Mucositis*—Stevens–Johnson syndrome, Behçet syndrome, pemphigus, epidermolysis bullosa
- *Systemic sclerosis*—often impaired esophageal motility with difficulty swallowing
- *Plummer–Vinson syndrome*—esophageal web, clubbed fingers, iron deficiency, and risk of carcinoma
- *Howel–Evans syndrome*—tylosis in childhood and high risk of esophageal carcinoma as an adult

Pancreas
- Liquefying panniculitis is a sign of pancreatic inflammation and tumors.
- Superficial migratory thrombophlebitis and other unexplained thromboses are associated with pancreatic carcinoma.

> **Note:** Always exclude pancreatic carcinoma in any patient with unexplained panniculitis or thrombophlebitis.

- Necrolytic migratory erythema is a marker for glucagonoma; differential diagnosis includes zinc deficiency (acrodermatitis enteropathica).
- Periumbilical (*Cullen sign*) and flank (*Gray–Turner sign*) hemorrhage may be a clue to pancreatic disease.

Gastrointestinal Tract
- *Gastrointestinal bleeding*—associated with vasculitis, hereditary hemorrhagic telangiectasia with perioral telangiectases, pulmonary arteriovenous fistulas, vascular tumors, both benign (blue rubber bleb nevus) and malignant (Kaposi sarcoma), connective tissue defects (vascular form of Ehlers–Danlos, pseudoxanthoma elasticum), systemic corticosteroids, and NSAIDs.
- *Polyposis*—several syndromes can be associated with GI polyps and skin disease, as shown opposite.
- *Malabsorption*—many nutrients are poorly absorbed, leading to dry scaly skin, pruritus, diffuse nonscarring alopecia, and slow-growing, brittle nails. Associated diseases may include celiac disease with dermatitis herpetiformis, acrodermatitis enteropathica with zinc deficiency, and collagen vascular diseases.

Rectum. Extramammary Paget disease may reflect underlying rectal carcinoma.

B. Cutaneous Signs of Gastrointestinal Malignancy

The gastrointestinal tract is the site of many tumors including the common carcinoma of the colon, as well as the most fatal human carcinoma—pancreatic carcinoma. There are both syndrome-related and acquired cutaneous markers of such malignancies, which can also metastasize directly to the skin:
- acanthosis nigricans (Ch. 27.9)

> **Note:** Always evaluate any adult with recent onset of acanthosis nigricans for GI tumors.

- Sister Mary Joseph nodule—metastasis to the umbilicus from an abdominal tumor
- vasoactive syndromes—ectopic hormone production may lead to flushing and diarrhea (Zollinger–Ellison syndrome)
- glucagonoma syndrome (Ch. 27.9).

C. Inflammatory Bowel Disease

There are two common inflammatory bowel diseases, with overlapping GI and skin features.

Crohn disease. Granulomatous inflammation of the bowel wall; a microorganism has long been suspected but never found. It may result from aberrant regulation of innate immunity; it usually starts in the small intestine. Skin findings include:
- perianal granulomatous inflammation with fissures; may extend to involve the genitalia
- "metastatic" Crohn disease—cutaneous granulomas not located in the perianal region
- erythema nodosum
- granulomatous cheilitis—lip granulomas similar to those found in the gut
- frequent or severe aphthae
- pyoderma gangrenosum.

Ulcerative colitis. This is a more intense inflammatory disease with a similar etiology; it almost always starts in the colon or rectum. Skin features include:
- pyoderma gangrenosum
- erythema nodosum.

— Gastrointestinal Diseases ——

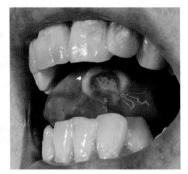

Behçet disease

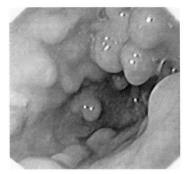

Polyposis in Peutz–Jeghers syndrome

Cutaneous syndromes associated with gastrointestinal polyposis

Syndrome	Cutaneous findings
Cowden syndrome	Acral and facial papules, multiple hamartomas
Gardner syndrome	Multiple epidermal cysts
Peutz–Jeghers syndrome	Lentigines on lips, hands, and feet

A. Cutaneous Signs of Gastrointestinal Disease

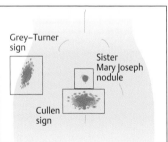

Grey–Turner sign

Sister Mary Joseph nodule

Cullen sign

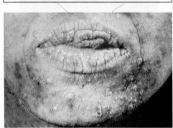

Acanthosis nigricans

B. Cutaneous Signs of Gastrointestinal Malignancy

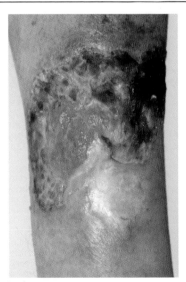

Pyoderma gangrenosum

C. Inflammatory Bowel Disease

A. Disorders of Lipid Metabolism

Patients with elevated cholesterol and/or triglycerides may present with *xanthomas*—cutaneous lipid deposits. Predisposing factors include genetic abnormalities, diet, and metabolic syndrome (DM, obesity, gout), as well as hypothyroidism. Not all xanthomas are associated with lipid abnormalities; sometimes normolipemic xanthomas are seen.

■ Types of Xanthomas

- *Xanthelasma*—yellow plaques about the eyes; the most common xanthoma but only associated with lipid disturbances in 50%; can be excised or laser-ablated.
- *Eruptive xanthoma*—small red-yellow papules appearing in crops, often over pressure points such as the digits or buttocks. It is a marker for familial hypertriglyceridemia.
- *Tendon xanthomas*—bulky deposits attached to tendons, especially Achilles, patellar, and back of the hand. Markers for familial hypercholesterolemia, familial defective apolipoprotein B-100, and familial dysbetalipoproteinemia; also seen in normolipemic xanthomas.
- *Tuberous xanthomas*—large symmetric nodules over knees, elbows, hands, and feet; associated with the same defects as tendon xanthomas.
- *Palmar crease xanthomas*—tiny yellow papules in the palmar creases are very suggestive of familial dysbetalipoproteinemia.

Therapy. When the lipid disturbance is treated, many xanthomas will resolve.

B. Gout

Gout is caused by an excess of uric acid, modified by diet, inflammation, medications, and associated diseases (leukemia). It affects the joints, especially the great toe (*podagra*), and kidneys (both stones with colic and renal damage). The urate crystals cause fever, leukocytosis, and elevated erythrocyte sedimentation rate (ESR), thus mimicking an infection. Acute disease is treated with NSAIDs; allopurinol, used to reduce uric acid levels, is one of the main causes of severe skin reactions.

Tophi are subcutaneous uric acid nodules, most common around joints (differential diagnosis rheumatoid nodule) and ear (differential diagnosis chondrodermatitis nodularis chronica helicis, Ch.22.1). Therapy is excision.

C. Hemochromatosis

This is the most common genetic disorder, with a prevalence of 500:100 000, caused by mutations in several genes that are important in iron uptake and transport. M:F ratio is 8:1, presumably because of the protective effect of menstruation. Secondary hemochromatosis occurs after multiple transfusions with iron overload.

There is a wide variety of problems all caused by tissue hemosiderin deposition, including arthritis, DM, cirrhosis, and hypogonadism. The skin is often darkened (*bronze diabetes*) because of increased melanin. Patients have severe pruritus, which is helped by broad-spectrum UVB therapy.

D. Calcification

Cutaneous calcification may be associated with elevated serum calcium levels secondary to parathyroid disease or malignancies. Any tissue that is damaged can become calcified. Subcutaneous calcification is very common in systemic sclerosis (Ch.17.4) where calcified tissues may be extruded through acral ulcers. Other commonly calcified lesions include pseudoxanthoma elasticum, trichilemmal cysts, pilomatricoma, and chronic stasis dermatitis. Calciphylaxis refers to sudden dramatic calcification and is discussed with renal disease (Ch.27.5).

E. Fabry Disease

Fabry disease is a rare disorder inherited in X-linked recessive fashion, with deficiency of α-galactosidase A leading to deposition of ceramide trihexoside in endothelial and muscle cells. The main clinical problems are renal failure, painful peripheral neuropathies, cardiac disease, and thromboses. Corneal opacities (cornea verticillata) aid in diagnosis. The first clinical finding is often angiokeratomas, small ruby red vascular tumors (Ch.22.6) around the umbilicus. Urine microscopy with polarized light may show a "Maltese cross" appearance (birefringent lipid molecules).

Therapy. Treatable by gene-replacement therapy; two replacement enzymes are available. In addition, stem cell transplantation can restore enzyme activity.

– Metabolic Diseases

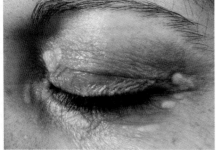

Xanthelasmas

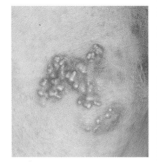

Xanthomas

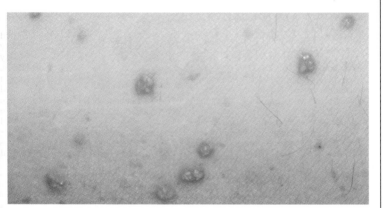

Eruptive xanthomas

A. Disorders of Lipid Metabolism

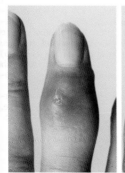

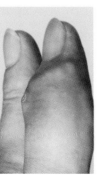

B. Gout

Histopathology: uric acid crystals

A. Neuropathic Skin Disease

Neuropathic changes result from loss of sympathetic and sensory cutaneous innervation, such as in a polyneuropathy or paraplegia.

Clinical features. Several unique findings help identify skin with neuropathic changes:

- *Madonna fingers*—long thin fingers with little subcutaneous fat
- failure to develop wrinkling following immersion of the hands in warm water
- loss of skin lines
- increased skin fragility
- changes in the temperature and color of the skin (due to vascular denervation and to disturbance of pigmentation)
- the nails develop striations and ridges and lose their luster
- both hyper- and hypotrichosis develop in denervated skin
- abnormalities of sweating resulting from autonomic damage or malfunction:
  - anhidrosis when the nerve supply is completely lost
  - hyperhidrosis with partial denervation or reinnervation
  - dyshidrosis with abnormal branching and reinnervation. *Frey syndrome* refers to erythema and sweating of the cheek with eating, following auriculotemporal nerve injury, usually through parotid gland surgery where the parasympathetic nerves previously serving salivary glands connect with sweat glands.

Neuropathic ulcer. Abnormally innervated skin is more likely to develop ulceration. Common causes of neuropathy include DM, alcoholism, tuberculoid leprosy, syphilis, and HIV/AIDS. A classic example is *diabetic foot ulcer*—a combination of both sensory and autonomic neuropathy with impaired perfusion and loss of pain sensation that facilitates the development of ulcers at pressure points and retards healing. Ulcers are most likely to occur under callus. Proper foot care and special shoes are most important.

Note: Loss of pain sensation produces a major defect in the body's protection. Failure to recognize damage may lead to severe ulcers.

B. Neurocutaneous Diseases

■ Inherited Diseases

- Several genodermatoses (neurofibromatosis, tuberous sclerosis—both Ch. 30.1) invariably involve both systems.

- Fabry disease (Ch. 27.7) may present with severe peripheral neuropathies.
- Ataxia-telangiectasia often starts with conjunctival telangiectases; patients soon develop severe ataxia (Ch. 30.1).
- Familial dysautonomia (*Riley–Day* syndrome) is an autosomal recessive disorder in Ashkenazi Jews, with defective tearing, skin flushing, and *total absence of pain sensation.*
- Some ichthyoses with lipid abnormalities also have CNS problems.
- Pigmentary disorders may be coupled with ocular or hearing problems.
- Midline hemangiomas may be associated with variety of CNS problems (*PHACE syndrome*) (Ch. 22.5).

Note: Any patient with midline skin lesions of the sacrum (even hypertrichosis) should be evaluated for possible underlying spinal column and cord defects.

■ Infectious Diseases

- Herpes simplex "hides" in sensory nerves; recurrences are preceded by tingling and pain.
- Herpes zoster follows dermatomal distribution, it always affects nerves, and may cause long-term severe pain (*postherpetic neuralgia*).
- Borreliosis may cause Bannwarth syndrome (lymphocytic meningoradiculitis) as well a a variety of other neurologic findings, including facial nerve paralysis, sensory and motor neuropathies, and meningeal signs.
- Late syphilis almost always has CNS and spinal neurological findings. In the secondary stage, CNS and peripheral nerves are occasionally affected; in HIV patients, changes may occur at an earlier stage.
- Tuberculoid leprosy has profound sensory defects, which lead to ulcers and mutilating injuries. Nerves in cooler body regions are most affected.
- *Neisseria meningitidis* causes septic purpuric vasculitis, often as a warning sign of impending meningitis.

■ Miscellaneous Disorders

- Angioedema may be associated with facial nerve palsy.
- Melkersson–Rosenthal syndrome features granulomatous cheilitis, plicated tongue, and facial nerve palsy.

Neurologic Diseases

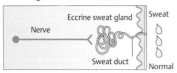

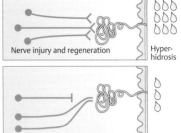

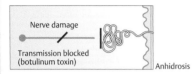

Disturbances in sweating

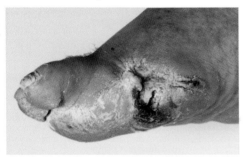

Neuropathic ulcer with callus in diabetes mellitus

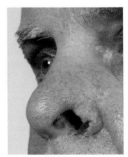

Neuropathic ulcer after stroke with hemiparesis

Clinical features

A. Neuropathic Skin Disease

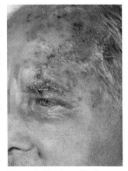

Zoster in first branch of trigeminal nerve

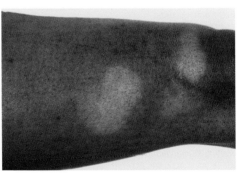

Hypopigmented anesthetic macules in leprosy

B. Neurocutaneous Diseases

27 Cutaneous Signs of Systemic Diseases

297

A. Cutaneous Signs of Internal Malignancy

A paraneoplastic sign is one that is associated with a malignancy but does not involve direct extension or metastasis. It must fulfil the following criteria:

- no other explanation for the disease
- statistical connection is shown
- skin changes appear at about the same time as the malignancy or they may precede any clinical manifestations of the underlying cancer
- skin changes improve with cancer treatment and may reappear if cancer recurs.

B. Obligate Paraneoplastic Markers

Some cutaneous findings almost always indicate an underlying malignancy.

Acanthosis nigricans. Velvety plaques are seen in the flexures, consisting of hundreds of tiny filiform papules, which, under the microscope, look like tiny seborrheic keratoses. It is associated with insulin resistance and obesity. It is caused by stimulation of epidermal or fibroblast growth factor receptor by insulin, tumor products, or other unknown triggers.

When an adult who is not overweight presents with acanthosis nigricans, he must be investigated for underlying GI malignancy. Variants of acanthosis nigricans include:

- *Leser–Trélat sign*—sudden appearance of multiple small seborrheic keratoses
- *florid cutaneous papillomatosis*—sudden appearance of many tiny human papillomavirus (HPV)-negative "warts"
- *tripe palms*—pebbly palms
- *florid oral papillomatosis*—similar changes in the oral mucosa.

Erythema gyratum repens. This is the most distinctive annular erythema; 1–2 cm wide bands create a "wood grain" pattern rapidly moving across the skin, changing over hours. There are much more complex patterns and rapid change compared to erythema annulare centrifugum.

Necrolytic migratory erythema. An annular scaly migratory erythema coupled with severe periorificial and periungual erosions (often confused with candidiasis); it is a marker for glucagonoma but occasionally seen with other pancreatic disease or zinc deficiency. There is a combination of acral and periorificial erosions and crusts with migratory erythematous patches on the trunk and thighs.

Hypertrichosis lanuginosa acquisita. Rapid appearance of fine, nonpigmented lanugo hairs covering the body.

Acrokeratosis Bazex. Dirty hyperkeratotic lesions on the digits, nose, and rim of the ears as a marker for airway carcinoma.

Paraneoplastic pemphigus. Bullous disease with features of both pemphigus and erythema multiforme; it usually presents with oral erosions and erythematous macules or patches. It is always associated with malignancy, usually lymphoma or Castleman tumor (Ch. 14.11).

Necrobiotic xanthogranuloma, diffuse normolipemic plane xanthoma. These are reliable markers for gammopathy (Ch. 27.4).

C. Possible Paraneoplastic Markers

There are many other situations where a search for associated malignancy is warranted even though the association is not as strong as in the above examples.

Dermatomyositis. 20–50 % of adults with rapidly progressive or refractory dermatomyositis have an underlying malignancy; ovarian tumors are especially common.

Thromboses. Unexplained thromboses may reflect an underlying tumor; the most common associations are prostate, cervical, and ovarian carcinomas.

Recurrent thrombophlebitis. Also known as *Trousseau sign*, this is a classic marker for carcinoma of the pancreas but can reflect a variety of internal malignancies.

Panniculitis. If above the knees or liquefying, it may be a sign of pancreatic carcinoma.

Pyoderma gangrenosum. Unexplained severe, rapidly enlarging ulceration with an undermined border. Marker for gammopathy, hematologic malignancy and inflammatory bowel disease (Ch. 25.1).

Sweet syndrome. Juicy red plaques full of neutrophils in a patient with fever; this is most often idiopathic but may be a sign of leukemia (Ch. 17.2).

Pachydermoperiostosis. A rare condition with thickening of the skin, nail clubbing, and hypertrophic osteoarthropathy. It is a marker for lung cancer or pulmonary disease.

Flushing. If no other explanation is available, flushing may reflect carcinoid tumor or pheochromocytoma.

Vitiligo. All adults with recent onset of vitiligo should be checked for possible malignant melanoma, especially one with signs of regression.

Paraneoplastic Disorders

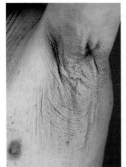
Acanthosis nigricans

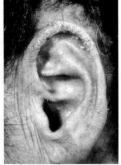
Acrokeratosis Bazex

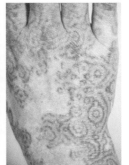
Erythema gyratum repens

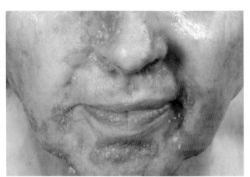
Glucagonoma syndrome

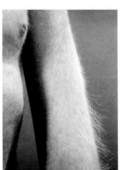
Hypertrichosis lanuginosa acquisita

B. Obligate Paraneoplastic Markers

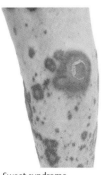
Sweet syndrome

Panniculitis

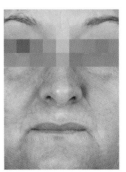
Dermatomyositis

C. Possible Paraneoplastic Markers

A. Unique Features of Infantile Skin

At birth the skin is covered by the vernix caseosa (cheesy varnish), a white mixture of sebum and shed scales that resembles a soft cheese. The skin adjusts rapidly to the extrauterine environment and most adult functions are present by 6 months. However, there are some important distinguishing features of infant skin:

- less mechanical resistance leads to more injuries and quicker blister formation. The epidermis is thinner and the keratinocytes are less well anchored to one another. The dermis is thinner and the collagen and elastic fibers thinner and shorter
- the barrier function is less developed so the skin is more sensitive to irritants
- the surface:volume ratio in an infant is unfavorable, increasing the risk of transcutaneous intoxication by absorption
- infants tend to sunburn easily, as they do not tan well
- thermoregulation is not as effective. The sweat glands are not functional in the first weeks of life and the autonomic regulation of vascular tone is poorly developed
- reduced defense against infections because both cellular and humoral immunity requires months to become functional. There is a gap as maternally transferred antibodies disappear and infant-made ones are slow to appear.

B. Skin Diseases in Infancy

■ Skin Findings at Birth

Almost every infant has some skin finding at birth. Some of the more dramatic ones include:

- widespread blisters or erosions may indicate epidermolysis bullosa (Ch. 16.1)
- sometimes an ulcer or scar is seen on the vertex; this represents *aplasia cutis congenita* where the skin has failed to fuse during embryologic life
- a firm papule anterior to the ear is a cartilaginous rest known as an *accessory tragus*, often associated with pits, fistulas, or sinuses, and reflects aberrations in the complex embryology of the head and neck
- vascular malformations such as port-wine stains are present at birth; the infant should be checked for associated anomalies (Ch. 22.4). Hemangiomas generally appear after a few weeks of life (Ch. 22.5)
- congenital melanocytic nevi (Ch. 24.2), especially large ones, should be evaluated for early therapy.

■ Neonatal Diseases

Erythema toxicum neonatorum. Between 30% and 70% of all newborns develop disseminated erythematous papules and sterile pustules. The palms of the hands and soles of the feet are spared and resolution is rapid and spontaneous.

Transient neonatal melanosis. At birth both intact pustules and ruptured crusted lesions with postinflammatory hyperpigmentation are seen. This also resolves spontaneously.

Neonatal cephalic pustulosis. *Malassezia*-associated pustules on the scalp and face that respond to topical imidazoles.

Acne neonatorum. About 20% of infants have comedones on the cheeks, more often in boys. It resolves spontaneously, in contrast to acne infantum (Ch. 26.1) which occurs later and carries more risk of severe acne later in life.

Milia. About 40% of newborns develop milia (tiny occluded follicular cysts) or have prominent sebaceous glands on the face.

> **Caution:** The classic childhood infections all follow a much more aggressive course in the neonatal period. Varicella, herpes simplex, and staphylococcal infections are the most dangerous and all require expert consultation and immediate systemic therapy.

■ Diseases of Infancy

Diaper dermatitis. The most common infantile skin disease results from occlusion of stool and urine between the skin and diaper. It is much less of a problem with superabsorbent diapers. When severe, infants may develop inverse psoriasis or atopic dermatitis.

Atopic dermatitis. Also very common, this affects up to 15% of infants and typically starts at 3–6 months of age. Typical features in this age group are intense pruritus, exudative, superinfected dermatitis, excoriations, and prominent scalp crusting (Ch. 14.4).

Infantile acropustulosis. Sterile acral pustules often confused with scabies, and in some cases the disorder may follow a true scabies infestation. It is often persistent and very difficult to manage.

Skin Diseases in Infancy

Easily
injured

Sensitive
to UV

Reduced
microbial
defenses

Impaired
thermo-regulation

Increased absorption
(large surface area for small weight)

Caution: Intoxication

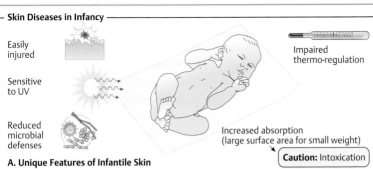

A. Unique Features of Infantile Skin

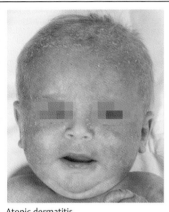

Atopic dermatitis

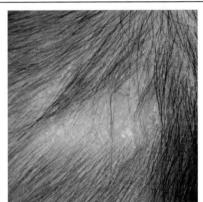

Aplasia cutis congenita

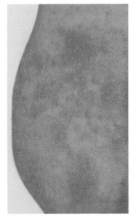

Erythema toxicum neonatorum

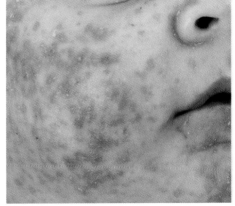

Neonatal cephalic pustulosis

B. Skin Diseases in Infancy

A. Physiologic Skin Changes

Hormonal or physiologic changes that occur in most pregnant women are:

- *hyperpigmentation*—darkened nipples, labia minora, the linea alba between the pubis and umbilicus becomes a linea nigra; also *melasma (chloasma)* as gray-brown patches on the cheeks and forehead are associated with pregnancy as well as oral contraceptives, sun exposure, and some cosmetics
- *hypertrichosis*—the anagen phase is prolonged; after pregnancy there is telogen effluvium
- *striae distensae*—better known as stretch marks, these result from a combination of stretching and hormonal factors
- *vascular changes*—the fetus impairs venous return causing hemorrhoids and pelvic varicosities
- *worsening of preexisting skin diseases*—atopic dermatitis is more likely to worsen than to improve, by roughly a 2:1 ratio. Psoriasis tends to improve but may relapse a few months after delivery. Acne and seborrhea generally get better.

B. Dermatoses of Pregnancy

Polymorphic exanthem of pregnancy. Also known as PUPPP = pruritic urticarial papules and plaques of pregnancy. Typically, pruritic erythematous papules appear within the striae in the 3rd trimester in the 1st pregnancy. It heals after delivery and poses no risk to the infant. The main differential is pemphigoid gestationis, as well as erythema multiforme.

Therapy. Topical corticosteroids; if severe, a systemic course.

Pemphigoid gestationis. This is a variant of bullous pemphigoid (Ch. 15.1) in pregnancy, also known as herpes gestationis. In >90% there are complement-fixing IgG1 autoantibodies (herpes gestationis factor) against BP180. Usually in 2nd half of pregnancy, it presents with pruritic urticarial plaques around the umbilicus and then spreading; there are often grouped blisters. It usually resolves with 6 months of delivery, but tends to recur with subsequent pregnancies or oral contraceptives. There is a risk of placental insufficiency.

Differential diagnosis. PUPPP, other autoimmune bullous diseases, erythema multiforme, drug eruption.

Therapy. Topical corticosteroids; sometimes systemic treatment is needed. Antihistamines for pruritus.

Impetigo herpetiformis. This is a rare variant of pustular psoriasis with reduced calcium level in the 2nd half of pregnancy. Management of the mother should include psoralen plus UVA (PUVA) or bath PUVA with consideration of systemic ciclosporin; corticosteroids should not be used (Ch. 14.5).

Intrahepatic cholestasis of pregnancy. Also known as pruritus gravidarum, this presents in 1%–4% of pregnancies with intense pruritus, worse at night, in the late 2nd to early 3rd trimester. There are no primary lesions, just excoriations. About 10% develop hepatic cholestasis 2–4 weeks later, with jaundice and risk of bleeding. Miscarriages and premature births are a threat. It improves after delivery, but often recurs with subsequent pregnancy. Ursodeoxycholic acid is only therapy shown to decrease fetal risk.

Other dermatoses. Atopic eruption of pregnancy has many names but presents with pruritus and prurigo nodules, as well as typical atopic changes or history. Pruritic folliculitis of pregnancy is usually a flare-up of acne. Erythema nodosum gravidarum usually occurs in the 1st trimester and heals spontaneously but is likely to recur in subsequent pregnancies.

C. Infections in Pregnancy

Herpes simplex or varicella zoster virus infections. Viral infections can cause miscarriages in the 1st trimester. Active *herpes genitalis* at the time of delivery is an indication for Cesarean section to reduce the risk of neonatal herpes. *Varicella* between 13 and 20 weeks can cause fetal varicella syndrome with many malformations, while varicella around delivery can lead to neonatal infection and increased risk of zoster in childhood. Thus if either herpes simplex virus (HSV) or varicella zoster virus (VZV) infection is suspected in pregnancy systemic aciclovir therapy should be started.

Other infections. *Erythema infectiosum* (infection with parvovirus B19) leads to hydrops fetalis with intrauterine death in 40% of cases. *Condylomata acuminata* can cause laryngeal papillomas in infants; thus they should always be removed prior to vaginal delivery. When the mother has syphilis or borreliosis, therapy should be started as quickly as possible to minimize fetal effects.

Skin Diseases during Pregnancy

Hypertrichosis

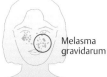

Melasma gravidarum

Telogen effluvium: 3 months after delivery

Hyper-pigmentation

Nipples

Genitalia

Linea alba

Striae distensae

Varicosities

Legs

Vagina

Hemorrhoids

A. Physiologic Skin Changes

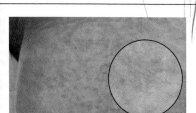

Polymorphic exanthem of pregnancy

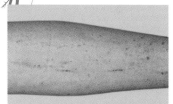

Excoriations and scattered prurigo nodules in intrahepatic cholestasis

B. Dermatoses of Pregnancy

Herpes genitalis at time of delivery

Caution: Neonatal herpes, do Cesarean section

Varicella during weeks 13–20

Caution: Fetal varicella syndrome

Prompt use of aciclovir mandatory

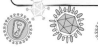

Caution

Condylomata acuminata at time of delivery

Caution: Risk of laryngeal papillomas in infant

Any rash during pregnancy always exclude syphilis, German measles, and erythema infectiosum

C. Infections in Pregnancy

A. Skin Aging

There are two types of skin aging—instrinsic and extrinsic.

- *Instrinsic aging*—the inevitable progression of the biologic clock with programmed loss of cell number, size, and function in all cutaneous systems. This physiologic aging process runs at variable rates, but affects everyone.
- *Extrinsic aging*—almost completely preventable, caused primarily by UV exposure, along with tobacco smoke. Both DNA mutations and free radicals are felt to play a pathogenic role.

The skin on the forearm or neck can be compared to that of the triceps region or buttock. Intrinsic aging leaves fine wrinkly skin, while extrinsic aging is associated with pigmentary, vascular, and keratotic alterations among others.

B. Features of Aging Skin

Some of the typical findings are:

- dry, slack, wrinkled skin because of loss of water-binding hyaluronic acid in the dermis. Loss of elastic fibers also contributes to wrinkling
- increased skin fragility and delayed wound healing as the thinned epidermis regenerates slowly and the ziplok effect between rete ridges and dermal papillae is reduced
- reduced sweat and sebum production contributes to dry skin and a weakened barrier effect. It also helps explain why heat stroke is more common in the elderly. In addition to androgenetic alopecia, hairs become thinner or do not replace themselves
- melanocytes cease to produce or transfer melanin, leading to graying of hairs and sometimes loss of pigment in melanocytic nevi. True gray hairs do not exist; they reflect a combination of dark and white hairs
- damage to connective tissue supporting vessels can lead to easy bruising, usually limited to sun-damaged skin of the forearm. Thermoregulation is also impaired
- chronic UV damage leads to irregular pigmentation, telangiectases, and the development of a variety of skin tumors. *Solar elastosis* refers to the deposits of increased amounts of damaged elastin fibers in sun-damaged skin.

C. Diseases of Aging Skin

Most of the skin changes in the elderly are not life-threatening, but all combine to greatly reduce the quality of life. Aging changes in other organs may also have an effect on the skin. Hepatic or renal disease often interferes with therapy for onychomycosis, which develops in almost every older individual. Similarly, a chronic venous ulcer is much harder to manage in a stroke patient whose ulcerated limb is paralyzed, or in a patient with extensive arterial occlusion.

■ Xerosis and Senile Pruritus

The most common skin problem in the elderly is dry skin, often associated with intense pruritus. The skin no longer tolerates prolonged water exposure (shower or tub) and cleansing as it previously did. Often the problem worsens in winter, as heating is turned on decreasing the humidity indoors. Treatment consists of avoiding drying agents and relubricating the skin, especially after water exposure. Products containing urea are useful as they are humectants trapping water in the skin. Patients with persistent pruritus should be evaluated for drug reactions, diabetes mellitus, hepatic and renal disease, and underlying tumors.

■ Intertrigo and Decubitus Ulcer

Intertrigo is common, often complicated by candidiasis especially in individuals with diabetes, which is extremely common among the elderly. Bedridden patients are at risk for pressure ulcers if they are not rotated regularly and given optimal care.

■ Skin Tumors

Aging skin should be monitored for neoplasms. While the two most common tumors—seborrheic keratosis and cherry angioma—are completely harmless, the many ultraviolet (UV)-induced tumors require attention. They include actinic keratoses, squamous cell carcinoma, basal cell carcinoma, and melanoma.

In the new age of aesthetic dermatology (Ch. 12.2), many individuals try to retard or alter the inevitable effects of cutaneous aging. The other option is to follow Mark Twain's advice:

"Age is a matter of mind—if you don't mind, it doesn't matter!"

Skin Diseases in the Elderly

Extrinsic Environmental factors

Photodamage   Lifestyle

Intrinsic

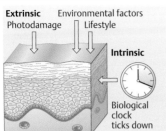

Biological
clock
ticks down

A. Skin Aging

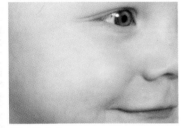

Skin of infant

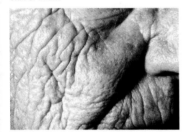

Solar elastosis

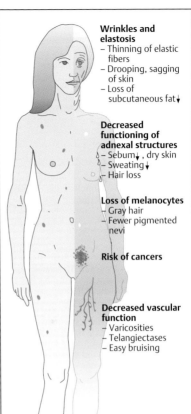

Wrinkles and elastosis
- Thinning of elastic fibers
- Drooping, sagging of skin
- Loss of subcutaneous fat↓

Decreased functioning of adnexal structures
- Sebum↓, dry skin
- Sweating↓
- Hair loss

Loss of melanocytes
- Gray hair
- Fewer pigmented nevi

Risk of cancers

Decreased vascular function
- Varicosities
- Telangiectases
- Easy bruising

B. Features of Aging Skin

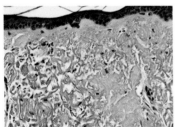

Histopathology: solar elastosis with blue-grey dermis

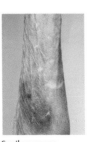

Senile purpura

Seborrheic keratoses

C. Diseases of Aging Skin

A. Overview

Epidemiology. Adverse drug reactions (ADRs) affect over 5% of hospitalized patients and cause 100 000 deaths yearly in the USA, making ADR the 4th leading cause of death. Statistics on outpatient ADRs are sparse, but the problem is immense.

Pathogenesis. ADRs are usually divided into three groups:

- *toxic*—dose-related changes reflecting the underlying mechanism of a drug
- *allergic*—not dose related; proven immunologic mechanism
- *idiosyncratic*—unexplained reaction.

> **Note:** Every drug can cause almost every reaction, but 80% of allergic reactions are caused by β-lactam antibiotics, aspirin, nonsteroidal anti-inflammatory drugs (NSAIDs), sulfonamides, allopurinol and antiepileptics.

Clinical features. The skin is often the first place where ADRs are noted. The classic reaction is a maculopapular exanthema that is usually difficult to distinguish from a viral exanthem. Other more distinctive types are considered below.

Diagnostic approach. The history is most important; make a detailed list of all medications (including nonprescription drugs, vitamins, and other supplements) and their time course. Allergy testing is mandatory.

> **Note:** Suspected drug reactions are the most common reason for dermatologic consultation in hospitalized patients.

Therapy. Withdrawal of suspected medication is the only proven approach. Systemic corticosteroids are often given, but not proven effective. Topical treatment is symptomatic.

B. Severe Skin Reactions

In most instances of severe skin reaction (SSR), skin findings are a clue to severe systemic ADR, but in rare instances the cutaneous drug reaction is itself life-threatening.

Epidemiology. The incidence in Germany is 2/1 000 000 and much higher in patients with human immunodeficiency virus/acquired immune deficiency syndrome (HIV/AIDS), organ transplantation, head injuries or brain tumors, and lupus erythematosus.

Pathogenesis. Altered drug metabolism is the most likely explanation; a small number of drugs cause most SSRs. The reactions are probably type II or type IV immune reactions to the medication or its metabolites. It is very likely that the underlying diseases modify the metabolism of the drugs or alter the immune reaction to foreign substances.

Clinical features. SSRs usually start with an erythema multiforme (EM)-like reaction, but then show increasing skin and mucosal involvement. The classification used by the German SSR Study Group is shown opposite. Stevens–Johnson syndrome (SJS) refers to patients with prominent mucosal involvement, while *toxic epidermal necrolysis* (TEN) describes those with widespread loss of skin resembling a burn patient. Of special importance are:

- the target lesions in EM-like drug reactions are usually atypical, without classic rings, and favor the trunk
- 90% of patients with SSR have mucosal involvement—oral, ocular, or genital.

> **Caution:** Any patient with a cutaneous drug reaction and mucosal involvement is at risk for SSR.

Histopathology. Full-thickness epidermal damage; early lesions show interface change.

Differential diagnosis. Staphylococcal scalded skin syndrome (SSSS) is similar, but there is only loss of stratum corneum. In transplantation patients, graft versus host disease and radiation dermatitis, or their combination, are impossible to separate. Other differential diagnoses are diffuse fixed drug eruption, DRESS (see below), autoimmune bullous diseases, and severe phototoxicity reactions.

Complications. Ocular scarring including blindness, urethral strictures, and nail and hair loss.

Therapy. Problems include temperature control, fluid loss, and susceptibility to infection. High-dose i.v. immunoglobulins 2–3 g/kg over 4–5 days seem promising but require further study. We avoid systemic corticosteroids.

C. Classic Drug Reactions

Maculopapular exanthema. Classic "rash" with erythematous macules, papules, and pruritus. Biopsy often shows eosinophils. *Causative agents*: penicillin, ampicillin, amoxicillin, allopurinol, barbiturates, benzodiazepines, carbamazepine, co-trimoxazole, phenytoin, and piroxicam.

Fixed drug eruption. Reaction that always recurs at same site—often on the genitalia—starts as a blue-red plaque, may blister and

Adverse Drug Reactions

Reaction	Trigger	Clinical features	% of skin surface affected	Mortality
Erythema multiforme	Herpes simplex	Classic, acral	<1%	0%
Erythema multiforme-like	Medications	Atypical, trunk, mucosa	<10%	1%
Stevens–Johnson syndrome	Medications (occasionally *Mycoplasma*)	Atypical, trunk, mucosa	<10%	6%
SJS/TEN	Medications	Atypical, trunk, mucosa	10–30%	25%
TEN	Medications	Atypical, trunk, mucosa	>30%	40%

Classification of severe skin reactions

Short exposure
Co-trimoxazole, sulfonamides, aminopenicillins, quinolone, cephalosporins

Long-term use
Carbamazepine, phenytoin, phenobarbital, valproic acid, lamotrigine, NSAIDs (especially oxicams) allopurinol

Causative drugs

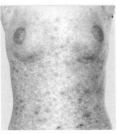
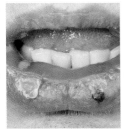
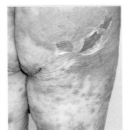

Stevens–Johnson syndrome TEN TEN

B. Severe Skin Reactions

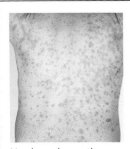
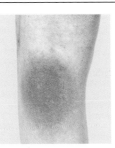

Maculopapular exanthem Fixed drug eruption Urticaria

C. Classic Drug Reactions

heals with red-brown hyperpigmentation *Causative agents*: ampicillin, aspirin, barbiturates, dapsone, metronidazole, NSAIDs, oral contraceptives, phenolphthalein, phenytoin, quinine, sulfonamides, and tetracyclines.

Urticaria and angioedema. Drugs must always be excluded. *Causative agents*: penicillin, related antibiotics, aspirin, captopril, NSAIDs, sulfonamides, insulin, contrast media. Angiotensin-converting enzyme (ACE) inhibitors are a common cause of angioedema; some tyrosine kinase inhibitors are also implicated (Ch. 17.1).

D. Unique Drug Reactions

Acneiform and rosacea-like lesions. Follicular papulopustular eruption different from acne because of sudden onset. *Causative agents*: androgens ACTH corticosteroids, oral contraceptives (especially progesterone dominant), ciclosporin, halogens, and lithium. Epidermal growth factor inhibitors cause rosacea-like eruption.

Acute generalized exanthematous pustulosis (AGEP). Small nonfollicular pustules on an erythematous background appear within 24 hours, sometimes with fever and neutrophilia. *Causative agents*: penicillin and macrolide antibiotics.

Allergic contact dermatitis. Patients are sensitized to a drug topically and then react severely when exposed systemically (Ch. 14.2). Called *baboon syndrome* when severe and prominent in the genital region. *Causative agents*: antihistamines, benzocaine, neomycin, penicillin (so common as to limit topical use), and sulfonamides.

Bullous reactions. Rarely, drugs may trigger autoimmune bullous diseases (Ch. 14.11, 15.1): vancomycin (IgA pemphigus) and penicillamine (bullous pemphigoid, pemphigus foliaceus and vulgaris).

Erythema nodosum. Drugs are a common cause of this common form of panniculitis (Ch. 18.1). *Causative agents*: oral contraceptives, antibiotics, amiodarone, hypoglycemic agents, NSAIDs, and sulfonamides.

Erythroderma. Drugs cause erythroderma (Ch. 13.3) after first producing a maculopapular exanthem or SSR. *Possible causative agents*: barbiturates, captopril, carbamazepine, cimetidine, NSAIDs, furosemide, sulfonamides, and thiazides.

Hyperpigmentation. *Causative agents*: ACTH, amiodarone, antimalarials, arsenic, chlorpromazine, estrogens, minocycline, phenytoin, phenothiazine, psoralens (with UVA), and che- motherapy agents (busulfan, 5-fluorouracil, cyclophosphamide).

Hypertrichosis. *Causative agents*: androgens, ciclosporin, minoxidil, phenytoin are most common (Ch. 26.4); others include diazoxide, streptomycin, corticosteroids, penicillamine, and psoralens.

Hypersensitivity syndrome. This is also known as DRESS (drug reaction with eosinophilia and systemic symptoms) and presents as severe persistent exanthem 3–4 weeks after the start of therapy. It is associated with lymphadenopathy (80%), fever, hepatitis, nephritis, and eosinophilia (90%) with atypical lymphocytes (50%). *Causative agents*: carbamazepine, phenobarbital, phenytoin; less often allopurinol, dapsone, gold salts, minocycline, sorbinil, and sulfonamides.

Lichen planus-like eruptions. Many drug eruptions have a lichenoid histologic pattern but few clinically mimic lichen planus (Ch. 14.8). *Causative agents*: β-blockers, gold salts, and developing solutions for color film.

Lupus erythematosus. *Causative agents*: hydralazine, procainamide and terbinafine are most common; perhaps isoniazid, minocycline and biologicals (Ch. 17.5). Associated with antihistone antibodies.

Photoallergic and phototoxic reactions. *Photoallergic causes*: benzodiazepines, griseofulvin, nalidixic acid, NSAIDs, phenothiazine, sulfonamides, sulfonylureas, thiazides, and triacetyl diphenyl isatin (laxative). *Phototoxic causes*: amiodarone, furosemide, nalidixic acid, NSAIDs (especially piroxicam, carprofen, diclofenac), psoralens, phenothiazine, and tetracyclines (especially doxycycline).

Psoriasiform reaction. Agents worsening psoriasis include ACE antagonists, β-blockers, antimalarials, gold, interferons, lithium, and some oral contraceptives (Ch. 14.5).

Purpura. Drug-induced antibodies cross-react with and damage platelets. *Causative agents*: heparin, co-trimoxazole, gold salts, quinidine, quinine, and sulfonamides (Ch. 25.1). Heparin-induced thrombocytopenia (HIT) occurs in around 5% of those receiving heparin.

Serum sickness. This is a type III hypersensitivity response to foreign proteins with deposition of circulating immune complexes leading to fever, urticaria, edema, and arthralgias. *Causative agents*: penicillin, hydralazine, NSAIDs, para-aminosalicylic acid, sulfonamides, thiazides, and biologicals.

Vasculitis. Drugs are overrated as cause but culprits include: ACE inhibitors, amiodarone, ampicillin, cimetidine, furosemide, NSAIDs, phenytoin, sulfonamides, and thiouracil.

Adverse Drug Reactions

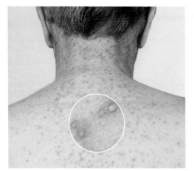

Acneiform exanthem

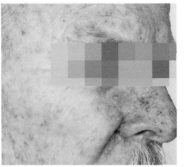

Rosacea-like reaction from anti-EGF therapy

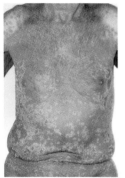

Acute generalized exanthematous pustulosis

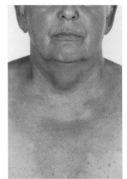

Phototoxic reaction

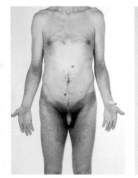

Baboon syndrome

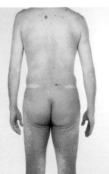

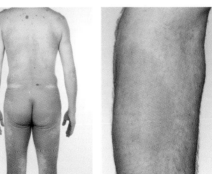

Phototoxic reaction from DTIC

D. Unique Drug Reactions

A. Neurofibromatosis

There are several variants of neurofibromatosis (NF); we will only discuss NF1 (*von Recklinghausen disease*) in detail.

Epidemiology. Common; prevalence 4:10 000.

Pathogenesis. Inherited in an autosomal dominant fashion; caused by mutations in neurofibromin which controls cell growth via guanosine diphosphate–triphosphate (GDP–GTP) cycling.

Clinical features. Major skin findings include:
- *café-au-lait macules*—tan macules that may be present at birth or appear in childhood; increased melanin, no increase in melanocytes
- *axillary freckling (Crowe sign)*—many tiny freckles in flexural areas
- *neurofibromas*—rubbery tumors, often pedunculated and can be invaginated (*doorbell sign*). They appear during childhood and can be so numerous as to be disfiguring
- *plexiform and subcutaneous neurofibromas*—deep bundles of thickened nerves; low risk of developing malignant peripheral nerve sheath tumor
- pruritus may be severe.

Other systemic findings include:
- Lisch nodule (iris hamartomas develop in almost all patients); also glaucoma
- skeletal problems (scoliosis, pseudoarthrosis, winged scapulas)
- mental retardation (usually mild)
- tumors: acoustic neuromas, optic gliomas, central nervous system (CNS) tumors, pheochromocytoma, leukemia, and a variety of sarcomas

Two relatively common variants are:
- segmental NF, which is mosaic (Ch. 20.2) with lesions following Blaschko lines
- NF2 involves mutation in neurofibromin 2 (merlin); patients have bilateral acoustic neuromas and fewer skin lesions than in NF1.

Histopathology. Neurofibromas are wavy spindle-cell tumors composed of Schwann cells and often rich in mast cells. Solitary and syndrome-related neurofibromas are identical.

Differential diagnosis. Solitary neurofibroma is of no significance; it may be clinically confused with papillomatous melanocytic nevus.

Complications. Optic glioma, acoustic neuroma, learning deficits, malignant peripheral nerve sheath tumors, pheochromocytoma.

Therapy. Genetic counseling, antihistamines for pruritus, individual lesions excised, close attention to complications.

B. Tuberous Sclerosis

Also known as Bourneville–Pringle disease.

Epidemiology. Common; prevalence 1:10 000

Pathogenesis. Inherited in an autosomal dominant fashion; caused by mutations in two different tumor suppressor genes (hamartin and tuberin).

Clinical features. Characteristic skin findings include:
- *ash-leaf macules*—depigmented ellipsoid macules present at birth

Note: Any infant with unexplained seizures should be examined for ash-leaf macules using a Wood light to enhance pigment differences.

- *connective tissue nevi*—pebbly plaque on the back (*shagreen patch*); also facial plaques
- *angiofibromas*—multiple facial papules concentrated about the nose, erroneously called adenoma sebaceum; the periungual version is known as *Koenen tumor.*

Differential diagnosis. Patients with multiple endocrine neoplasia (MEN)1 have similar skin changes; all of the lesions can appear in sporadic form.

Complications. Systemic problems are protean but a major concern is CNS involvement with seizures and mental retardation. Other complications are renal angiomyolipomas, cardiac rhabdomyomas with conduction defects and pulmonary lymphangiomas.

Therapy. Genetic counseling, anticonvulsants as needed; facial lesions can be laser ablated; regular imaging to monitor for systemic tumors. Rapamycin may block tumor formation.

C. Ataxia-telangiectasia

Rare disorder (1:50 000 prevalence) caused by mutation in the *ATM* gene involved in cell-cycle control and DNA repair and inherited in an autosomal recessive fashion. Patients develop conjunctival and later cutaneous telangiectases, coupled with ataxia, other CNS problems, severe infections, and an increased number of malignancies, especially lymphomas. An unusual skin finding is ulcerated plaques of necrobiosis lipoidica. An impaired immunoglobulin switch enhances susceptibility to pneumococcus. They are extremely sensitive to ionizing radiation.

Note: Carriers of the *ATM* gene (such as parents or relatives) are also at risk for increased malignancies.

— Neurocutaneous Genodermatoses —

Major criteria (two or more must be present)
• Six or more café-au-lait macules over 5 mm in greatest diameter in prepubertal individuals and over 15 mm in greatest diameter in postpubertal individuals • Two or more neurofibromas of any type or one plexiform neurofibroma • Freckling in the axillary or inguinal regions • Optic glioma • Two or more Lisch nodules (iris hamartomas) • Distinctive osseous lesion such as sphenoid dysplasia or thinning of the long bone cortex with or without pseudarthrosis • A first-degree relative (parent, sibling, or offspring) with NF1 by the above criteria

Diagnostic criteria for neurofibromatosis 1

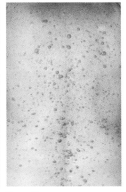

Neurofibromas

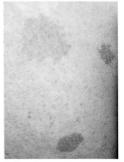

Café-au-lait macules

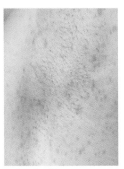

Axillary freckling

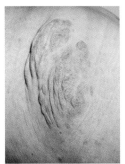

Plexiform neurofibroma

A. Neurofibromatosis

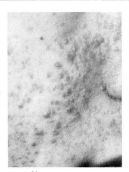

Angiofibromas

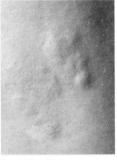

Connective-tissue nevus (shagreen plaque)

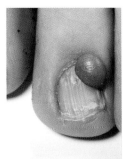

Koenen tumor

B. Tuberous Sclerosis

A. Porphyria

Porphyria is a group of diseases characterized by defects in hemoglobin metabolism and clinically presenting with varying degrees of photosensitivity and neuropsychiatric problems.

Pathogenesis. Acute attacks of porphyria are a life-threatening emergency. They are triggered by drugs (as shown opposite), alcohol, hormones, diet, and infections, but often unexplained. Photosensitivity is caused by the ability of many porphyrins to absorb 400 nm ultraviolet (UV) light in the skin.

Clinical features

- *Porphyria cutanea tarda (PCT)*—the only common form. Presents with photosensitivity, fragile skin, milia and blisters on the backs of hands, and facial hirsutism. There is often a history of alcoholism, hepatitis C infection, or hormone use. Treated with blood letting or low-dose antimalarials.
- *Hepatoerythropoietic porphyria*—a variant of PCT presenting in childhood with more severe photosensitivity.
- *Acute intermittent porphyria (AIP)*—no cutaneous findings; only neuropsychiatric emergencies with nausea, vomiting, and poorly explained signs like paralysis or severe unexplained pain, which are often misdiagnosed.
- *Variegate porphyria* (large pedigrees in Sweden, South Africa, Chile) and *coproporphyria* combine features of PCT and AIP.
- *Erythropoietic protoporphyria*—presents with photosensitivity, and often solar urticaria, in childhood. Later there is typical waxy or cobblestone scarring on the nose and dorsal hands. Treated with UVA blockers and β-carotene (must take enough to get discolored skin: 120–180 mg daily).
- *Erythropoietic porphyria*—probably represents the werewolves of legend: patients have extreme photosensitivity mandating night-time activity, as well as blisters with marked scarring, hirsutism, and even fluorescent teeth. The only therapy is total light avoidance.

Diagnostic approach. All are diagnosed by identifying porphyrin metabolites in erythrocytes, urine, or stool.

Differential diagnosis. *Pseudoporphyria* refers to patients who clinically resemble porphyria patients but have normal porphyrin levels. Patients with chronic renal disease, often on dialysis, develop lesions on their hands that resemble PCT, but have normal porphyrin values. Some patients with epidermolysis bullosa acquisita may also mimic PCT.

B. Xeroderma Pigmentosum

Xeroderma pigmentosum (XP) refers to a group of disorders with marked photosensitivity and enormous risk of cutaneous malignancies.

Epidemiology. Prevalence of 1:1 000 000 worldwide; higher in Japan, Turkey and Mediterranean basin.

Pathogenesis. Inherited in an autosomal recessive pattern, at least eight different mutations in various DNA repair enzymes (called complementary subtypes XPA–XPH).

Clinical features. Features vary markedly depending on the exact mutation.

- Photosensitivity is the most striking feature; children burn with their first sun exposure and soon have severely sun-damaged skin with actinic keratoses, telangiectases, atrophy, and pigmentary changes.
- Multiple skin cancers occur in XPA, XPC and XPD in early childhood, including basal cell carcinomas, squamous cell carcinomas melanomas, and sarcomas (angiosarcoma atypical fibroxanthoma). The first skin cancers appear very early; lifetime risk is 1000 × normal.
- Patients also have increased risk of systemic malignancies.
- Ocular problems common, with photophobia, corneal scarring, and cancers.
- Neurological manifestations present in 30%; *DeSanctis–Cacchione syndrome* refers to severe neurologic problems and dwarfism.

Differential diagnosis. There are some overlaps with Cockayne syndrome and trichothiodystrophy, which involve the same genes, but have no increased risk of skin cancer. Other childhood diseases with photosensitivity include erythropoietic protoporphyria, Bloom syndrome, and Hartnup syndrome.

Therapy. The mainstay is absolute sun avoidance, becoming night people, and maximum-protection sunscreens. Actinic keratoses are treated with topical 5-fluorouracil or imiquimod. Monitoring and prompt excision of tumors is essential. Routine ophthalmologic care is also important. Bacterial DNA repair enzyme in a topical liposome-containing preparation may reduce the number of new actinic keratoses and basal cell carcinomas.

Light-sensitive Genodermatoses

- Barbiturates
- NSAID (phenylbutazone)
- General anesthetics (halothane)
- Antiseizure medications
- Hormones (oral contraceptives, estrogens, androgens)
- Antibiotics (sulfonamides)
- Griseofulvin
- Ergot derivatives

Medical triggers of AIP

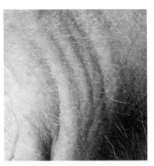

Hypertrichosis in PCT

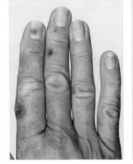

Blisters, erosions, scars, phototoxic onycholysis in PCT

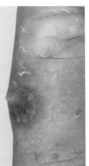

Blister with peripheral erythema in PCT

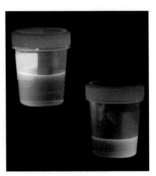

Fluorescent urine in porphyria (above); normal urine below

A. Porphyria

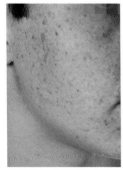

Multiple lentigines in young XP patient

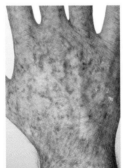

Light-damaged skin in young XP patient

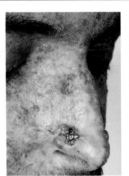

Multiple carcinomas in XP

B. Xeroderma Pigmentosum

There are several syndromes that are usually inherited in an autosomal dominant fashion with distinctive cutaneous markers and predictable underlying malignancies. Most involve mutations in tumor suppressor or growth control genes; peculiarly, the cutaneous tumors are usually benign and the systemic ones malignant. In most instances, the skin changes precede the malignant tumors by years, making monitoring for or prophylactic treatment of systemic malignancies possible.

A. Cancer-associated Syndromes

■ Gardner Syndrome

Pathogenesis. Mutation in the *APC* tumor suppressor gene.
Systemic tumors. Colonic polyposis with 100% lifetime risk of colon carcinoma, as well as hepatic and other malignancies.
Skin. Multiple epidermoid cysts, jaw cysts, hyperdontia (excessive numbers of teeth), and aggressive fibrous tumors (desmoids) in surgical sites.

■ Muir–Torre Syndrome

Pathogenesis. Mutations in several DNA repair genes, associated with hereditary nonpolyposis colon carcinoma syndrome (Lynch syndrome).
Systemic tumors. Patients have colon, other gastrointestinal, pulmonary, and urogenital carcinomas.
Skin. Multiple peculiar sebaceous tumors, often carcinomas, and keratoacanthomas. Lack of repair gene product can be demonstrated in the skin tumor with immunohistochemical stains.

■ Cowden Syndrome

Pathogenesis. Mutations in the *PTEN* gene, an important tumor control gene.
Systemic tumors. High risk of breast carcinoma; also thyroid and gastrointestinal, as well as uterine leiomyomata.
Skin. Multiple facial, oral, and acral papules with features resembling both warts and trichilemmoma (benign hair follicle tumor); conflicting evidence for human papillomavirus (HPV) involvement. Pigmented macules on the penis, lipomas, hemangiomas, and neuromas are also seen.

■ Carney Complex

Pathogenesis. Mutations in two different genes produce a similar clinical picture.

Systemic tumors. Cardiac myxomas (benign but potentially fatal), Sertoli cell testicular cancers, pigmented neural tumors, pigmented adrenal hyperplasia with Cushing syndrome.
Skin. Myxomas, especially about the eyes and ears; diffuse lentigenes and epithelioid blue nevi.

■ Nevoid Basal Cell Carcinoma Syndrome (Gorlin Syndrome)

Pathogenesis. Mutation in the *PTCH* gene, part of a complex growth-control pattern. Frontal bossing, bifid ribs, calcification of falx cerebri, and other dysmorphologic signs.
Systemic tumors. Medulloblastoma in childhood; ovarian and breast tumors.
Skin. Multiple basal cell carcinomas, many of which look like skin tags or small melanocytic nevi; (Ch. 21.4). Palmar pits. Extreme radiation sensitivity.

■ Multiple Endocrine Neoplasia 2B (MEN 2B)

Pathogenesis. Mutation in the *RET* proto-oncogene.
Systemic tumors. Medullary carcinoma of the thyroid in 85%; pheochromocytoma in 50%.
Skin. Multiple mucosal neuromas usually on the lips, eyelid neuromas causing *everted lid sign*.

■ Peutz–Jeghers Syndrome

Pathogenesis. Mutation in *STK11*, a serine-threonine kinase growth-control gene.
Systemic tumors. Intestinal polyposis with risk of intussusception; genital tumors.
Skin. Periorificial and acral lentigines.

■ Birt–Hogg–Dubé Syndrome

Pathogenesis. Mutation in folliculin; function not established.
Systemic tumors. Unusual bilateral renal cell carcinomas; also spontaneous pneumothoraces.
Skin. Multiple fibrofolliculomas and benign hair follicle tumors with fibrous reactive stroma.

■ Howel–Evans Syndrome

Pathogenesis. Mutation located on chromosome 17 but the gene is poorly defined.
Systemic tumors. 75% develop carcinoma of the esophagus by age 60 years.
Skin. Diffuse palmoplantar keratoderma (tylosis) appears in childhood, along with leukokeratosis (white hyperkeratotic oral plaques).

Cancer-associated Genodermatoses

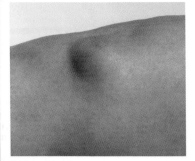

Epidermoid cyst
Gardner syndrome

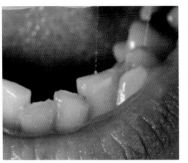

Hyperdontia

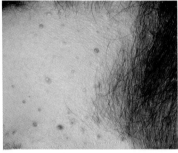

Multiple nevoid basal cell carcinomas

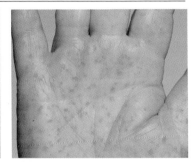

Palmar pits

Nevoid basal cell carcinoma syndrome

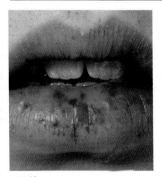

Labial lentigines

Peutz–Jeghers syndrome

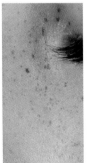

Lentigines

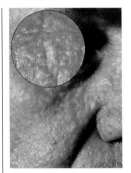

Multiple fibrofolliculomas

Birt–Hogg–Dubé syndrome

A. Cancer-associated Syndromes

A. Primary Psychiatric Disorders

All these disorders are primarily psychiatric in origin but the patients tend to present to dermatologists, who must be astute enough to recognize the underlying problem and help the patient obtain expert help from a psychiatrist or dermatologist with special training in psychodermatology.

■ Factitious Disorders

There are several variants on self-induced disease. They include:
Artifacts. Self-induced lesions in patients with borderline personality disturbance. Lesions on accessible sites (face, left arm in right hander) with hard-to-reach sites like the interscapular area spared. Typical artifacts include unexplained pyodermas, bizarre wounds, and thermal or chemical burns (round small burns from cigarettes).

Artifact is a diagnosis of exclusion; often the first clue is that the skin changes do not fit any recognizable disease. If lesions clear under occlusive dressing, this is a good clue.
Para-artifacts. Also known as *impulse control disturbance.* Features are repetitive acts such as trichotillomania (tugging at the hair), nail chewing, lick dermatitis around the lips, or acne excoriée (picking at minimal acne). Patients are somewhat aware of the nature of their disease.
Malingering. Deliberate skin damage for external gain; this varies from inducing a lesion to avoid work to not taking medication so disease flares.

■ Münchhausen Syndrome

A form of malingering; patients feign illnesses, visit multiple hospitals, and provide fantastic histories to attract attention. In *Münchhausen by proxy,* an adult induces illness in a child—a peculiar form of child abuse.

■ Delusions of Parasitosis

Irrational perception of infestation, also known as acarophobia. Patients pick excessively, causing scratch artifacts and usually present with matchbox sign (small container full of scales and lint, but offered as evidence of bugs).

■ Delusion of Bromhidrosis

The patient is convinced that they smell so bad no one can be near them, while in fact they smell normal.

■ Dysmorphophobia

Although physically normal, the patient has delusions of facial asymmetry or other appearance defects. They are often a compulsive mirror user, with special attention to grooming and cosmetics.

■ Somatoform Disorder

Patients present repeatedly with physical symptoms (not signs) and stubbornly demand medical evaluation, despite previous negative results and assurance that nothing is physically wrong. Patients perceive their symptoms as real; they are not malingering. Examples include ecological syndrome, hypochondriasis (fear of infection, acquired immune deficiency syndrome [AIDS], cancer or other phobias), cutaneous dysesthesias (glossodynia, vulvodynia), and some forms of pruritus.

B. Psychosomatic Disorders

Psychosomatic is often used to describe symptoms without an immediate physiologic cause. We use it slightly differently, referring to chronic skin conditions with multifactorial causes that can be triggered or worsened by emotional influences. Included in this group are the two most common chronic inflammatory skin diseases—psoriasis and atopic dermatitis. In atopic dermatosis, there are subgroups of patients in whom stress plays a triggering role. Addressing emotional trigger factors can greatly facilitate overall treatment.

C. Secondary Psychiatric Disorders

Skin diseases can cause considerable emotional distress. Individuals with serious or disfiguring skin lesions (severe acne, psoriasis on readily seen sites, metastatic melanoma, hemifacial atrophy) are often depressed (*somatopsychic disease*). The combination of pruritus, stigmatization, impaired performance at work and recreation, limitations on what clothing one can wear, and many similar issues may lead to depression, loss of self-esteem, and feeling of rejection. Treatment is aimed at the skin disorder, with psychiatric support to help in coping.

In a completely different sense, allergic reactions, severe infections, and other noxious agents can lead to acute alterations in the mental status, including agitation or confusion, but also reduced consciousness.

Psychocutaneous Diseases

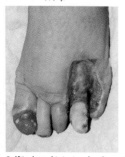

Psychiatric factors ⟶ Skin disease

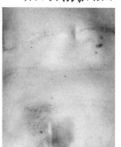

Self-induced injuries; healing while on psychotherapeutic agents

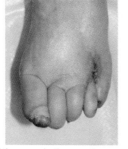

Injections of ink

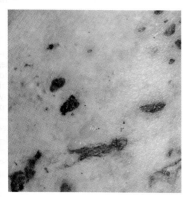

Scratch artifacts

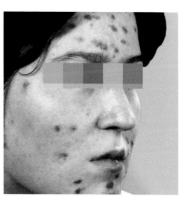

Acne excoriée

A. Primary Psychiatric Disorders

Skin disease ⟶ Emotional distress

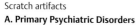

Chronicity

Pain

Pruritus

Disfigurement

Social deprivation

Loss of self-esteem

Aggression

Depression

C. Secondary Psychiatric Disorders

31 Psychocutaneous Disease

Over 100 genotypes of human papillomavirus (HPV) can infect the skin or mucosa. Several can be present simultaneously and little resistance develops. With high-risk HPV types, viral DNA can be integrated into the host genome with immortalization of keratinocytes and a likelihood of malignant change.

A. Clinical Features

Verrucae vulgares. These are generally multiple and very often acral; they are usually caused by HPV1–4 and 26–29 and are more common in children with atopy. Patients have hyperkeratotic papules. When trimmed, tiny black points—papillary dermal vessels—are seen. The appearance varies with location: on the fingers and back of hand, classic dome-shaped warts are seen; between the digits they are more papillomatous; beneath the nail plate, they are painful and often eroded; on the eyelids they are long and delicate (filiform); and in the anogenital region, there are smoother skin-colored or brown plaques. Lesions usually heal spontaneously over weeks to years. Warts in adults or extensive facial involvement in children are clues to possible immunosuppression. Butchers are particularly susceptible to warts on their hands, but they are caused by HPV, not bovine viruses. In addition to HPV1–4, a unique HPV7 is also found.

Verrucae plantares. Plantar warts can be solitary or multiple; they tend to hurt when at weight-bearing points. Bleeding points are prominent. When confluent, they are called *mosaic wart*.

Verrucae planae. Plane or flat skin-colored papules most often occurring on the face of younger patients.

Condylomata acuminata. Common sexually transmitted viral disease caused by HPV6 and 11, presenting with white-red, sometimes stalked, papules that are often macerated. In women they occur from the labia to the introitus, in men around the glands and on the shaft. The patient's partner should be checked.

> **Note:** HPV6 and 11 cause over 90% of genital warts but high-risk types 16 and 18 cause cervical carcinoma. Vaccines are available against both groups.

Bowenoid papulosis. Flat dark genital papules in young adults; almost always HPV16 and 18. Histological changes of squamous cell carcinoma in situ are seen, but not all behave aggressively; some regress. Sometimes they are not pigmented; then they are known as *condy-lomata plana.* Because they are caused by high-risk HPV, patients should be followed, even if regression occurs, and partners also monitored.

Condylomata gigantea. Large destructive tumor caused by HPV6 and 11 typically involving the prepuce or perianal region; best regarded as verrucous squamous cell carcinoma (Ch. 21.5).

Oral florid papillomatosis. Oral variant of verrucous carcinoma. Linked to several HPV types.

Focal epithelial hyperplasia. Hundreds of perioral and intraoral papillomas caused by HPV13 and 32 are present in infancy, primarily in Native American, Inuits.

Epidermodysplasia verruciformis. Abnormal inherited susceptibility to HPV via *EVER1* or *2* genes. The main HPV types are 5 and 8. There are two types of lesions: small verrucae, planar-like; and larger pityriasis, versicolor-like. There is little tendency to spontaneous regression; instead there is a likelihood of progression to squamous cell carcinoma (SCC).

Warts in immunocompromised patients. Warts can be very widespread and uncontrollable (*verrucosis generalisata*), but more importantly, especially in sun-exposed sites, HPV types 5 and 8 can lead to SCC. Rarely, diffuse spread occurs in atopic children.

B. Therapy

In children, the basic rule is do not harm (no scarring or very painful procedures), as most warts are self-limited. In contrast, when dealing with high-risk lesions, aggressive therapy then monitoring are essential. One view is that all therapeutic measures when applied long enough induce an immune response against HPV.

Hyperkeratotic warts need to be débrided first with keratolytic agents (salicylic acid plasters or varnishes) coupled with trimming or sanding. Then cytostatic agents (5-fluorouracil) or immunomodulators (imiquimod) can be used. Cryotherapy is another option; it must be localized, sparing normal skin, and aggressive enough to cause a blister. For plane warts, light cryotherapy, topical retinoids, or imiquimod are useful. Condylomata are usually treated with podophyllotoxin, now available for home application, or imiquimod as an immunomodulator. Warts can also always be anesthetized and then destroyed with electrosurgery, curettage, excision, or laser ablation. Recurrences are surprisingly common, indicating that the HPV is not eliminated.

Human Papillomaviruses

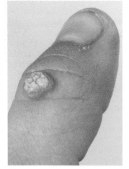

Common wart

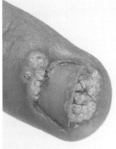

Periungual and subungual warts

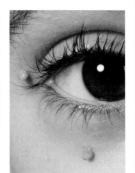

Filiform warts

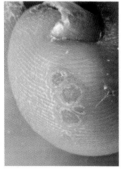

Plantar warts

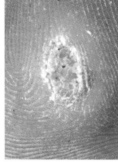

Plantar wart

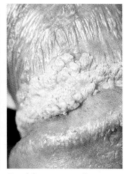

Condylomata acuminata

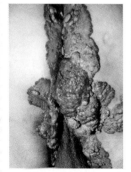

Condylomata gigantea

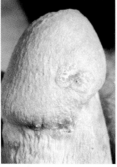

Bowenoid papulosis

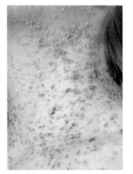

Epidermodysplasia verruciformis

A. Clinical Features

A. Herpes Simplex Virus

Herpes simplex virus (HSV) types 1 and 2 are neurotropic and epidermotropic; they remain latent in ganglia and can be reactivated.

Primary oral HSV infection. *Herpetic gingivostomatitis* usually occurs in children after incubation of 7–14 days, with painful oral blisters and erosions, fever, malaise, and difficulty eating. The fingers may be secondarily inoculated (*herpetic whitlow*). Infection is usually caused by HSV1 and is generally self-limited. In immune-compromised patients it is far more severe, with skin, mucosal, and genital involvement (*aphthoid of Pospischill–Feyrter*).

Recurrent oral infection. More than 90% of adults carry HSV1, causing "cold sores" or "fever blisters"—*herpes simplex labialis.* There is a burning feeling as a warning sign, followed by grouped blisters and polycyclic erosions. It is often triggered by ultraviolet (UV) light or fever and can be the site of entry for recurrent erysipelas with lymphatic damage (*elephantiasis nostras*). It persists for more than a week only in patients with leukemia, lymphoma, acquired immune deficiency syndrome (AIDS), and other immunosuppression.

Eczema herpeticatum. This is an endogenous activation and then dissemination of HSV in patients with atopic dermatitis, Darier disease, or Hailey–Hailey disease. Multiple tiny erosions are seen, and, rarely, blisters along with fever and malaise. It may also progress to herpetic keratitis, pneumonia, or central nervous system (CNS) disease.

Herpes genitalis. Caused by HSV 2 in 80%–90% of cases, the primary attack is usually not as dramatic as with oral disease; 20% of adults carry HSV2 and develop painful genital ulcers on an erythematous base.

Herpes neonatorum. This is an acute primary infection of the newborn, usually acquired during passage through a HSV-positive birth canal. There is a risk of CNS involvement. Transplacental transmission is also possible and leads to spontaneous abortion in 25% of cases.

■ Therapy

Topical drying measures are used for mild cases, and systemic antiviral agents for all others, used intravenously in sick patients. Options include aciclovir, famciclovir, valaciclovir, or brivudine. For recurrent disease, either long-term suppression or short-term treatment starting at first warning.

B. Varicella Zoster Virus

The first infection with varicella-zoster virus (VZV) is *chickenpox* or *varicella.* It affects 90%–95% of the population before 15 years. Transmission is via droplets, with an incubation period of 2–3 weeks. Patients have disseminated red macules and then small blisters with an erythematous rim. Lesions in different stages are seen together, in contrast to smallpox where they are synchronous. The scalp and hard palate are frequently involved. Lesions are pruritic and thus excoriated; they usually heal with small punched-out scars. VZV also remains latent in dorsal root ganglia.

In adults or immunocompromised patients, there is a more severe course, with CNS involvement or varicella pneumonia (fatal in 10% of cases). Infections in the 1st half of pregnancy lead to fetal varicella syndrome (limb hypoplasia, scarred ulcerations, ocular malformations, CNS damage). In the 3rd trimester, varicella pneumonia in the fetus can lead to spontaneous abortion or premature birth. If the mother has varicella 5 days before to 2 days after birth, the infant is at great risk of disseminated varicella, with a mortality rate of 30%. If infection occurs sooner, protective maternal antibodies are transferred.

Zoster. Around 20% of individuals experience reactivation of VZV with damage to the ganglion, dermatomal nerve, and skin. Segmental grouped vesicles on an erythematous base become pustules, then crust and scar. Sometimes patients have *zoster sine herpete* (pain but no skin lesions). Nerve damage is painful. Postherpetic neuralgia is the persistence of the pain 4 weeks after skin lesions have healed.

Zoster ophthalmicus. About 15% of zoster involves the 1st branch of the trigeminal nerve, with ocular complications (keratitis, conjunctivitis). Involvement of the tip of the nose indicates that eye disease is likely. It is managed with ophthalmology to avoid late complications (scleritis, acute retinal necrosis).

Zoster of the 2nd and 3rd trigeminal branches. Grouped ulcers on half of the hard palate for 2nd branch and on one side of the chin for 3rd branch. Ear involvement is associated with facial nerve paralysis in 50% of cases. If the vestibulocochlear nerve is affected, tinnitus, vertigo, and hearing loss can follow (*Ramsay–Hunt syndrome*).

Generalized zoster. VZV infections are more severe in immunocompromised patients. Patients may have zoster involving multiple dermatomes, zoster with dissemination, or recurrent varicella (disseminated from the start with rapid onset and monomorphic blisters).

Human Herpes Viruses

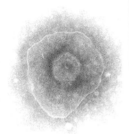

Electron microscopic image of herpes simplex virus

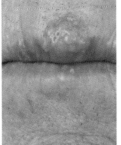

Herpes labialis

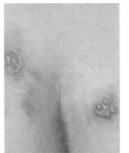

Recurrent herpes simplex

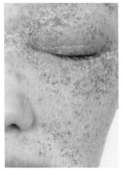

Eczema herpeticatum

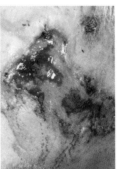
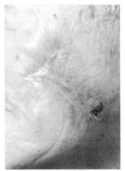

Persistent ulcerated herpes simplex in HIV/AIDS and healing while on aciclovir

A. Herpes Simplex Virus

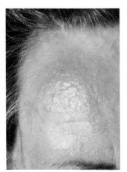

Early zoster of the 1st trigeminal branch

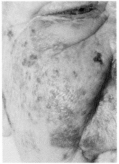
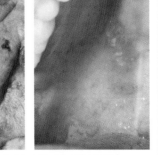

Zoster of the 2nd trigeminal branch with oral mucosal involvement

B. Varicella Zoster Virus

Lesions are often hemorrhagic and necrotic. Most common systemic problems are pneumonia and encephalitis; less, often myocarditis, hepatitis, pancreatitis.

■ Therapy

For uncomplicated *varicella*, drying measures such as shake lotions usually suffice. Systemic antiviral therapy slightly shortens the course. A vaccine is available.

For *zoster*, drying lotions are also useful. Promptly instituted systemic therapy with the same agents listed under herpes simplex but in higher doses softens the course and reduces the risk of post-herpetic neuralgia. Immuno-compromised patients require immediate intravenous acyclovir. Acute pain is treated with analgesics. Carbamazepine is the treatment of choice for zoster neuralgia with pulsating severe pain. Other choices for chronic pain include tricyclic antidepressants, gabapentin and pregabalin. A zoster booster vaccine is available for adults.

C. Epstein–Barr Virus

Epstein–Barr virus (EBV) causes infectious mononucleosis as well as Burkitt lymphoma; in immunocompromised patients it also causes also lymphoproliferative diseases, oral hairy leukoplakia, and leiomyosarcomas.

Infectious mononucleosis is a disease of adolescents; it is asymptomatic in 50%. It is spread by droplets with an incubation period of 2–3 weeks. EBV remains in the salivary glands and is excreted for life. Findings include fever, angina, myalgias, lymphadenopathy, splenomegaly (monitor with sonography), and atypical lymphocytes. Complications include hepatitis with jaundice, thrombocytopenia, and cold agglutinin disease. Maculopapular exanthems occur in 3%–15%; a few develop oral or genital ulcers. When treated with amoxicillin for presumed bacterial pharyngitis, almost 100% develop drug-induced exanthem. The recovery period can be prolonged, with myalgias and malaise.

Diagnosis is based on clinical findings, heterophile antibody test, and specific anti-EBV antibodies. Therapy is symptomatic.

D. Cytomegalovirus Virus

Cytomegalovirus (CMV, human herpes virus [HHV]5) usually causes asymptomatic infection or less often a mononucleosis-like picture. It then remains latent in the body. In human immunodeficiency virus (HIV)/AIDS, it causes oral and skin ulcers, chorioretinitis, and pneumonia. It is a common intrauterine infection; if the mother has primary infection, the newborn is at risk (microcephaly, optic nerve atrophy, cataracts, and intracerebral calcifications; a major cause of mental retardation). It is the most common infectious agent after bone marrow or solid organ transplant and can help trigger a rejection reaction. Ganciclovir i.v. or valganciclovir p.o. are the mainstays for preventative regimens and to treat ocular disease (ganciclovir is usually injected into the eye). Both are considerably more toxic than aciclovir.

E. Human Herpes Virus 6

HHV6 causes *exanthem subitum*, also known as *roseola infantum* or *sixth* disease. This is a disease of infants with droplet transmission and almost 100% seropositivity after 2 years. After an incubation period of 1–2 weeks, patients have high fever (39–40.5 °C) for 3–4 days. As the fever breaks, exanthem appears on the chest and arms, with small erythematous macules and papules that may reach the neck but almost never the face; enanthem with red blotches on the palate is seen. Other problems include gastroenteritis, lid edema, and respiratory symptoms. It is reactivated in 50% of transplant patients and can also contribute to initiating rejection. It can also trigger graft versus host disease after bone marrow transplantation.

F. Human Herpesvirus 8

Human herpesvirus 8 (HHV8) can be identified in 98% of all Kaposi sarcoma (KS) (Ch. 22.6), as well as HIV-associated primary effusion lymphoma and multicentric Castleman disease. How HHV8 causes KS is unclear, but the best guess is that vGPCR (viral G-protein-coupled receptor) turns on angiogenic agents such as vascular endothelial growth factor (VEGF). HHV8 LNA (latent nuclear antigen) can be identified in skin biopsy of KS patients, confirming the diagnosis.

Human Herpes Viruses

Polymorphic appearance of varicella

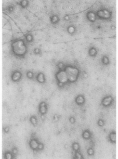

Varicella with lesions in varying stages

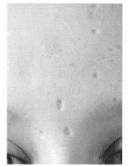

Varicella scars

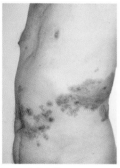

Zoster in beltlike pattern on the thorax

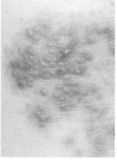

Confluent grouped blisters

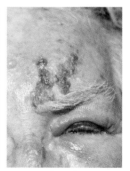

Zoster involving the eye

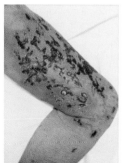

Necrotic zoster in an immuno-compromised patient

B. Varicella Zoster Virus

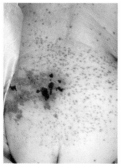

Hemorrhagic zoster with generalization in an immuno-compromised patient

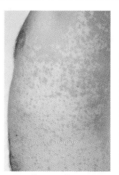

Ampicillin exanthem in infectious mononucleosis

C. Epstein–Barr Virus

A. Pox Viruses

■ Orthopoxviruses

Smallpox (*variola vera*) was declared extinct by the World Health Organization (WHO) in May 1980. The last endemic pockets were in India and Africa. It was caused by poxvirus variolae, spread by droplets or direct contact, with a 2-week incubation period. Patients then developed fever (41 °C), malaise, and generalized monomorphic exanthem which progressed in synchronous fashion through papules, vesicles, pustules, and crusts with an overall mortality of 33 % and distinctive scarring in survivors. The virus is maintained in at least two laboratories in Russia and USA. Even the suspicion of smallpox must be promptly reported.

Cowpox virus can be transmitted to humans by cows, cats (most common source), and rodents. Several outbreaks have been caused by infected rats and prairie dogs kept as pets. Cowpox poses a threat to atopic and immunocompromised patients. Two weeks after inoculation, erythema, vesicles, pustules, and ulcers develop. Negative staining electron microscopy is the quickest way to identify the organism. It is a self-limited disease that only requires topical disinfectants.

Poxvirus officinalis or the vaccina virus is a separate species. Normal individuals develop erythema, pustules, and crusts at the vaccination site, with distinctive scar. When atopic or immunocompromised patients are vaccinated or exposed to virus by vaccinated contacts, they may develop widespread cutaneous disease (*eczema vaccinatum*) and even systemic findings.

■ Parapox Viruses

Milker's nodule. Milker's nodule virus (MNV), also called paravaccinia virus, is found in cows. Formerly seen on the hands of milkmaids, it is now more of a problem for butchers. Blue-red nodules develop 5–7 days after inoculation. It is diagnosed with negative-image electron microscopy. Only symptomatic care is needed.

Orf. Orf is also called ecthyma contagiosum. *Parapoxvirus ovis* is a virus of sheep and goats, either identical to or closely related to MNV. It too is best identified by negative-staining electron microscopy. Shepherds may be inoculated directly by contact with the weeping facial lesions of animals. After an incubation period of 4–10 days, erythematous nodules develop, which are identical to milker's nodules. They heal spontaneously after a few weeks.

Molluscum contagiosum. This is a common pox virus spread by direct skin contact. It is seen in children, usually on the trunk and extremities. It is quite uncommon in immunocompetent adults where it presents primarily with genital lesions. It can be widespread and recalcitrant in atopic, immunocompromised, and HIV/AIDS patients. After incubation of weeks to months, white-pink 2–10 mm broad-based glassy papules with a central dell appear. In HIV/AIDS, they are often large and deep. Locally destructive measures such as curettage are simplest; in children first use EMLA anesthetics. Cryotherapy or a variety of irritants can also be tried.

B. Picorna Viruses

Hand foot and mouth disease. This is usually caused by Coxsackie-A1 virus, less often by Coxsackie-A2, -B2, -B3, and enterovirus 71. After an incubation period of 3–5 days, patients present with sore throat and oral ulcers, as well as tense blisters surrounded by an erythematous ring on the palms of the hands soles of the feet, and buttocks. It clears spontaneously. Epidemics in Asia with enterovirus 71 have had a 20 % mortality rate from pulmonary hemorrhage and CNS disease.

> **Note:** Do not confuse with hoof and mouth disease—another picorna virus disease affecting hoofed mammals; even in large epidemics with cattle, human infections are rare.

Herpangina. Also known as *Zahorsky disease* this is caused by Coxsackie A viruses. It primarily affects infants and small children; after incubation of 2–9 days, 3–5 mm vesicles with an erythematous rim develop on the tonsils and hard palate, along with marked fever. It is typically confused with HSV or aphthae by the uninitiated, and is self-limited.

Coxsackie-virus exanthems. Many other exanthems are caused by this common group; they are hard to separate from drug exanthems and rubella.

Other Viruses

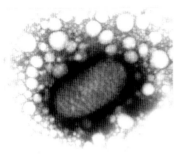

Parapox virus in negative contrast electron microscopy, showing "ball of wool" pattern

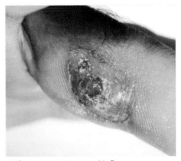

Ecthyma contagiosum (Orf)

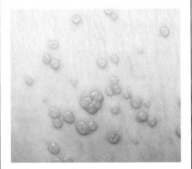

Mollusca contagiosa

A. Pox Viruses

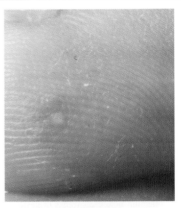

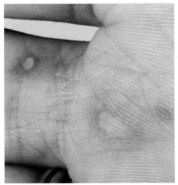

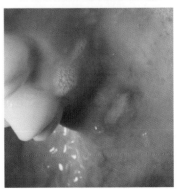

Hand foot and mouth disease

B. Picorna Viruses

C. Classic Viral Infections of Childhood

Measles. Measles is caused by *Morbillivirus*, a paramyxovirus. It is carried by droplet spread with an incubation period of 10 days, and is highly infectious during the acute phase (3 Cs = cough, coryza (runny nose), and conjunctivitis, as well as high fever and photophobia). Typical white buccal mucosal macules (*Koplik spots*) appear transiently on the 2nd–3rd day. Macular exanthem starts in the face and behind the ears and spreads to the trunk and extremities; it is initially erythematous but later red-brown. Complications include severe secondary bacterial infections, especially pneumonia, otitis media, and encephalitis; *subacute sclerosing panencephalitis* is a long-term risk

Prior to immunization, the mortality rate was < 3:1000 in healthy individuals, but up to 30% in poor countries or immunocompromised patients. Measles became rare but increasing parental rejection of immunizations has increased community susceptibility and mini-epidemics have occurred.

Rubella. Also known as German measles, this is caused by togavirus. The incubation period is 2–3 weeks. Diffuse fine macular exanthem starts in the face in a butterfly distribution but rapidly disseminates. There is lymphadenopathy, especially over the mastoids, with modest fever (38 °C) and malaise. In adults, rubella may cause a significant and persistent inflammatory arthritis, which also can be a complication of immunization in this age group.

There is a risk of congenital syndrome as high as 50% in unprotected mothers who contract infection before 20 weeks of gestation. There is also a risk of spontaneous abortion or severe fetal malformations with deafness, cardiac anomalies (50% patent ductus arteriosus), and cataracts (*Gregg syndrome*), as well as thrombocytopenic purpura (blueberry muffin rash). A vaccine is available. All women should be checked for protective status prior to getting pregnant.

Erythema infectiosum. Also known as *fifth disease*, this is caused by parvovirus B19 and is a disease of young children. It presents with diffuse erythema on the cheeks (*slapped cheeks disease*), later, transient lacy or wreath-like patterns of erythema appear on the inner aspects of the limbs. Patients are no longer infectious by the time the rash appears.

It is also a troublesome virus during pregnancy. If an unprotected mother is infected in the first 20 weeks, there is a 10% risk of fetal damage with anemia, myocarditis, and hydrops fetalis. It can also trigger aplastic crisis in patients with sickle cell anemia or thalassemia and cause arthritis in adults. Symptomatic therapy suffices for skin findings.

> **Caution:** Always consider measles, rubella and parvovirus B19 when a rash occurs in pregnancy. The greatest risk occurs when a woman contracts a primary infection before the 20th week.

D. Other Viral Exanthems

Gianotti–Crosti syndrome. This presents with distinctive non-pruritic lichenoid papules on the cheeks, hands, and feet; it is seen almost exclusively in children and occurs as a secondary reaction to a wide variety of viral infections. In developing countries, most cases are triggered by hepatis B infection, but often in subclinical form. In western countries there is a greater variety of triggers, including cytomegalovirus, EBV, and even immunizations. It is self-limiting but may last for months. Therapy is symptomatic.

Purpuric gloves and socks syndrome. This is primarily caused by parvovirus B19, less often by Coxsackie, HHV6, or CMV. Initially pruritic papules evolve into edematous petechial erythema, affecting almost exclusively the hands and feet, hence the name. Sometimes there is amazingly sharp delineation between diseased and normal skin. There is often mucosal involvement with vesicles, erosions, and aphthae. Systemic complaints may include fever, lymphadenopathy, arthralgias, and myalgias. Therapy is symptomatic.

Asymmetric periflexural exanthem. While a viral agent is suspected, none has been identified for this puzzling disorder. It usually appears at the age of 2–3 years, sometimes following a respiratory tract infection. Initially there is a unilateral distribution, as erythematous papules start around the axilla, less often inguinally, then coalesce and spread to cover the side of the chest or down the leg. Later contralateral involvement is possible. Therapy is symptomatic.

Eruptive pseudoangiomatosis. This is almost exclusively a disease of childhood, with eruptive red-brown papules on the cheeks and extremities, following typical prodromal findings. Both ECHO viruses 25 and 32, as well as parvovirus B19 have been incriminated. On histology, a mixture of superficial blood vessels and lymphocytic infiltrate is seen. It resolves spontaneously.

— **Other Viruses** —

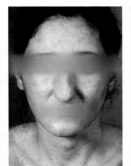

Measles on the face

Measles on the trunk

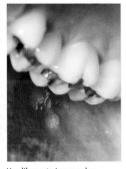

Koplik spots in measles

Rubella

C. Classic Viral Infections of Childhood

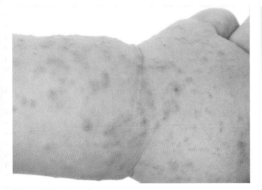

Gianotti–Crosti syndrome

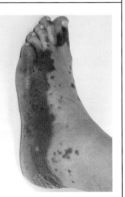

Purpuric gloves and socks syndrome

D. Other Viral Exanthems

■ Staphylococci

Staphylococci are a common Gram-positive group of bacteria. The main pathogen is coagulase-positive *Staphylococcus aureus*; in contrast, *S. epidermidis* is part of normal flora. There are increasing problem with meticillin-resistant *S. aureus* (MRSA). Between 10% and 20% of *S. aureus* tested in Germany are MRSA. In the past, most MRSA were acquired in hospital, but there has been a disturbing trend in recent years to community-acquired MRSA, with epidemics for example among a professional American football team. The other great significance of staphylococci is that some of them produce dangerous toxins.

■ Streptococci

There are numerous species of Gram-positive catalase-negative cocci that have different lysis patterns on sheep blood agar.

A. Impetigo

Impetigo is most often caused by *S. aureus* but also by *Streptococcus pyogenes* (group A). It most commonly occurs on the face in children, starting with tiny macules, which become vesicles, pustules, and then form a honey-colored crust. Staphylococci secreting exfoliative toxins can cause larger blisters (*bullous impetigo*). Some of the streptococci causing impetigo also cause glomerulonephritis, so patients' renal status should be checked initially then 2–4 weeks later. Topical therapy with disinfectants produces healing about as fast as systemic penicillinase-resistant penicillins, but the systemic therapy helps reduce the spread of bacteria. Also check for nasal carriers of staphylococci.

B. Folliculitis, Furuncle, and Carbuncle

All these are staphylococcal infections of hair follicles and are treated with penicillinase-resistant penicillins.

Ostiofolliculitis. *S. aureus* causes superficial follicular infection with tiny pustules. It is more common in warm moist areas, usually on the face, scalp, or axillae.

Furuncle. Deeper infection involving the entire hair follicle, with inevitable scarring. It is known colloquially as a "*boil*."

Carbuncle. Confluence of multiple furuncles; the patient is often sick and may require bed rest, as well as incision and drainage.

Recurrent folliculitis. Common and difficult problem, often the result of reinfection from nasal or perianal carrier sites. Epidemics occur in sport teams with close contact. Therapy is with disinfectants plus penicillinase-resistant antibiotics.

Hordeolum. *S. aureus* folliculitis of the eyelid. There is initially a foreign body sensation, and later a painful nodule involving the eyelash.

Chalazion. Granulomatous inflammation of the Meibomian gland that is slow growing and relatively asymptomatic. It may resolve; otherwise it must be excised.

Paronychia. Painful infection of the nail fold with *S. aureus*, often because of damaged protective cuticle. It causes nail dystrophy. Deeper paronychia is known as *felon* and carries the risk of infecting the tendon sheath, so immediate surgical management and systemic antibiotics are required.

Bulla repens. Acral firm blister contained by thick volar skin. Treament is to drain and then use systemic antibiotics.

C. Staphylococcal Scalded Skin Syndrome (SSSS)

Following staphylococcal conjunctivitis, otitis, or pharyngitis, usually young patients develop a perioral or intertriginous exanthem that progresses to large flaccid blisters that rupture rapidly. This is caused by exfoliative *S. aureus* toxins which split desmoglein 1, the same molecule that is attacked by autoantibodies in pemphigus foliaceus (Ch. 14.11). Light microscopy reveals subcorneal separation in contrast to full-thickness destruction and separation in toxic epidermal necrolysis. Immediate antibiotic treatment is life-saving and stops production of toxin, but does not influence existing toxins.

D. Erysipelas

Erysipelas is a potentially life-threatening lymphangitic infection usually caused by *S. pyogenes*, or, rarely, by other organisms. It starts from an entry portal on the feet (usually interdigital tinea pedis or a minor injury) or on the face following herpes simplex infection, or in tiny cracks and fissures.

Clinically, there is a rapidly spreading warm edematous erythema, with flame-like extensions. It is accompanied by ascending lymphangiitis, lymphadenopathy, and fever over 40°C with chills. There is a markedly elevated erythrocyte sedimentation rate (ESR) and neutrophilia. On the shin and in immunocompromised patients, there is a risk of hemorrhagic blisters with necrosis. With facial erysipelas there is also a risk of spread to the orbit and

Staphylococci and Streptococci

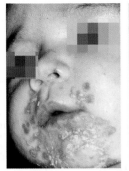
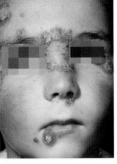
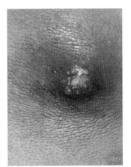

Perioral impetigo caused by *S. aureus* in two children; on the left, massive honey-colored crusts

Staphylococcal pyoderma of the axilla

A. Impetigo

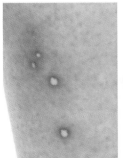
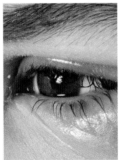

Ostiofolliculitis

Furuncle

Carbuncle

B. Folliculitis, Furuncle, and Carbuncle

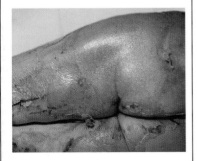
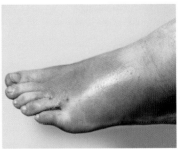

C. Staphylococcal Scalded Skin Syndrome (SSSS)

Erysipelas of the foot with interdigital entry point and ascending lymphangitis

D. Erysipelas

then cavernous sinus thrombosis. In recurrent erysipelas, chronic damage to the lymphatics leads to persistent lymphedema but milder acute infections.

■ Therapy

Benzyl penicillin 10 million IU i.v. t.i.d. is the therapy of choice: 10–14 days for initial infection and 21 days for recurrent infection. In penicillin allergy, clindamycin is the alternative. Prophylaxis against recurrence uses phenoxymethyl penicillin 1 g p.o. daily or depot penicillin G (benzathine penicillin G) 2.4 million IU i.m. every 3 weeks over years.

E. Other Deep Infections

Cellulitis. Deeper infection involving at least the subcutaneous fat, often associated with trauma or surgical wounds, and caused by wide variety of organisms. Streptococci are the most common cause; staphylococci usually require an obvious wound. Human or animal bites can cause aggressive cellulitis with a wide mixture of organisms. Patients are generally ill with fever and pain. Erythema, swelling, and pitting edema can progress to draining abscesses and sepsis, along with marked tissue damage.

Necrotizing fasciitis. There are two types—streptococcal gangrene caused by group A streptococci, and synergistic gangrene caused by mixed infections with an anaerobic component. Many patients are immunocompromised. There is a sudden onset of erythema and edema with rapid development of bullae and a necrotic eschar resembling a deep burn. Dramatic destruction of subcutaneous tissue and fascia is seen, with high mortality—hence the lay expression of "*meat-eating bacteria.*" Both surgical débridement and antibiotics (usually penicillin and clindamycin) are mandatory.

F. Other Infections

Ecthyma. Ecthyma usually starts as a streptococcal infection which, in moist climates and with reduced hygiene, leads to punched-out crusted dermal ulcers that heal poorly. It often starts on the shins and later becomes mixed infection. It responds slowly to systemic antibiotics and topical disinfectants.

Perineal streptococcal dermatitis. Pruritic anogenital infection caused by streptococci in young children; it may present with pain on defecation. There is a sharply circumscribed erythematous patch around the anus or genitalia. It is often misdiagnosed and responds rapidly to penicillin or macrolides; it should be treated for 2 weeks.

Subacute bacterial endocarditis. *Osler nodes* are a sign of subacute endocarditis usually from *Streptococcus viridans*, with seeding of bacteria causing tiny painful acral hemorrhagic nodules. *Janeway macules* have the same basis but are flat.

G. Toxic Shock Syndromes

Both *S. pyogenes* and *S. aureus* cause toxic shock syndrome (TSS) by secreting toxins that cause fever, nausea, diarrhea, and hypotension, followed by myositis, pneumonia, or meningitis. The mortality rate for TSS is up to 20%. *S. aureus*-TSS is usually associated with subclinical infections or superabsorbent tampon overuse, while *S. pyogenes*-TSS is linked to acute symptomatic soft-tissue infections.

■ Therapy

Treatment depends on the cause—either anti-staphylococcal agents or high-dose penicillin G combined with clindamycin.

H. Scarlet Fever

Scarlet fever is a streptococcal infection with production of erythrogenic toxin; it is usually but not always associated with pharyngitis ("strep throat").

■ Clinical Features

After a short incubation period of 3–5 days, it presents with fever, headache, sore throat, and fine exanthem starting in the flexure but rapidly spreading to the trunk. There are fine follicular lesions compared with rough sandpaper and facial erythema with sparing of the perioral region. Oral findings include macular enanthem on the hard palate and a denuded tongue with prominent papillae (strawberry tongue). There are often tiny petechiae and later there is desquamation of the tips of the fingers and toes. Complications include pneumonia, meningitis, glomerulonephritis, and rheumatic fever. Three different toxins are involved, so multiple infections are possible.

■ Therapy

Penicillin p.o. for 10 days, with monitoring of cardiac and renal status.

Staphylococci and Streptococci

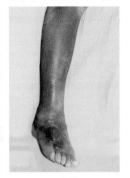

Hemorrhagic bullous erysipelas

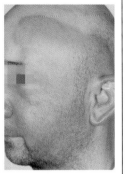

Facial erysipelas

D. Erysipelas

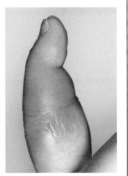

Digital cellulitis

E. Other Deep Infections

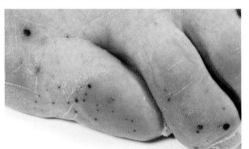

Osler nodes and Janeway macules

F. Other Infections

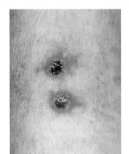

Ecthyma

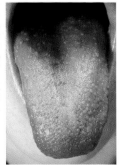

Strawberry tongue

H. Scarlet Fever

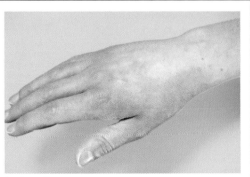

Acral exanthem

33 Bacterial Diseases

331

A. Corynebacteria

Corynebacteria are Gram-positive rods and part of the normal flora. They can cause disease when combined with excess sweating, obesity, and inadequate hygiene. They are all difficult to culture.

■ Erythrasma

This is a common intertriginous or vulvar infection with *Corynebacterium minutissimum.* Asymptomatic red-brown macules and patches are often mistaken for tinea but usually fluoresce with Wood light examination because of coral-red endogenous porphyrins. There is a high recurrence rate. Topical antimycotic agents work well (they also have antibiotic properties). Systemic erythromycin 250 mg daily for 1 week is also effective.

■ Trichomycosis Axillaris

This is a superficial white-yellow to red infection of axillary hairs by *C. tenuis*, with irregular concretions that adhere to the shaft. It causes bromhidrosis (foul-smelling rancid sweat). Regular cleansing or topical erythromycin is curative, as is shaving axillary hairs.

■ Pitted Keratolysis

Flat pits in the stratum corneum of the palms of the hands and soles of the feet are caused by corynebacteria and *Dermatophilus congolensis.* Cofactors include hyperhidrosis, occlusive shoes, and humid climate. It is occasionally painful, and is treated with topical antiseptics and by addressing the heat/moisture issue.

B. Other Gram-positive Bacteria

■ Erysipeloid

This is an infection with *Erysipelothrix rhusiopathiae* acquired from pigs, salt water fish, shellfish, and poultry, and after contact with animal products like bones and skin. It is typically seen in butchers, fishermen, and housewives with animal contact. After incubation of 3–7 days, a painful erythematous boggy plaque develops at the site of skin injury (usually the finger). It usually heals spontaneously after 2–3 weeks. Rare complications include endocarditis and sepsis.
Therapy. Penicillin G 3×10^6 IU p.o. daily for 6 days. Immunization is available for high-risk groups.

■ Meningococcal Infection

Neisseria meningitidis typically causes subclinical infections of the nose and pharynx in winter and spring. About 5% of the population are asymptomatic carriers. Endotoxin release may cause vessel damage and purpura. *Waterhouse–Friderichsen syndrome* is the virulent form, with disseminated intravascular coagulation (DIC). Chronic meningococcemia presents with pustules or leukocytoclastic vasculitis, often in crowded conditions such as military training.
Therapy. Mortality is 80% if untreated but most patients respond well if identified promptly; those with DIC still have a 50% mortality rate. Treatment combines high-dose penicillin G i.v. with appropriate measures for the DIC. Chronic forms respond well to penicillin p.o. Rifampicin is recommended for prophylaxis. Splenectomized patients are at special risk and should be immunized

■ Actinomycosis

Actinomyces israelii are gram-positive anaerobic-microaerophilic bacteria that are part of normal oral flora and usually found in mixed infection with *Actinobacillus actinomycetemcomitans*; only the combination is pathogenic. There is a *cervicofacial* form with woody induration of the soft tissues of the neck or cheeks. Fistulas are common and often drain yellow granules (called sulfur granules, but they are masses of organisms). Abdominal and thoracic actinomycosis usually follows trauma or surgical procedures, while IUDs predispose to genitourinary infections.
Therapy. High-dose, long-term penicillin G combined with débridement.

■ Nocardiosis

Nocardia spp. are Gram-positive soil pathogens that can be inoculated, causing local infection with draining sinuses and sulfur granules as well as often sporotrichoid lesions with lymphangitic spread. This is more common in immunocompromised patients. *Nocardia* spp. also cause mycetoma, a chronic granulomatous foot infection (Ch. 34.3).
Therapy. Long-term sulfonamides and débridement.

Corynebacteria and Other Gram-positive Bacteria

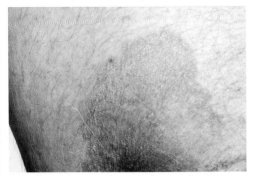

Erythrasma in the groin, where it is often mistaken for tinea inguinalis

Brick-red fluorescence under a Wood light

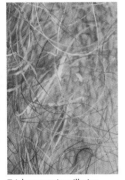

Trichomycosis axillaries

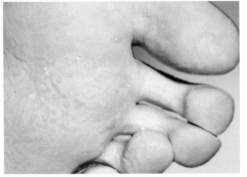

Keratoma sulcatum

A. Corynebacteria

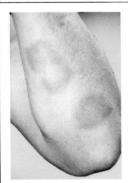

Erysipeloid

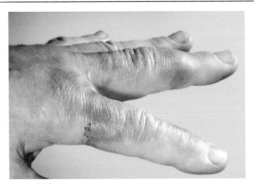

Erysipeloid

B. Other Gram-positive Bacteria

A. Gram-negative Folliculitis

Recurrent paranasal and perioral pustules occur as a complication of long-term antibiotic use, mainly for acne. Superficial lesions are usually caused by *Klebsiella*, and deeper nodules suggest *Proteus*.
Therapy. Culture-directed antibiotics and low-dose isotretinoin, as well as benzoyl peroxide topically.

B. Whirlpool Dermatitis

Pseudomonas aeruginosa can multiply in improperly maintained whirlpools and then cause a superficial skin infection with pruritic papules and pustules in those who use the facility. Systemic symptoms are uncommon. The course is self-limiting once exposure has stopped. Topical antipruritic measures suffice; there is no need for systemic antibiotics.

C. Gram-negative Toe-web Infection

Common problem for those with hyperhidrosis or who must wear occlusive shoes in a moist environment. Initially there is interdigital erythema, erosions, and maceration through mixed Gram-negative infection. Interdigital tinea can serve as an entry point. Secondary problems can include erysipelas, cellulites, and even sepsis. Subungual infections with *P. aeruginosa* have a green discoloration, suggesting the organism most likely to cause sepsis.
Therapy. Drying and antiseptic measures must be combined with systemic antibiotics.

D. Cat Scratch Disease

This is a worldwide infection caused by *Bartonella henselae* in children, adolescents, and immunocompromised patients. Bacteria are found in 25%–50% of urban cats; 10 days after cat-induced injury, malaise, fever, regional lymphadenopathy, and often macular exanthem develop. It is the most common cause of reactive lymphadenopathy in children. It heals spontaneously in normal hosts but in immunocompromised patients, *B. henselae* causes *bacillary angiomatosis* (benign vascular tumors) and peliosis (hemorrhagic cystic liver disease).
Therapy. Erythromycin or ciprofloxacin.

E. Yersiniosis

Yersinia enterocolitica causes colicky diarrhea, but in patients who are HLA (human leukocyte antigen) B27 positive, it often causes reactive arthritis (Reiter syndrome). It is also a common trigger for erythema nodosum in Europe and has been implicated in Sweet syndrome.
Therapy. Antibiotic therapy is generally unnecessary; in severe cases or with secondary disease, tetracyclines, cephalosporins, or gyrase inhibitors for 2 weeks are recommended.

F. Clostridia Infections

Clostridia are anaerobic Gram-negative bacteria that make a variety of toxins. Their spores are very resistant and widely distributed in soil and water.

Clostridium perfringens causes gas gangrene. Following a wound that introduces spores, toxins produce tissue damage (myonecrosis), crepitance, and shock. High-dose penicillin and prompt débridement are required.

C. difficile causes pseudomembranous colitis; it is facilitated by clindamycin therapy. Mild cases can be treated with metronidazole, while vancomycin is reserved for severe forms.

C. tetani causes tetanus or lockjaw, also following wound inoculation of spores through a puncture wound. The spores release tetanospasmin, a neurotoxin. Everyone should maintain immunization against tetanus toxoid. Nonimmunized victims are treated with tetanus immune globulin, which inactivates free toxin, but does not affect that attached to nerve endings. Penicillin kills organisms but this produces little clinical effect.

C. botulinum is the source of botulinum toxin used in aesthetic dermatology and against hyperhidrosis. Improperly canned or preserved food may also accumulate the bacteria and toxin.

G. Bite Injuries

Dog bites are more dramatic but generally superficial tears, while cat bites involve deep puncture wounds, often endangering the tendons of the hand through a closed-space infection. The most common pathogen is *Pasteurella multocida*. Bacteria in animal bites are usually extremely sensitive to antibiotics.

Human bites are far more dangerous. More common is clenched fist–tooth conflict where the fist usually loses out. Hand infections are the common result. Many bacteria are found in the mouth but the most common are streptococci, staphylococci, *Eikenella corrodens*, and *Haemophilus* spp.
Therapy. Tetanus prophylaxis and broad-spectrum antibiotic coverage.

Gram-negative Bacteria and Bites

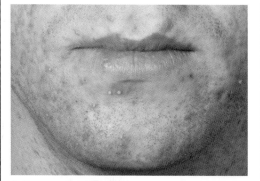
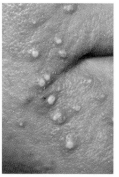

A. Gram-negative Folliculitis

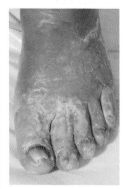
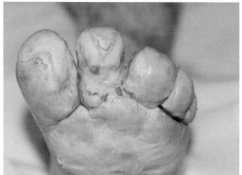

C. Gram-negative Toe-web Infection

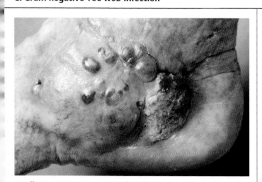

Bacillary angiomatosis in HIV/AIDS

D. Cat Scratch Disease

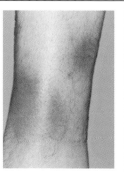

Erythema nodosum caused by *Yersinia*

E. Yersiniosis

33 Bacterial Diseases

335

A. Lyme Borreliosis

■ Epidemiology and Pathogenesis

Borrelia burgdorferi sensu-lato complex is a family of mobile corkscrew-like spirochetes and includes four human pathogens:
- *B. burgdorferi sensu stricto*
- *B. afzelii*
- *B. garinii*
- *B. spielmanii.*

It is transmitted in Europe by the wood tick *Ixodes ricinus*. In Germany there are 50 000 new cases each year. Not only adult ticks but also the tiny nymphs and larva can also transmit the disease if they manage to remain attached to the host for >24 hours; 5%–35% of ticks in Germany carry *Borrelia*. After a bite, 1.5%–6% of patients are infected and only 0.3%–1.4% develop overt disease.

■ Clinical Features

Clinical features are very variable depending on which species is transmitted and the immune status of the host. In the early stage, the first sign after about 10 days is usually *erythema migrans*, an annular lesion with an expanding erythematous border and pale center. Often the tick or a sign of the bite is in the center.

In early disseminated infections, there are a variety of symptoms, including flu-like illness, meningoradiculitis (*Bannwarth syndrome*), facial nerve paralysis, acute arthritis, and carditis. Skin findings may include multiple or coalescent areas of erythema.

Borrelial lymphocytoma can occur early or late; it is a red-brown nodule, usually on the ear, nipple, or genitalia, and by far the most common pseudolymphoma in Europe.

Late systemic manifestations include chronic arthritis, peripheral neuropathy, and encephalopathy. *Acrodermatitis chronica atrophicans (ACA)* develops, after months to years, starting as a puffy erythema over the joints and evolving into atrophic cigarette-paper-like skin through which the veins can be easily seen. Fibrous nodules may also develop around the joints.

Both morphea and anetoderma have been linked to *Borrelia* but this has now been excluded. Another rare late manifestation is cutaneous B-cell lymphoma.

■ Histopathology

Erythema migrans shows perivascular infiltrate with plasma cells, while ACA has extreme atrophy, with a bandlike lymphocytic infiltrate early on.

■ Diagnostic Approach

Culture is possible but not practical for routine use. Polymerase chain reaction (PCR) can be used to identify borrelial DNA in the skin in erythema migrans; it is reliable and sensitive. Serologic diagnosis with enzyme-linked immunosorbent assay (ELISA) and immunoblotting is the method of choice. The big problem is that in endemic areas many patients are seropositive but no longer in need of therapy. Thus, the clinical picture must determine the therapy. Control serologies are useless.

■ Therapy and Prevention

Early infections (localized and disseminated) should be treated for 2–3 weeks and late infections for 3–4 weeks. The treatment of choice for erythema migrans is doxycycline 100 mg b.i.d. for 2 weeks; alternatives for children <8 years and in pregnancy are amoxicillin 500 mg q.i.d. or cefuroxime 500 mg b.i.d. In disseminated or late disease with neurological symptoms, i.v. therapy with penicillin G or 3rd-generation cephalosporins (ceftriaxone or cefotaxime) is needed. If there is no neurologic disease, then doxycycline 100 mg b.i.d. for 30 days is adequate.

Protective clothing and insect repellants should be combined with prompt removal of ticks. Prophylactic antibiotics are not recommended. No vaccine is available.

B. Other Spirochetal Infections

■ Leptospirosis

Leptospira interrogans is contracted in contaminated water. After 1–2 weeks, patients have fever, macular exanthem, purpura, and malaise. The maximal variant is Weil disease with jaundice and renal disease.

■ Relapsing Fever

Body lice transfer *Borrelia recurrentis*; this is most common in African highlands. Ticks transmit other *B. hermsii* and *B. parkeri* in Africa, Spain, Middle East, and Western USA and Canada. The main clinical sign is relapsing courses of fever with a variety of systemic complaints. Sometimes there is a hemorrhagic rash. Relapsing fever should be remembered when evaluating travelers with tick bites.

Borrelia and Other Spirochetes

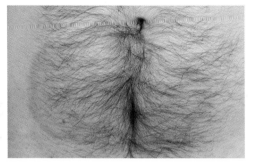

Erythema migrans

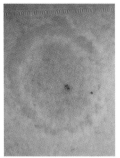

Urticarial erythema migrans

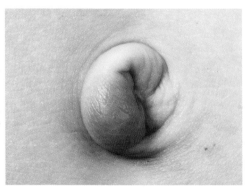

Borrelial lymphocytoma

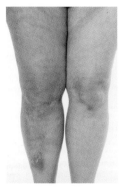

Acrodermatitis chronica atrophicans

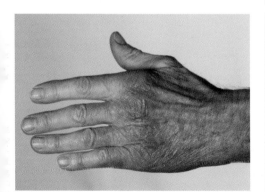

Acrodermatitis chronica atrophicans

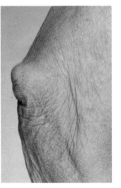

Fibrous nodule on elbow

A. Lyme Borreliosis

The World Health Organization (WHO) estimates that 8–9 million people worldwide develop tuberculosis (TB) each year. About 2 million die from the disease, especially in Africa where coinfection with HIV is common and facilitates spread. Causative organisms are *Mycobacterium tuberculosis* and, rarely, *M. bovis*. In Germany the incidence is 7.3:100 000. The incidence is 5-fold higher in Eastern European immigrants. There is a disturbing spread of multiresistant strains. Skin TB is uncommon; its clinical presentation varies depending on the host immune status.

A. Skin Tuberculosis in Anergic Patients

■ Primary Cutaneous Complex

M. tuberculosis is inoculated into a patient with no previous contact. After incubation of several weeks, changes analogous to primary complex in the lung develop, with an erythematous ulcerated papule and regional lymphadenopathy, which also may ulcerate and drain. It heals spontaneously but with scarring. Further development depends on immune status; in some patients the disease advances.

B. Skin Tuberculosis in Patients with Normal Resistance

Once resistance to *M. tuberculosis* has developed, usually following pulmonary infection, the tuberculin test is positive and lesions have few viable organisms. In severely immunocompromised patients, tuberculosis leads to disseminated papules and nodules rich in pathogens. This is a particular problem in patients with HIV and *M. tuberculosis*.

■ Lupus Vulgaris

This is the most common skin TB; it often results from inoculation following prior sensitization in other organs, but hematogenous or lymphatic spread is also possible. The classic lesion is a 2–3 mm red-brown papule which on diascopy has an apple-jelly color. Over years the papule slowly develops into a red-brown, usually ulcerated, plaque which destroys adjacent tissue. The name *lupus* comes from the Latin word for wolf and describes the destructive capacity. In addition to mutilation, the tight scarring is a fertile ground for the development of a squamous cell carcinoma.

The organism is identified via culture and PCR. Biopsy shows tuberculoid granulomas but only rarely acid-fast bacilli.

■ Tuberculosis Cutis Verrucosa

This is a butcher's or prosector's wart, which results from inoculation in a host with good resistance. There is usually a single verrucous red-brown papule, typically on the hands. It is often caused by *M. bovis* and chronic.

■ Tuberculids

A tuberculid is a disseminated reaction to mycobacteria in a patient with a vigorous immune response. The organism cannot be cultured but is sometimes identified with PCR. The best established is *erythema induratum Bazin*, which is a nodular vasculitis and panniculitis of the calf, often symmetrical, and usually in women. *Papulonecrotic tuberculid* has chronic recurrent necrotic papules that heal with varioliform scars.

Therapy. Skin TB and tuberculids should be treated exactly as TB in internal organs. WHO recommends isoniazid and rifampicin for at least 6 months, combined with ethambutol and pyrazinamide in the first 2 months. Therapy must be monitored closely to ensure compliance and identify resistant strains as soon as possible. Monotherapy can only be condemned. Small lesions of lupus vulgaris can be excised; once therapy is finished, considerable reconstruction can be needed.

C. Leprosy

Leprosy is a feared disease caused by *M. leprae*, which has shown a marked decrease in the past 15 years. The goal of elimination worldwide is unrealistic because of animal reservoirs. Leprosy is divided clinically into two major forms, based once again on the patient's immune status.

- *tuberculoid leprosy* (TL) has good resistance and few organisms and is usually asymmetrical.
- *lepromatous leprosy* (LL) has poor resistance and many organisms and is symmetrical.

There are transitional forms (borderline leprosy, BL) as well as an initial or indeterminate stage. *M. leprae* favors cooler body regions.

■ Indeterminate Leprosy

Initial infection is limited to the skin and nerves. There are usually single or few asymmetric hypopigmented macules. Sometimes there is associated impairment of sensation, but sweating is generally normal. A single nerve may be swollen. The lesions have few

┌─ **Mycobacteria** ─────────────────────────

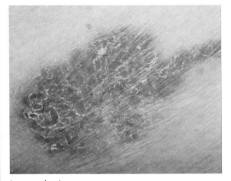
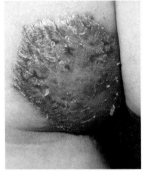

Lupus vulgaris

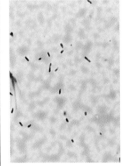
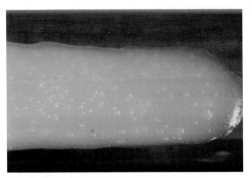

Histopathology: acid-fast rods Growth of *Mycobacteria* on Löwenstein–Jensen agar

B. Skin Tuberculosis in Patients with Normal Resistance

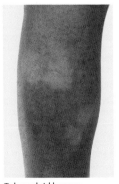
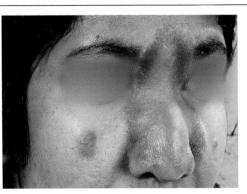

Tuberculoid leprosy

C. Leprosy

organisms and the histopathology may show granulomas but is frequently not helpful; the lepromin reaction to killed *M. leprae* is weak. Indeterminate leprosy lasts for weeks or months and then may heal spontaneously.

■ Lepromatous Leprosy

Pathogen-rich variant with impaired immune response to bacteria, negative lepromin test, no tendency to resolution, and grim prognosis. Symmetrical macules, elevated erythematous plaques, and eventually brown nodules develop. Facial infiltration produces a leonine facies. The nasal septum may be damaged. Typically, sensation is retained, in contrast to tuberculoid leprosy. The nasal mucosa, eyes, lymph nodes, liver, and spleen are also affected. On biopsy, foamy granulomas with large macrophages rich in acid-fast bacilli are seen.

■ Tuberculoid Leprosy

Noninfectious, slowly progressive form with little systemic involvement, and a tendency to spontaneous regression and a T_{H1}-mediated control of the organism with a positive lepromin reaction. Sharply bordered papules and macules are seen, with an erythematous border and central atrophy and hypopigmentation. The lesions are often anesthetic.

Peripheral nerves are thickened and damaged by granulomatous inflammation; superficial distal nerves like the ulnar and radial are most often affected, resulting in motor as well as sensory and autonomic defects. Histopathology shows granulomas with multinucleated giant cells and few if any organisms. The loss of sensation predisposes patients to trauma, whose sequelae may be overlooked, and then lead to mutilation, escpecially of the hands and feet.

■ Borderline Leprosy

Unstable stage between LL and TL. If untreated it tends to go to BL, and with treatment toward TL. Clinical features of both poles overlap.

■ Leprosy Reactions

Leprosy reactions make disease management difficult. *Type 1* reactions result from a change in immune status. Upgrading toward TL occurs with therapy and is often accompanied by severe nerve damage, while downgrading toward LL may reflect lack of therapy and produce new skin lesions. *Type 2* reactions are immune-complex reactions which occur when BL or LL is treated, and present with painful subcutaneous nodules, *erythema nodosum leprosum.* *Type 3* reaction is necrotic vasculitis, which occurs in patients with Lucio leprosy, a form of LL with diffuse cutaneous infiltrates and swelling.

■ Diagnostic Approach

The key to diagnosis is finding acid-fast bacilli in slit-skin or nasal smear using Ziehl–Neelsen stain. PCR can find organisms in secretions or tissue; it is helpful in TL where organisms are sparse. A serologic test against phenolic glycolipid 1 in the cell wall is positive in most LL, and 50% of TL.

■ Therapy

LL is treated with dapsone, rifampicin, and clofazimine for 2 years. In TL, dapsone and rifampicin for 6 months is sufficient. Systemic corticosteroids are the mainstay for leprosy reactions; thalidomide is added in type 2 reactions.

D. Atypical Mycobacteria

Ubiquitous mycobacteria cause localized infections in healthy individuals but disseminated disease in immunocompromised patients.

■ Swimming Pool Granuloma

M. marinum is found in fresh water as well as in aquaria. Minor injuries lead to inoculation and then after 2–4 weeks, a slow-growing papule that may ulcerate and often shows sporotrichoid (lymphangitic) spread. Histopathology shows tuberculoid granulomas, and organisms are found with PCR.

Therapy. A variety of antibiotics are recommended (clotrimazole, minocycline, clarithromycin, or ciprofloxacin), all for 6 weeks.

■ Other Infections

M. avium-intracellulare is a feared pathogen in HIV/AIDS. It causes pneumonia, osteomyelitis, and lymphadenopathy. When disseminated, cutaneous papules and nodules may appear. Treatment is with extremely complex regimens of multiple antibiotics.

M. chelonae is a frequent contaminant of tap water and may occasionally cause surgical-wound and other hospital-based infections. It, too, is far more troublesome in HIV/AIDS infections.

Mycobacteria

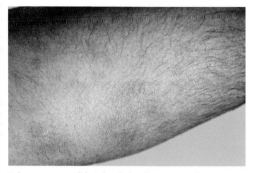

Subcutaneous nodule in borderline-lepromatous leprosy

C. Leprosy

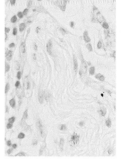

Histopathology: Fite–Faraco stain shows bacteria inside macrophages

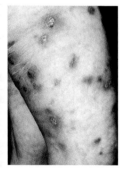

Disseminated *Mycobacterium chelonae* infection

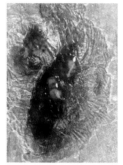

Pus-laden nodule caused by *Mycobacterium chelonae*

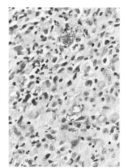

Immunohistopathology: intracellular rods seen with anti-BCG staining

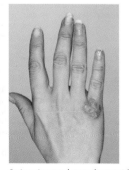

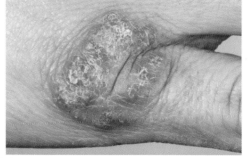

Swimming pool granuloma with close-up

D. Atypical Mycobacteria

These infections are very common; every 2nd adult aged >50 years has a dermatophyte infection. They are known as tinea (Latin for a larva or worm, so a completely incorrect designation) and then further named based on location. Scalp infection is tinea capitis, for example.

Typical for tinea is an annular spreading erythema with tiny papules and pustules and scale is prominent at the advancing edge. For this reason, it is often called "*ringworm.*" Dermatophytes can come from other humans, (anthrophilic), from animals (zoophilic), or from the soil (geophilic). Those from animals and soil elicit a far greater host immune response that those acquired from other humans. There are only three species—*Trichophyton*, *Microsporum*, or *Epidermophyton*.

A. Tinea Capitis

Pathogenesis. Usually caused by *Microsporum canis*, *Trichophyton soudanense*, and *T. verrucosum* in Europe; *T. tonsurans* is common in the USA and Japan.

Clinical features. It occurs most often in children, with patches of alopecia with erythema, scale, and pustules. *T. verrucosum* and related zoophilic species tend to cause intense boggy inflammation with pustules and scarring. Such intense first infections are known as *kerion*, and are often misdiagnosed as bacterial. *T. tonsurans* grows within hairs, damaging the shafts so they break off close to the scalp, leaving stubble (*black dot fungus*). In contrast, *M. canis* causes fine scale and little inflammation, but is very contagious and tends to fluoresce green under a Wood light.

Favus is caused by *T. schoenleinii*, the first infectious agent to be identified, and leads to armor-like plates of scale (scutula). Fungi can be identified in easy-to-pull hairs, scales, or pustules on direct examination in KOH solution, but should be confirmed with culture.

Therapy. Combined systemic and topical therapy is required for several months. Topical agents do not penetrate enough and are ineffective alone. Because of the risk of contagion, patients should be treated until KOH and culture are negative. The only systemic medication officially approved for children is griseofulvin, but more modern antifungals such as terbinafine and itraconazole are safer and more effective. Topically, imidazole creams and shampoos are useful. Often a domestic pet is the source of the tinea; it too may require treatment.

B. Tinea Barbae

Tinea barbae is infection of the beard area among young farmers after first intensive contact with large animals, usually caused by *T. verrucosum*. There is marked host reaction, with initially scaly macule advancing to deep pustulonodular follicular lesions, known as kerion. Undermined abscesses with lymphadenopathy and malaise develop; the end result is scarring alopecia. Diagnosis can be proved with KOH and culture on scales, pus, or hairs. Bacterial folliculitis can appear similar, but is usually not so severe.

Therapy. Systemic antifungals are required for several months.

C. Tinea Pedis and Manus

Pathogenesis. These are most often caused by *T. rubrum* or *T. interdigitale*, or less often *Epidermophyton floccosum*. Risk factors include diabetes mellitus, chronic venous insufficiency, foot deformities, and immunosuppression. In younger individuals, athletic activity is a factor because of occlusive footwear, sweaty feet, group showers, and minor trauma—thus it is known as "*athlete's foot.*" The fungi are widespread and can survive for months in shoes, as well as on carpets and bath mats.

Clinical features. This is the most common dermatophyte infection. Surprisingly, it is often unilateral, although both feet are exposed to same conditions. The *squamous-hyperkeratotic* (or moccasin) type has circumscribed scaly areas that are relatively asymptomatic. The *dyshidrotic* type presents with pruritic erythematous vesicles on the instep. The most common form is the *intertriginous* type, with interdigital (usually between 4th and 5th toes) fissures and maceration with white scales. The fissures and maceration serve as an entry point for erysipelas and Gram-negative toeweb infections. Secondary involvement of the nails is very common in all forms.

A typical but unusual situation is the "*one hand-two feet*" syndrome; why just one hand is affected is a great, if unimportant, mystery.

Therapy. Prophylaxis with meticulous foot hygiene and drying is essential. Generally, topical therapy should be tried first. If it fails, systemic agents can be employed. Once a cure has been achieved, intermittent prophylactic topical therapy is reasonable.

Dermatophytes

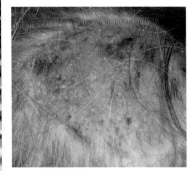

Kerion with pustules and alopecia

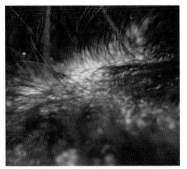

Green-yellow fluorescence of *M. canis* seen with a Wood light

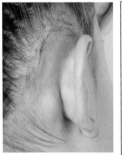

Tinea capitis with lymphadenopathy

A. Tinea Capitis

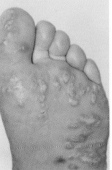

B. Tinea Barbae

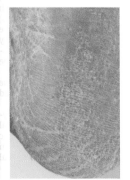

Squamous-hyperkeratotic type

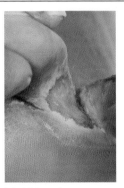

Dyshidrotic type

Intertriginous type

C. Tinea Pedis and Manus

D. Tinea Corporis and Faciei

Common in children and adolescents, this is usually caused by *M. canis*, contacted from cats (despite the name, it is less common in dogs). Often the contact occurs when children sleep with pets. On the trunk, the classic annular lesions with an advancing scaly erythematous pustular border are seen. On the face, the many curves and angles often mask the annular nature, making the diagnosis harder. Lesions are often pruritic. In immunocompromised patients, spread can be rapid or extend more deeply with granulomatous inflammation (*Majocchi granuloma*).

■ Therapy

If localized, topical therapy may suffice. With more widespread disease, systemic itraconazole or terbinafine is needed for 4 week. Once again, if a pet is the source, it must also be treated.

E. Tinea Inguinalis

Common dermatosis in older men, in whom it is a marker for tinea pedis and unguium. It typically involves the groin and inner aspects of the thigh; thus is often called "*jock itch*." There are pruritic circumscribed red-brown macules and patches that often have scale or tiny pustules at the periphery, explaining the old name of *eczema marginatum*. It can extend towards the anus, but the scrotum and penis are rarely affected. Almost all patients have tinea unguium—thus the old advice of "put on your socks before your underwear," to avoid inoculating the groin region.

■ Therapy

Improves rapidly with topical measures, but tends to relapse as long as tinea unguium is present.

F. Tinea Unguium

Tinea unguium implies a dermatophyte infection of the nail, while onychomycosis also includes yeasts and molds that cause nail disease. The most common cause is *T. rubrum* and usually the toe nails are involved. The nails may be discolored, deformed, or markedly destroyed. Four clinical subtypes are identified:

- distal subungual
- proximal subungual
- white superficial
- dystrophic.

Fungal hyphae can be identified in nail clippings with routine histological processing and then periodic acid–Schiff (PAS) stain. Culture is also essential before embarking on long, expensive therapy.

■ Therapy

Topical treatment with a medicated nail polish containing a potent antifungal agent can only succeed for mild distal subungual disease. Systemic therapy with an imidazole or terbinafine for 6–9 months, until the nail has been completely replaced, is otherwise required. After a cure, predisposed patients may benefit from prophylactic use of a medicated nail polish at intervals.

Mechanical nail extraction is no longer needed. Concentrated urea formulations can soften a dystrophic nail so it can be easily removed. This may facilitate therapy.

G. Special Variants

■ Tinea Incognita

Sometimes when tinea is treated with topical corticosteroids, its clinical appearance becomes masked. The inflammation and scale is initially suppressed, making the diagnosis difficult, but the organisms thrive, are easily identified on KOH examination, and later the disease flares when corticosteroids are stopped.

■ Fungal Id Reaction

An id is a secondary reaction involving an immunologic response to microbes at sites where no organisms are seen. The classic is the development of dyshidrotic hand dermatitis with pruritic vesicles—free of hyphae—at a time when tinea pedis is flaring.

A related variant is when a fungal infection seems to flare during the early stages of therapy, as an immune response is triggered by the damaged organisms. The inflammation clears as therapy progresses.

Dermatophytes

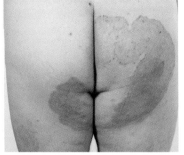

Tinea corporis

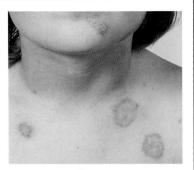

Tinea corporis and faciei

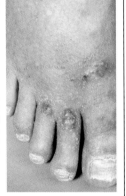

Granulomatous tinea

D. Tinea Corporis and Faciei

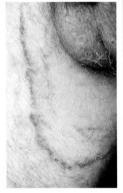

E. Tinea Inguinalis

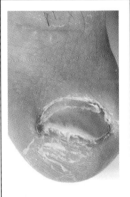

Distal subungual type

F. Tinea Unguium

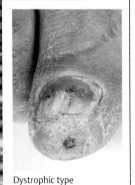

Dystrophic type

F. Tinea Unguium

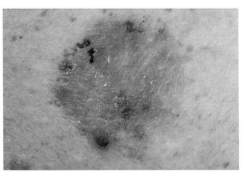

Tinea incognita

G. Special Variants

Yeasts of dermatologic importance includes the lipophilic *Malassezia* and many different species of *Candida*. Both yeasts belong to the normal flora of the skin or mucosa, but with changes in milieu, they can grow more easily and become pathogens.

A. Malassezia

Several *Malassezia* spp. are found in humans; most often *M. globosa* and *M. sympodialis*, and less often *M. furfur*. The genus was formerly called *Pityrosporon* and confusion still exists. These yeasts are part of normal flora, but with sweating, oily skin, or obesity, they tend to thrive and produce clinical disease.

Pityriasis versicolor. This is often called *tinea versicolor*, but is not caused by a dermatophyte. In temperate climates, pityriasis versicolor is more common in the summer, while in tropical areas it shows little seasonal variation. Clinically, asymptomatic circumscribed macules with a fine scale are seen. As the name versicolor suggests, the patches can range from white to pink to tan to brown. *M. furfur* can produce pigments that together with the scales inhibit melanogenesis (hence the white spots) and also fluoresce green-yellow with Wood-light examination. In the summer, the macules are paler than the surrounding tanned skin, while in the winter they tend to be darker than the now paler skin.

Malassezia folliculitis. This presents as small follicular papules and pustules, usually on the chest and upper back and frequently intensely pruritic. It affects young adults most often.

Confluent and reticulated papillomatosis. This is a confusing disorder with reticular papules and patches on the chest and back (Ch. 21.1). Some cases appear to be triggered by *Malassezia*, but others reveal no microbes.

■ Diagnostic Approach

A patient with pityriasis versicolor is ideal for learning how to do a KOH examination. The lesions are much more scaly than the naked eye would suggest, so that the scale is easily removed with a tongue blade. In addition, the scales are full of spores and hyphae (*spaghetti and meatballs*). They fluoresce yellow-green on Wood-light examination. Culture on lipid-rich media is possible but rarely needed.

■ Therapy

The diseases tend to recur once therapy is stopped, which makes sense as *Malassezia* are part of the normal flora and only controlled,

not eliminated. Antimycotic shampoos, lotions, or creams are usually sufficient; once clinical improvement has been obtained; intermittent therapy is useful for prophylaxis. If the disease is widespread or recurrences frequent, systemic therapy with an imidazole is indicated, such as itraconazole 200 mg daily for 7 days and then 400 mg in a single dose once monthly.

B. Candida

A variety of *Candida* species populate our mucosal surfaces as harmless commensals. Thus, a positive culture without associated clinical findings is never an indication for treatment. In immunocompromised patients or when the local milieu is altered (obesity, maceration, antibiotics, dental prostheses, hormonal therapy, or changes in bacterial flora through antibiotics), both local and even life-threatening systemic infections can develop. The most common species is *Candida albicans*. Recent years have seen a dramatic increase in the incidence of other species, such as *C. glabrata*, *C. tropicalis*, *C. krusei*, and *C. dublinensis*. Some of them are primarily resistant to imidazoles, while secondarily resistant strains of *C. albicans* are also becoming more common.

Oral candidiasis. The classic finding in acute candidiasis is easily removed white pseudomembranes (*thrush*); erythematous patches are also common. In more chronic disease, there may be erythematous, atrophic, or hyperkeratotic lesions; the latter are usually firmly adherent. Markedly therapy-resistant oral candidiasis is a clue to immunosuppression, while severe oral or esophageal candidiasis is an acquired immune deficiency syndrome (AIDS)-defining illness. *Candida* is also frequently involved in angular stomatitis (perlèche), with white patches in the corners of the mouth and median rhomboid glossitis with an atrophic patch on the mid-central dorsal aspect of the tongue.

Vulvovaginal candidiasis. Over 75% of women have at least one episode. Around 5% have chronic infections or four or more recurrences in a year. Infection is often secondary to oral contraceptives or antibiotic therapy suppressing normal bacterial flora that otherwise help control *Candida*. It presents with cheesy white discharge with pseudomembranous plaques on the vagina as well as vulvar erythema. The most common organism is *C. albicans*, followed by *C. glabrata*.

Candidal balanitis. This presents as erythema, erosions, and white patches on the glans, which, under a foreskin, provides an ideal

Yeasts

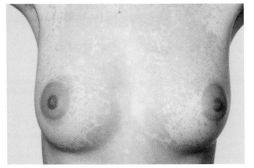

Pityriasis versicolor with circumscribed brown macules and patches

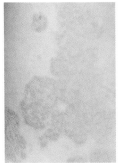

Pityriasis versicolor: close-up

Erythematous form

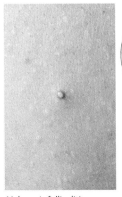

Malassezia folliculitis

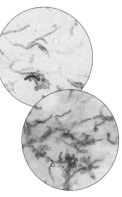

Spaghetti and meat balls

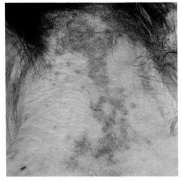

Confluent and reticulated papillomatosis

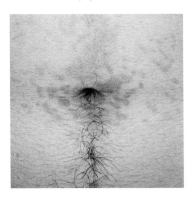

A. *Malassezia*

growth milieu. It is most common in old, obese men, often with diabetes mellitus, or phimosis, which inhibits proper hygiene. Circumcision is the treatment of choice, demonstrating that altering the environment, in this case drastically, is required to combat candidiasis.

Candidal intertrigo. Although *Candida* does not grow on normal glabrous skin, when an area is warm, moist, and macerated, the yeast feels at home. Predisposing factors are once again obesity (skin folds touching), increased sweating, and occlusive clothing; with recurrences, diabetes mellitus should be excluded. Clinical features are circumscribed erythematous erosions beneath the breasts, in skin folds, or especially in the groin. Lesions tend to have peripheral scale like a dermatophyte infection, but distinguishing features are central superficial erosions, satellite pustules, and involvement of the scrotum.

Candidal folliculitis. Immunocompromised patients can develop follicular pustules and furuncle-like nodules of the beard hairs; a sure clue to immune deficits—never seen in normal hosts.

Candidal paronychia. If the cuticle is damaged, usually by excessive soap and water exposure, then *Candida* can insinuate into the nail fold, where it causes painful swelling with discharge of pus.

Candidal onychomycosis. This is usually secondary to candidal paronychia. Initially there are just irregular grooves and ridges but it can progress to crumbly destruction of the entire nail.

Chronic mucocutaneous candidiasis (CMC). This is a group of etiologically unrelated disorders with immune and barrier defects that predispose to chronic candidal infection of the skin, mucosa, and nails, often starting in childhood. The causative organism is usually C. *albicans*. Acquired imidazole resistance is very common because the patients are treated for months to years. Variants include:

- autoimmune polyendocrinopathy-candidiasis-ectodermal dystrophy (APECED) with several patterns of inheritance, associated with hypoparathyroidism, Addison disease and gonadal defects
- autosomal recessive CMC, which presents in childhood with persistent oral, mucosal and nail candidiasis without other problems
- those with autosomal dominant CMC are similar, but also have trouble with dermatophyte infections
- diffuse granulomatous CMC that has widespread cutaneous granulomas, especially on the scalp, and systemic infections like cryptococcosis and miliary tuberculosis, as well

as iron deficiency and bronchiectasis; the mortality rate is high
- acquired or late-onset CMC presents in middle-age with thymoma and myasthenia gravis.

C. Therapy

Cutaneous candidiasis can usually be managed with topical antimycotic therapy, accompanied by drying measures such as blow-drying after bathing and laying absorbent cotton strips between touching skin layers. Mucosal candidiasis can be treated with nystatin, imidazoles, or ciclopirox olamine suspensions or troches. Underneath a denture, a cream is useful. Care must be taken not to choose products containing sugar, especially in edentate patients whose problems are complicated by xerostomia. Systemic therapy with fluconazole or itraconazole is more convenient and rapidly effective.

Chronic-recurrent vaginal candidiasis can be treated initially with fluconazole 150–300 mg and then with fluconazole 150 mg every 1–4 weeks for a long period of time, coupled with topical therapy as needed. Candidal paronychia and onychomycosis must be treated for systemically for several months, while CMC requires lifelong treatment. Many new antifungal agents including voriconazole, posaconazole, and caspofungin show promise in CMC, but they are very expensive and only time will tell if they help avoid the development of resistant strains.

Yeasts

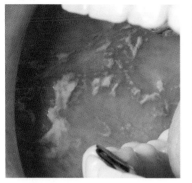
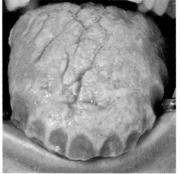

Oral candidiasis involving the buccal mucosa and tongue

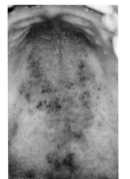
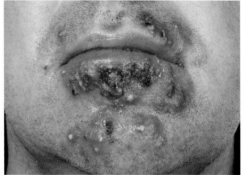

Erosive candidiasis

Candida folliculitis

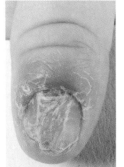
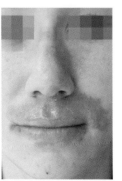
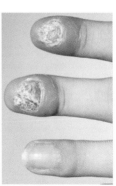

Candida onychomycosis

Chronic mucocutaneous candidiasis, autosomal recessive form

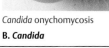
B. Candida

A. Subcutaneous Mycoses

These infections typically occur following inoculation injury (splinter, plant thorn); they are more common in the tropics because of barefoot exposure.

■ Sporotrichosis

Sporothrix schenckii is a dimorphous fungus (mold at 25 °C, yeast at 37 °C). Classic injury is from a rose thorn in gardeners. An innocent papule develops at the injury site, then ulcerates and heals over months with scarring. Lymphangitic spread generally occurs. This pattern is called *sporotrichoid* (also seen with *Nocardia*, atypical mycobacteria, and many other infections). Disseminated sporotrichosis results when the fungus spreads to internal organs. It is diagnosed with culture from biopsy material or drainage.
Therapy. Itraconazole is the most convenient therapy; potassium iodide solution is effective but hard to use.

■ Chromoblastomycosis

Papillomatous or verruciform nodules develop following splinter injuries from a variety of molds.
Therapy. Small lesions should be excised; larger ones require systemic therapy with itraconazole, flucytosine, amphotericin B, and combinations.

■ Mycetoma

Destructive, tumorlike process of the foot with sinus tracts and discharge of fluid with granules, also known as Madura foot. It is a chronic mixed infection involving bacteria (*Actinomyces* or *Nocardia*) along with fungi (*Madurella* and *Pseudallescheria*).
Therapy. Surgery and long-term antifungal or antibacterial therapy are needed.

B. Systemic Mycoses

■ Cryptococcosis

Cryptococcus neoformans is a yeast found worldwide in pigeon droppings. After inhalation, it initially infects the lungs but can spread to the skin, presenting as erythematous papules and nodules. It is primarily seen in immunosuppressed patients.
Therapy. Systemic voriconazole or amphotericin B.

■ Blastomycosis

Blastomyces dermatitidis is a geophilic saprophyte found primarily in North America. Once again, primary infection is usually pulmonary, with secondary cutaneous spread—typically with poorly healing ulcerated papules, nodules, and plaques. It also spreads, often to the prostate and bone.
Therapy. Systemic itraconazole, voriconazole, or in severe cases amphotericin B.

■ Coccidioidomycosis

Disease of the deserts of Southwestern USA and Mexico. *Coccidioides immitis* is limited to the San Joaquin Valley, while *C. posadasii* has a wider range. Either is inhaled with dust, leading to primary pulmonary infection; most are asymptomatic. Also a frequent trigger of erythema nodosum. There is a problem in HIV/AIDS with disseminated cutaneous papules resembling mollusca contagiosa. The main threat from dissemination is central nervous system (CNS) disease. It is far more aggressive in black individuals and during pregnancy.
Therapy. Most early pulmonary cases require no therapy; disseminated disease needs systemic itraconazole, voriconazole, or amphotericin B.

■ Histoplasmosis

Histoplasma capsulatum is a dimorphic fungus that is a mold in the environment (bird or bat droppings, barnyard soil) and converts to pathogenic yeast in humans. It is present in the Americas and Asia, mainly in the Ohio Valley. Initial infection is pulmonary and often subclinical. Extremely aggressive in HIV/AIDS.
Therapy. Systemic itraconazole, voriconazole, or amphotericin B.

■ Fusaria Infections

Fusaria are molds that produce toxins. Tissue damage is required in normal hosts (burns, trauma). In immunosuppressed patients, there is a risk of dissemination with ulcerated skin nodules.
Therapy. Systemic voriconazole, posaconazole, or amphotericin B combined with flucytosine.

Subcutaneous and Systemic Mycoses

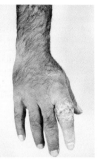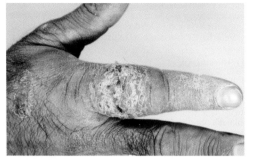

Sporotrichosis with close-up following injury from tropical wood

A. Subcutaneous Mycoses

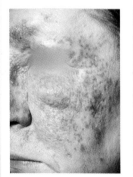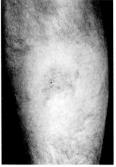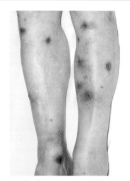

Coccidioidomycosis

Coccidioidomycosis

Multiple necrotic nodules caused by *Fusarium*

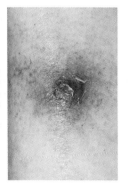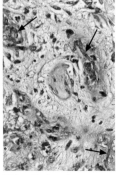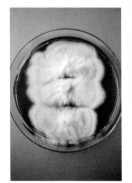

Close-up of *Fusarium* necrosis

Histopathology: hypnae (arrows) with PAS stain

Culture

B. Systemic Mycoses

Protozoa are unicellular eukaryotes, which are generally mobile (amoeboid, flagellate, ciliate) and do not engage in photosynthesis. They occur in several branches of the phylogenetic tree. Some have evolved as human parasites.

A. Leishmaniasis

Leishmaniasis occurs in the tropics and subtropics, and in Europe south of the 10°C yearly isotherm. In Germany, most infections are brought back from Mediterranean holidays. *Leishmania* exist as intracellular immobile amastigotes in humans and animal reservoirs (dogs, rodents) and as flagellated promastigotes in *Phlebotomus* sandflies.

■ Localized Cutaneous Leishmaniasis

Sandflies are low fliers and feed in the evening, typically biting an uncovered area like the face or arms. After 2–4 weeks, a helper T cell (T_{H1}) immune response develops; a red papule appears and over weeks to months expands and ulcerates. In the Old World, *Leishmania tropica* is usually responsible; spontaneous resolution with scarring is the rule. *L. infantum* is likely to cause multiple lesions, while *L. major* from the Near and Middle East causes multiple ulcers and lymphadenopathy, but seldom remains active for more than 24 months. In parts of Africa, Asia, and the New World, *L. tropica* and others elicit a T_{H2} response which fails to control the parasite and leads to a more aggressive course, attacking the nose and ears, with damage to cartilage, and can affect mucosae.
Diffuse anergic cutaneous leishmaniasis. *L. aethiopica* or *Viannia brasiliensis* may produce multiple nonulcerated papules and nodules rich in organisms in a host with no previous exposure or with impaired resistance.
Chronic hyperergic cutaneous leishmaniasis. In those with a good immune response, persistent red-brown infiltrates develop, resembling sarcoidosis or tuberculosis, sometimes with keloids.
Mucocutaneous leishmaniasis. This usually occurs in the New World from *V. brasiliensis*, less often in the Old World through *L. aethiopica*. There is marked mucosal damage following hematogenous or lymphatic spread (not local advancement to mucosa), with high morbidity.
Visceral leishmaniasis. This is present in all tropical zones except Australia; it is caused by the *L. donovani* group and causes hepatosplenomegaly, anemia, fever, and many other problems. The best-known local name is *kala-azar*. It also occurs in AIDS.

■ Diagnostic Approach

Leishmania can be identified in histological sections as 2–4μm intracellular organisms. Immunofluorescent antibodies against amastigotes are more sensitive, while polymerase chain reaction (PCR) or culture on Novy–McNeal–Nicolle (NMN) medium allows speciation, which helps determine therapy.

■ Therapy

Old World infections are usually self-limited. Nodules can be frozen, excised, or treated with 15% paromomycin ointment under occlusion. If lesions fail to respond, progress, or are caused by high-risk species, then antimony compounds are the treatment of choice. Alternatives include amphotericin B, dapsone, and metronidazole.

B. Trichomoniasis

This is a common sexually transmitted infection caused by *Trichomonas vaginalis*. It is both more frequent and more symptomatic in women and is not uncommonly combined with gonorrhea.
Clinical features. The most common complaints in women are vaginal discharge, burning, dysuria, and dyspareunia. Men are usually asymptomatic or may have dysuria or urethral discharge. *T. vaginalis* is easily recognized under the microscope by its flagellate motion. Culture is confirmatory.
Therapy. Metronidazole 1.5–2.0 g as a single dose. Sexual partners should be treated at the same time.

C. Amebiasis

While many different amebas can infect man, the term amebiasis is restricted to disease caused by *Entamoeba histolytica*. Infection is usually via a fecal–oral route. Most are asymptomatic, but bloody mucus-laden diarrhea sometimes develops. Complications include invasive mucosal disease, hepatic abscesses, and perianal nodules and draining sinuses. In homosexuals, it is considered a sexually transmitted disease.
Therapy. Metronidazole, tinidazole, or ornidazole.

Protozoa

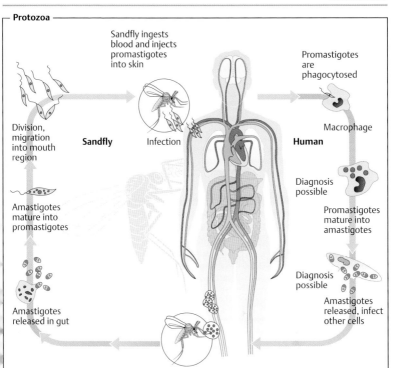

Sandfly ingests
blood and injects
promastigotes
into skin

Promastigotes
are
phagocytosed

Division,
migration
into mouth
region

Sandfly

Infection

Macrophage

Human

Amastigotes
mature into
promastigotes

Diagnosis
possible

Promastigotes
mature into
amastigotes

Diagnosis
possible

Amastigotes
released in gut

Amastigotes
released, infect
other cells

Sandfly feeds again, takes up
infected macrophages

Life cycle of *Leishmania*

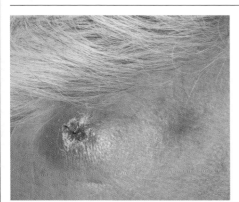

Ulcerated erythematous nodule on scalp after vacation
in Italy

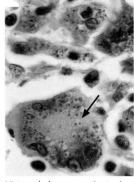

Histopathology: amastigotes in
macrophage

A. Leishmaniasis

Worm infections are often overlooked in temperate climates. They can cause both direct skin involvement and allergic and pruritic reactions secondary to systemic infection. Eosinophilia and elevated immunoglobulin (Ig)E are often signs of a worm infection.

A. Cutaneous Larva Migrans

This widespread tropical and subtropical infection is caused by different nematodes (roundworms) of the species *Ancylostoma*, *Strongyloides*, or *Necator*. They are typically inoculated from soil or sand contaminated by animal feces. In Europe, infection is generally a travel souvenir.

Clinical features. The larva penetrates the skin but finds itself in an inhospitable host where it cannot complete its life cycle. Instead it is confined to skin, where it migrates causing pruritic worm-like burrows (*creeping eruption*, *ground itch*), sometimes with secondary impetiginization. It usually occurs on the feet and is self-limited over weeks to months.

Therapy. The simplest approach is cryotherapy or topical thiabendazole 5%–15% in occlusive vehicle b.i.d. for 4 days. Systemic choices are albendazole 400 mg daily for 2–3 days or a single dose of ivermectin (200 µg/kg).

B. Cercarial Dermatitis

This is a worldwide problem in freshwater lakes. In Germany and Northern USA, it is limited to the summer months when bathing is possible. Infection occurs through a variety of nonhuman schistosomes (primarily *Trichobilharzia* and *Gigantobilharzia*) that normally cycle between snails and aquatic birds. Human swimmers are "mistaken" for the latter. Usually the first exposure is clinically asymptomatic but serves to sensitize the swimmer for subsequent exposures.

Clinical features. Shortly after bathing, the swimmer notices an intense itch. Soon a macular exanthem develops and evolves over the course of a day into fluid-filled pruritic papules that heal over 1–2 weeks. Anticercarial antibodies are present in the serum.

Therapy. Topical corticosteroids. On rare occasions, a short course of systemic corticosteroids is required.

C. Subcutaneuos Dirofilariasis

Dirofilaria repens is a subcutaneous parasite of dogs and cats in most of the world. It can be transmitted by mosquitoes to man as an accidental host. At the bite site, there is a slowly expanding subcutaneous nodule containing a growing worm; this is often accompanied by angioedema. It can be excised or treated as cutaneous larva migrans.

D. immitis causes dog heartworm disease and is less often transmitted to humans but can cause a similar picture.

Therapy. Incision or excision of the mass.

D. Onchocerciasis

Onchocerciasis is common in equatorial Africa as well as Central and South America. It is one of the leading causes of preventable blindness in the world (*river blindness*). *Onchocerca volvulus* is transferred from human to human by black flies (*Simulium* spp.). Larvae reach the subcutis, where they grow in a fibrous capsule. They then release microfilariae, which can be transmitted by another black fly bite, but move through the lymphatics eliciting an aggressive immune response, especially when they die and release antigens from *Wolbachia* symbiotic bacteria. They cause urticaria, intensely pruritic papules, erysipelas and lymphadenopathy, leading to hypopigmentation and skin atrophy (*leopard skin*). They also cause intense inflammatory eye disease with scarring.

Therapy. A worldwide campaign over past two decades has greatly impacted on onchocerciasis. The breeding sites of black flies in fast streams have been treated with insecticides. Ivermectin once yearly has been supplied free of charge; it does not kill the worms but prevents them from breeding. Doxycycline kills symbiotic *Wolbachia* bacteria, reducing the inflammatory reaction.

E. Schistosomiasis

This is a common disease, with 200 million infected humans in tropical lands. In Europe it is usually imported from Africa. Following contact with contaminated water, cercariae of the genus *Schistosoma* once again penetrate the skin, and pass through the veins and lymphatics to the urogenital veins where they develop into mature worms. Some primarily affect the genitourinary tract, others the gut.

Clinical features. Initial infection is accompanied by fever, urticaria, and eosinophilia (*Katayama fever*). Later, there are chronic anogenital warty papules, nodules, and fistulas with slowly healing ulcers that can evolve into squamous cell carcinoma.

Therapy. Widespread treatment programs with praziquantel are in place.

Worms

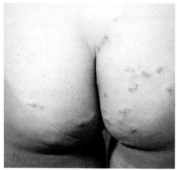
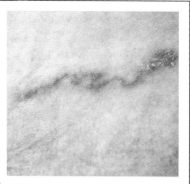

Larval tracks on buttocks: overview and close-up

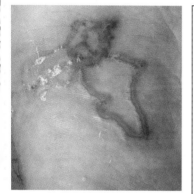

A. Cutaneous Larva Migrans

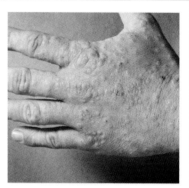

B. Cercarial Dermatitis

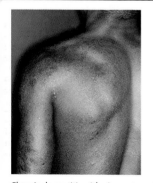
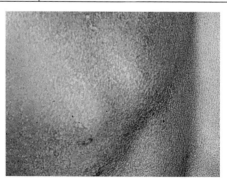

Chronic dermatitis with pigmentary changes; overview and close-up

D. Onchocerciasis

A. Pediculosis

■ Pediculosis Capitis

The head louse (*Pediculus humanus capitis*) is 3–4 mm long and transferred from person to person, most often among children, or via combs and headwear.
Clinical features. Head lice feed every 2–3 hours, inducing pruritic papules. Untreated, they evolve into severe crusted dermatitis especially on the nape. They attach the larva as nits to hairs, often in the warm retroauricular region. The 0.8 mm oval nits are easily seen but the lice are hard to find. Epidemics are common in daycare centers and schools.
Therapy. Permethrin is the usual first-line choice, as it is extremely safe. Unfortunately, resistance is an increasing problem. There are many options; none are effective against nits, so application should be repeated in 1 week. Nits can also be removed with fine-toothed combs. Contacts should also be treated.

■ Pediculosis Corporis

The slightly larger body louse (*Pediculus humanus corporis*) lives in clothing and lays its eggs there, jumping to the body only to feed. It is only seen when hygienic measures are lacking and is a disease vector.
Clinical features. Bites are intensely pruritic (*vagabond's itch*) and become lichenified and secondarily infected.
Therapy. The only treatment is washing clothes at high temperature. Attempts should be made to improve hygienic standards.

■ Phthiriasis

The pubic louse (*Phthirus pubis*) is crab shaped and prefers the genitalia. It is often sexually transmitted, so other STD should be excluded.
Clinical features. In adults, the lice are usually noticed moving about on the pubic hairs. Bites are pruritic and typically evolve into blue macules (*maculae coeruleae*). In children it favors the eyebrows and eyelashes.
Therapy. The same as for head lice but there is little problem with resistance.

B. Cimicosis

The bedbug (*Cimex lectularius*) spends its days in dark cracks but comes out at night once weekly, looking for a blood meal. Bedbugs can live for months without feeding. They typically feed with several bites in the same area. Symptomatic treatment and a visit from the exterminator are required.

C. Pulicosis

The human flea (*Pulex irritans*) is 2–4 mm long but capable of jumping 50 cm high or wide. A flea can eat several times daily or fast for months. Flea bites are usually multiple and linear—*breakfast, lunch, and dinner*. Fleas transmit plague and murine typhus. They must be killed with insecticides while the bites are treated symptomatically. Dog and cat fleas may also bite humans.

D. Tungiasis

The sand flea (*Tunga penetrans*) is common in tropical Africa and America. Its larva attaches to a beachgoer, and burrows into the skin between the toes or beneath a toenail. In 7–14 days, a pea-sized nodule develops, with the abdomen of the flea extruding in the center. The lesion is pruritic or painful and can become infected. The flea can be excised or, if one is lucky, removed with tweezers.

E. Myiasis

Many different flies occasionally lay their eggs on necrotic tissue, where the maggots hatch and then feed. A few species are obligate parasites causing furunculoid myiasis. Eggs are introduced from feces into a minor wound or bite, or larvae wander from contaminated clothes to the skin. The larva lives in the subcutis, releases enzymes to digest its meals, and emerges occasionally for air, leaving after a week to enter its pupal stage. Larvae must be removed mechanically.

The enzymatic activity of larvae from the sterilely bred greenbottle flies (*Lucilia sericata*) is used to débride chronic wounds (biosurgery).

F. Caterpillar Dermatitis

Caterpillars of the oak processionary moth and related species have fine hairs with toxic substances such as histamines and kinins. These caterpillars can fall onto a passerby in the woods and then cause intensely pruritic urticarial papules and plaques known as erucism. Systemic features such as fever, asthma, or anaphylaxis may develop. Epidemics have been reported where the caterpillars got into air-conditioning systems and their hairs were thus distributed through a building.
Therapy. Treatment is symptomatic. Systemic corticosteroids may be required.

Arthropods

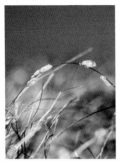

Nits on hairs

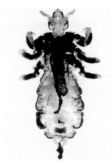

Pediculus humanus capitis

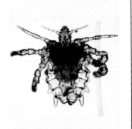

Phthirus pubis

A. Pediculosis

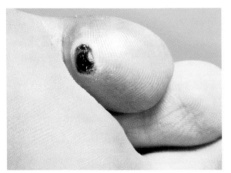

Rear end of sand flea protruding from skin

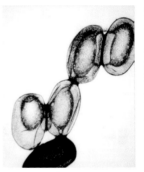

Eggs of sand flea

D. Tungiasis

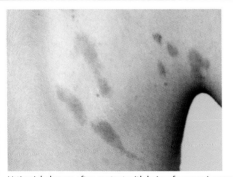

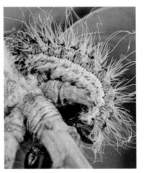

Urticarial plaques after contact with hairs of processionary moth caterpillar

F. Caterpillar Dermatitis

G. Scabies

■ Pathogenesis

The tiny 0.4 mm scabies mite (*Sarcoptes scabiei varietas hominis*) can only affect humans. The female is transferred by close personal contact. In the first infestation, it takes 3–6 weeks before the host becomes sensitive to the scabies mite and experiences intense pruritus, especially at night. With reinfestation, itching occurs within 24 hours. Usually only 10–15 mites are on the body.

> **Note:** Always think of scabies when a patient complains of night-time pruritus or when multiple family members are itching.

■ Clinical Features

The most distinctive feature is the itch. Often only excoriations and pruritic papules can be seen; common sites are the interdigital folds, nipples, and glans penis. If scratching has not been excessive, the burrows of the female may be seen, especially between the fingers. Papules develop as an allergic type IV reaction to the mite feces and parts. Secondary impetiginization is common, especially in children. In scabies of the cleanly, there are very few clinical signs—just a mysterious pruritus that is often overlooked for months.

■ Diagnostic Approach

Mites can often be identified at the end of the tunnel, either directly by scraping and examining under microscope, or with dermatoscopy.

■ Therapy

All contact individuals must be treated. Choices include topical permethrin, benzyl benzoate, or crotamiton. All should be repeated after a week. Resistance is a problem, but nowhere near as dramatic as with head lice. An option is ivermectin 200 µg/kg on days 1 and 7; this is especially helpful in epidemics in nursing homes or daycare centers.

■ Clinical Variants

Often itching following treatment is an irritant effect from overtreatment or excessive washing. Patients should never be retreated just for pruritus without finding the organism again.

Post-scabietic persistent papules are often seen in children as a hyperergic reaction. Persistent *nodular scabies* is seen most often on male genitalia and a common type of pseudolymphoma.

Crusted scabies (*Norwegian scabies*) is an uncommon variant in immunosuppressed patients as well as in nursing home patients. Thick crusts with thousands of mites are present. One such person can start an epidemic in a care facility. Treatment is ivermectin plus keratolytic agents.

H. Demodicosis

Demodex folliculorum and *Demodex brevis* are 0.3 mm mites that favor the sebum-rich facial area of older individuals. They cause a rosacea-like eruption with pruritic follicular papules, often asymmetrically distributed (Ch. 26.2). Infection is treated with permethrin or crotamiton.

I. Accidental Parasitic Mites

Dogs can have sarcoptic or demodectic mange; the mites are transferred to humans by direct contact. They cannot proliferate on the accidental host but cause intensive self-limited pruritic reactions. Treating the pet solves the problem. *Cheyletiellidae* cause "walking mange," and when transferred produces multiple tiny pruritic bites. Bird mites can cause similar problems.

Neotrombicula autumnalis and other harvest mites worldwide can transfer from plants to exposed skin and cause *trombidiosis*. They generally bite at sites where their progress is restricted by tight clothing, and then fall off again. They cause pruritic urticarial papules, which itch for about a week and may persist for 2 weeks. Treatment is symptomatic.

J. Ticks

The European wood tick (*Ixodes ricinus*) is a significant carrier of diseases. In Southern Germany, 5%–35% are infected with *Borrelia burgdorferi* (Ch. 33.4), while, with marked regional variation, 1%–5% carry the arbovirus responsible for tickborne meningoencephalitis. Ticks require some time to transfer *Borrelia*, so prompt removal by gradual twisting extraction with a tweezers is advisable.

In other parts of the world, ticks transfer Rocky Mountain spotted fever, ehrlichiosis, relapsing fever, babesiosis, and many other disorders.

Arthropods

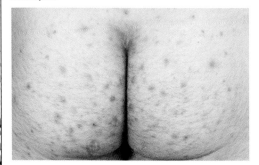

Pruritic dermatitis secondary to *Sarcoptes scabiei*

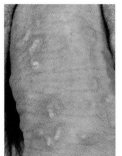

Papules on penis

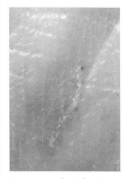

Burrow on sole with mite (dark dot) at end

Sarcoptes scabiei with white eggs, as seen with dermatoscopy

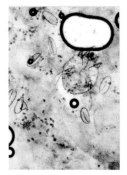

Sarcoptes scabiei with empty eggs and feces (scybala) seen under microscope after unroofing burrow

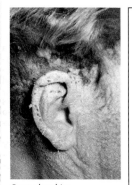

Crusted scabies

G. Scabies

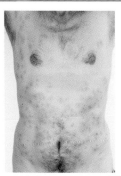

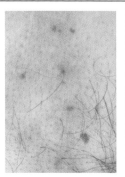

Trombidiosis: overview and close-up

I. Accidental Parasitic Mites

A. Gonorrhea

Neisseria gonorrhoeae causes a broad spectrum of clinical reactions, mostly affecting the anogenital mucosa.

Gonorrhea in men. Following direct inoculation of the urethral mucosa during intercourse, marked discharge (*clap* or *drip*) and extremely painful dysuria appear after about 5 days. Rarely there is mild discharge or it is asymptomatic. If the urethral glands are infected, abscesses can develop. Ascending infections can involve the prostate and epididymis.

Gonorrhea in women. In women there is a yellow vaginal discharge and dysuria following sexual transmission; 50% of infected women are asymptomatic but can transmit gonorrhea. The urethral and vaginal glands are often affected, sometime with Bartholin gland swelling. Ascending infections cause salpingitis and adnexitis, with infertility as a common sequela. In the most severe form, there is abdominal involvement with perihepatitis (*Fitz-Hugh–Curtis syndrome*). In pregnancy, there is a risk of septic abortion.

Rectal and pharyngeal forms. About 50% of women have asymptomatic rectal gonorrhea via direct contamination from vaginal fluid. In homosexual men, the rectum is a common primary site, with proctitis. Similarly, pharyngeal gonorrhea should also be excluded.

Conjunctivitis. Gonorrhea infections of the eyes in newborns can be contracted on passage through the birth canal or afterwards from an infected mother. Marked lid swelling accompanies pus-laden discharge. Untreated blindness is a serious risk. Thus, prophylaxis with antibiotic ointment is routine around the world. Conjunctivitis is also seen in adults but is much less common.

Disseminated gonorrhea. Disseminated disease occurs mostly in women, affecting 0.5%–3% of patients with local disease. Dissemination is more common during menses. The classic triad is fever, acute polyarthritis, and pustular vasculitis, usually overlying the joints, especially of the hands. The clinical spectrum ranges from purpuric macules to inflammatory papules to hemorrhagic pustules with central necrosis.

■ Diagnostic Approach

Paired Gram-negative diplococci lie within neutrophils. They can be seen with Gram or methylene blue stain, and confirmed on culture. Smears are taken from the urethra in men and the cervix and urethra in women; anal and pharyngeal smears increase the yield.

■ Therapy

There has been a marked increase in resistant strains worldwide. Current recommendations for uncomplicated gonorrhea include ceftriaxone 250 mg i.m. once, cefixime 400 mg p.o. once, or cefotaxime 500 mg i.m. once. For more advanced disease, i.v. therapy for 2–3 weeks is usually required. Consult guidelines for rapidly-changing resistance and new therapies.

B. Chlamydial Infections

Chlamydiae are bacteria that cause airway, urogenital, and ocular infections. *Chlamydia trachomatis* serovars D–K cause 30% of urethral cases in men. Other serovars cause trachoma and lymphogranuloma venereum (Ch. 36.3).

■ Clinical Features

After an incubation of 1–3 weeks, there is a yellow discharge and dysuria. An asymptomatic course is possible. Ascending infections can cause epididymitis, with a risk of oligospermia. In women, there is cervical infection but with additional risk of infection of ascending routes, and sterility. Transfer to a newborn is possible, via the birth canal, with conjunctivitis and pneumonia. Diagnosis is made with direct immunofluorescence antigen identification, cell culture, or polymerase chain reaction (PCR).

■ Therapy

Either azithromycin 1.0 g in single dose or doxycycline 100 mg b.i.d. for 7 days. Sexual partners should be treated,

C. Nongonococcal Nonchlamydial Urethritis

Both gonococcal and chlamydial urethritis can be diagnosed with specificity. Mixed infections are not uncommon. In around 50% of patients, neither microbe is found. Such cases are referred to as nongonococcal nonchlamydial urethritis (NGNCU). *Ureaplasma urealyticum* and *Mycoplasma genitalium* cause most of the rest. NGNCU cannot be separated clinically from chlamydial disease. Treatment is usually doxycycline or azithromycin. Other rare causes of urethritis include other bacteria, *Candida*, herpes simplex virus, and trauma.

Gonorrhea and Chlamydial Infections

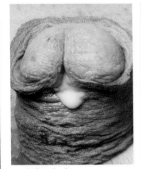

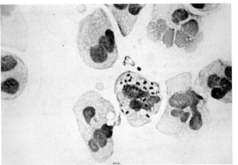

Pus-laden discharge in
gonorrhea

Intracellular diplococci with Gram stain

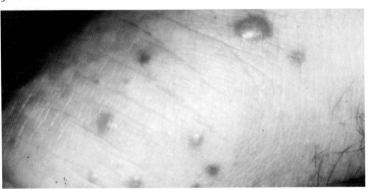

Gonococcal sepsis
A. Gonorrhea

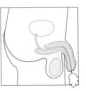

Risk of epididymitis

Salpingitis

Caution: Infertility

Pus laden, 3–5 days
Gonorrhea

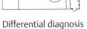

Watery, 14–21 days
Chlamydia,
Mycoplasma

B. Chlamydial Infections

Differential diagnosis

The word syphilis first appeared in 1530 in the title of a poem by the Veronese physician Fracastorius (1483–1553)—*Syphilis, sive Morbus Gallicus* (Syphilis or the French disease).

■ Epidemiology

Syphilis (also known as lues) occurs worldwide; it is a bacterial disease, which, if left untreated, becomes chronic and goes through characteristic stages but often clears spontaneously. *Treponema pallidum* is a Gram-negative 15 μm corkscrew-like spirochete that is a facultative anaerobe.

While syphilis is most often acquired through sexual contact, it can also be transmitted by blood transfusion or transplacentally. In Germany there was a huge post-World War II epidemic, another peak in the late 1970s, and then a gradual decline. In the 1990s the incidence was 1.4:100 000. The rate has increased in recent years, primarily in Eastern Europe and among homosexual men, who have apparently relaxed their caution as human immunodeficiency virus/acquired immune deficiency syndrome (HIV/AIDS) appears less threatening. Reduced use of condoms and increased numbers of partners in high-risk situations are the main factors.

> **Note:** Always investigate a patient with syphilis for other sexually transmitted diseases. HIV serology should be repeated in 3 months.

A. Early Syphilis

■ Stage I

The primary lesion in syphilis develops after 3 weeks, at the entry site, which is usually genital. A firm papule evolves into an ulcer, known as a *chancre* or *ulcus durum* (hard ulcer in contrast to chancroid with ulcus molle): only 10% of chancres are extragenital; then they are usually found in the anus, mouth, or nipples. Both the chancre and accompanying unilateral lymphadenopathy are painless. It heals with scarring over 6 weeks. In 60%–70% of patients, the disease heals spontaneously at this stage.

> **Note:** The presence of a chancre facilitates the transmission of HIV.

■ Stage II

The secondary stage starts about 9 weeks after infection, and follows a stuttering course with symptom-free latent periods. The cutaneous lesions or syphilids take many forms, almost never itch, and are rich in spirochetes and often highly infective.

Macular syphilid is the most common, presenting with pale pink discrete symmetrical macules on the trunk as well as the palms of the hands and soles of the feet. Papular, lichenoid, papulosquamous, and even, on rare occasion, papulonecrotic exanthems can all develop. In black individuals, annular (*nickel and dime*) syphilids are common. All can be confused with drug reactions, viral exanthems, and diseases such as psoriasis and lichen planus—making clear why syphilis is known as the *great imitator.*

Condylomata lata are broad-based moist plaques found in anogenital sites; they are teeming with organisms.

Patches at the corner of the mouth can mimic angular stomatitis. *Mucous patches* develop on the oral mucosa; after they acquire a gray-white membrane, they are known as *opaline plaques.* Syphilis involvement of the tonsils was formerly known as *specific angina*, while all other forms of angina were considered nonspecific.

The palmoplantar lesions can become hyperkeratotic *(clavi syphilitici).* Alopecia also occurs; initially the hair loss may be diffuse but the classic finding is a moth-eaten alopecia resembling alopecia areata, which occurs late in stage II. All syphilids can heal with hypo- or hyperpigmentation.

More than 50% of patients develop generalized lymphadenopathy known as *polyscleradenitis* because the nodes are so firm. A typical site is the epitrochlear nodes. Arthralgias and bone pain can also occur, as well as iritis, meningitis, and nephritis, but all are rare.

Symptom-free latent periods alternate with active disease, which tends to be milder with each relapse.

Syphilis

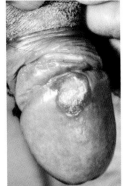
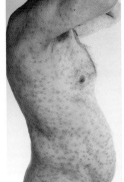

Chancre

Macular syphilid: overview and close-up

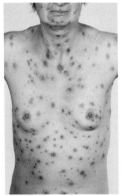
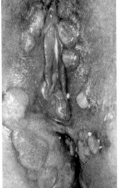
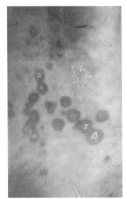

Papulonecrotic syphilid

Condylomata lata

Clavi syphilitici

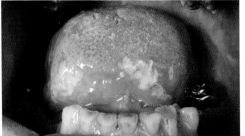
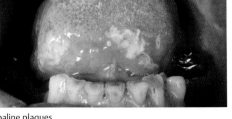

Opaline plaques

Mucous lesion at the corner of the mouth

A. Early Syphilis

B. Late Syphilis

If stage II lasts more than 1 year, it is considered late syphilis for therapeutic purposes, as longer treatment is needed. Two-thirds of untreated latent patients remain symptom free; one-third advance to tertiary disease.

■ Stage III

The interval between primary and tertiary infection can last 1–10 years. The clinical distinction between late stage II and stage III is not sharp. A typical skin finding in stage III is *tubero-serpiginous syphilid*, slow-growing infiltrative, ulcerated nodules arranged in a serpiginous pattern. *Gumma* is a painless subcutaneous nodule, which becomes matted to skin and deeper tissues, ulcerates, and then heals with a distinctive scar. Gummata typically involve the nasal septum and palate.

Optic nerve atrophy can follow direct infection of the nerve or be secondary to syphilitic lesions pressing on the nerve. The classic clinical finding is a pupil that fails to respond to light, but still accommodates—*Argyll–Robertson pupils*.

Permanent bony changes are a prominent part of stage III. The bones undergo massive destruction and regeneration at the same time. Areas where the bones are close to skin seem at greatest risk; examples include bowed tibias (*saber shins*), bossed forehead (*Olympic forehead*), and *saddle nose*, following destruction of the bony bridge.

About half of patients with stage III have relatively benign skin and bone changes; the other half develops life-threatening cardiac and central nervous system (CNS) disease. *Cardiovascular syphilis* primarily affects the aorta, with dilation, aneurysms, and possible rupture; the coronary arteries are also affected.

■ Neurosyphilis

Gummata can cause focal neurologic damage, while *meningovascular syphilis* develops after 4–7 years, with symptoms such as headaches, personality changes, or even strokes. *Tabes dorsalis* is the result of demyelinization of the posterior columns and dorsal roots, leading to paresthesias, shooting pains, and a peculiar *foot-slap walk*. Neuropathic ulcers may develop, and joint damage is common because of lack of feedback sensation (*Charcot joins*). Patients with *general paresis* formerly filled mental institutions; they have a wild mixture of neurologic and psychiatric symptoms.

C. Congenital Syphilis

Congenital syphilis can be avoided by prenatal screening. If primary infection accompanies conception, many spirochetes cross the placenta, the fetus is damaged, and it usually aborts at 7–8 months. If the mother has secondary syphilis at conception, a viable infant is born but with a spectrum of clinical findings resembling stage II or III disease. Finally, infection may occur via a spirochete-laden birth canal; then the newborn develops a chancre, usually on the presenting part.

Maternal IgG crosses the placenta, but IgM does not. Finding antitreponemal antibodies in the newborn with the 19S-IgM-FTA-ABS (IgM fluorescent treponemal antibody-absorption) test proves that in-utero infection has occurred.

■ Early Congenital Syphilis

This is defined as disease in the first 2 years of life. Typically, there is failure to thrive, *sniffles* (massive nasal discharge interfering with eating and breathing), and hepatosplenomegaly with fibrosis and jaundice (*flint liver*). *Parrot pseudoparalysis* follows epiphyseal dislocation of the ulna, leaving a useless forearm. The cutaneous findings are very similar to secondary syphilis; one difference is that neonatal lesions may be bullous—something never seen in adults.

■ Late Congenital Syphilis

Lesions appear after 2 years of age and resemble tertiary disease. Gummata may develop, as well as neurosyphilis; there is no congenital cardiac disease. A typical finding is *Hutchinson triad*, with interstitial keratitis, deafness from auditory nerve damage, and dental abnormalities (*moon molars* and screwdriver-shaped *Hutchinson incisors*). There is symmetrical joint swelling and synovitis, usually of the knees, known as Clutton joints. Additional stigmata include saddle nose, *Parrot lines* (deep radial furrows around mouth, crossing the vermilion), saber shins, and Olympic forehead—all discussed under late syphilis.

D. Syphilis in HIV

Syphilis has an atypical, accelerated, and more severe course in patients infected with HIV. In homosexual men, syphilis must always be excluded when confronted with oral or anal ulcers, as well as pharyngitis. Primary syphilis may feature multiple primary chancres that

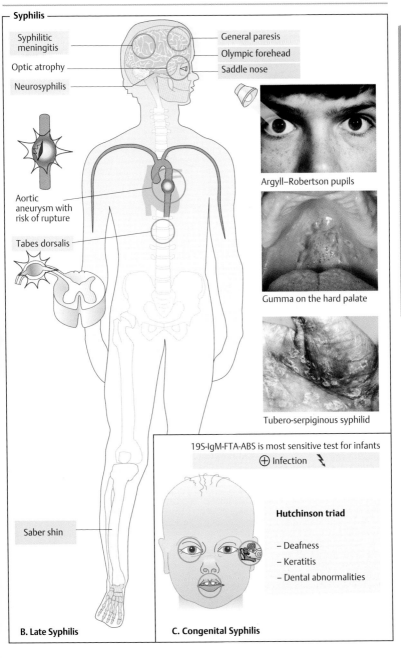

Syphilis

- Syphilitic meningitis
- Optic atrophy
- Neurosyphilis
- General paresis
- Olympic forehead
- Saddle nose

Argyll–Robertson pupils

- Aortic aneurysm with risk of rupture
- Tabes dorsalis

Gumma on the hard palate

Tubero-serpiginous syphilid

- Saber shin

19S-IgM-FTA-ABS is most sensitive test for infants

⊕ Infection

Hutchinson triad

– Deafness
– Keratitis
– Dental abnormalities

B. Late Syphilis

C. Congenital Syphilis

heal slowly. Systemic signs and symptoms are more common with overlapping features of primary and secondary disease such as fever, headache, and malaise, as well as generalized lymphadenopathy, splenomegaly, and elevated liver function tests.

Neurologic problems are of special concern, as the brain is a privileged site where the spirochetes are poorly cleared. In addition, the CD4+ cell count appears critical. As it falls, a latent, less than optimally treated syphilis may be reactivated. *Lues maligna* is an uncommon variant, seen most often in association with HIV. Papulopustular lesions rapidly evolve into necrotic ulcers in patients with many systemic findings.

E. Diagnostic Approach

■ Direct Identification

T. pallidum can be found in the tissue fluid from primary and early secondary lesions. Darkfield microscopy on carefully obtained blood-free fluid reveals the characteristic corkscrew motion of the spirochete. *T. pallidum* can be separated from the many normal oral spirochetes using direct immunofluorescence with labeled monoclonal antibodies. The organisms can also be identified in tissue sections, using immunoperoxidase techniques. Specific nucleic acids can be identified in smears, tissues, blood, cerebrospinal fluid (CSF), amniotic fluid, or other sites, with PCR.

■ Serologic Diagnosis

It is important to distinguish between nontreponemal and treponemal methods. The former are used for screening; the latter, for confirmation. The *nontreponemal tests* include the venereal disease research laboratory (VDRL) and the rapid plasma reagin (RPR) tests. These antibodies appear 4–6 weeks after infection, reach a peak during secondary syphilis, and decline during the latent periods. Their titers generally decline or disappear after successful therapy. In contrast, *T. pallidum-specific tests* include the *T. pallidum* particle-agglutination (TPPA) test and the fluorescent-treponema-antibody-absorption (FTA-ABS) test, which remain positive lifelong, also after therapy, as they recognize IgG antibodies. The 19S-IgM-FTA-ABS test is a modification to identify fetal IgM and clarify the diagnosis of congenital syphilis or a re-infection. IgM antibodies indicate a new identification and have almost 100% specificity; they disappear years after therapy and sometimes also in latent syphilis.

Practical approach. If syphilis is suspected, a TPPA test should be done. If it is negative, no further tests are required. VDRL or RPR may also be used for screening, but the false-positive rate is much higher. If the TPPA is positive or borderline, then FTA-ABS is done. If it too is positive, then the diagnosis of syphilis is confirmed. Then the quantitative VDRL and the *T. pallidum-specific* IgM should be determined to assess disease activity and monitor the response to therapy.

The decision on therapy is determined by the history, clinical findings, and presence of IgM antibodies. If IgM is negative but IgG titers are positive and appropriate therapy has not been provided, then treatment is indicated. The 19S-IgM-FTA-ABS test can also be used to follow response to therapy.

F. Therapy

Penicillin remains the treatment of choice, as resistance has not become a problem over the past six decades. *T. palladium* has a long generation time, so a bactericidal serum level must be maintained for several weeks. Thus, the mainstay of therapy is long-acting intramuscular depot preparations. Current therapeutic recommendations are shown opposite. The recommendations change frequently; the latest guidelines should always be followed.

Caution: Always be alert to the possibility of Jarisch–Herxheimer reaction when treating secondary syphilis with potentially large numbers of organisms!

When the spirochetes are killed in large numbers, enough toxins are released after 2–8 hours to cause fever, chills, headache, and worsening of any syphilids. When the aorta is involved, there is a real risk of iatrogenic-facilitated rupture. Prednisolone 0.5.0 1.0 mg/kg p. o. should be given for prophylaxis 30–60 minutes before the first dose of penicillin.

Since HIV patients with secondary syphilis have an increased risk of neurosyphilis, the approach must be modified slightly. Benzathine penicillin G is only used with a negative CSF serology and then once weekly for 3 weeks. If a CSF diagnosis is not possible, then the patient should be treated as though they have neurosyphilis.

Patients with syphilis should have repeat serology at 6, 12, and 24 months after conclusion of treatment. Syphilis is a reportable disease and partner tracing should be performed whenever feasible. HIV serology should also be checked and monitored.

Syphilis

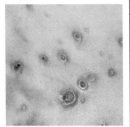

VDRL	19S-IgM-FTA-ABS	19S-IgM-FTA-ABS
RPR	(IGB)-FTA-ABS	IgM ELISA
TPPA	TPPA	(enzyme-linked immunosorbent assay)
		VDRL titers
Screening tests	Confirmatory tests	Control tests

Lues maligna

D. Syphilis in HIV

Appropriate use of serologic tests

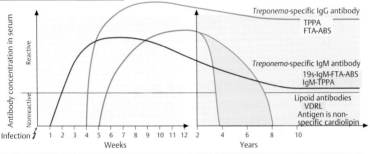

Antibody concentration in serum — Reactive / Nonreactive

Treponema-specific IgG antibody
TPPA
FTA-ABS

Treponema-specific IgM antibody
19s-IgM-FTA-ABS
IgM-TPPA

Lipoid antibodies
VDRL
Antigen is non-specific cardiolipin

Infection

Weeks: 1 2 3 4 5 6 7 8 9 10 11 12
Years: 2 4 6 8 10

Clinical course

Chancre — Recurrent exanthems or early latency — Late latency 30%

First exanthem

Primary syphilis — Secondary syphilis — Tertiary stage

3 weeks | 3 months | 5 years | 30 years

Antibody patterns in the course of syphilis

E. Diagnostic Approach

Guideline	Early syphilis	Late syphilis	Neurosyphilis
First choice	Benzathine benzylpenicillin 2.4 million units i.m. (1.2 million in each buttock)	Benzathine benzylpenicillin 2.4 million units i.m. (1.2 million in each buttock) on days 1, 8, 15	Penicillin G crystalloid solution 6x3–4 million units i.v. daily for at least 14 days or 3x10 or 5x5 million units i.v. daily for 2–3 weeks or ceftriaxone 2 g i.v. once daily for 10–14 days (first dose 4 g)
Allergic to penicillin	Doxycycline 100 mg b.i.d. p.o. for 14 days or erythromycin 500 mg q.i.d. p.o. for 14 days	Doxycycline 100 mg b.i.d. p.o. for 28 days or erythromycin 500 mg q.i.d. i.v. for 28 days	Doxycycline 200 mg q.i.d. p.o. for 28 days (not in children or pregnancy)
Alternative	Ceftriaxone 1.0 g daily i.v. over 30 minutes for 10 days or 1.0 g daily i.m. for 10 days or tetracycline 500 mg q.i.d. p.o. for 14 days	Ceftriaxone 2.0 g daily i.v. over 30 minutes for 14 days	

F. Therapy

A. Lymphogranuloma Venereum

Infection with *Chlamydia trachomatis*, serovars L1–L3, and is more common in tropical lands. In Germany it is primarily a problem in returning travelers and prostitutes, and as a cause of proctitis in homosexual men.

Stage I. Two to six days after infection, a tiny papule develops on the genitalia with rapid transition to a pustule and then flat ulcer. The primary lesion is painless and heals spontaneously within 14 days.

Stage II. Infection is often first noticed at this stage, with unilateral painful lymphadenopathy with breakdown, abscess formation, and draining fistulas. An enlarged inguinal lymph node, generally associated with a sexually transmitted disease, is known as a *bubo*. Sometimes associated with malaise and weight loss.

Stage III. Strictures and fibrosis lead to lymphedema and swelling of the external genitalia (*elephantiasis*). The anal–rectal symptom complex is limited to women and homosexuals; marked inflammation leads to rectal and anal strictures with draining sinuses.

■ Diagnostic Approach

There is a 4-fold increased titers of antichlamydial antibodies (greatly exceeds titers seen in chlamydial urethritis). Chlamydia can be detected in primary lesion or lymph node with culture or PCR. Syphilis and HIV should be excluded.

■ Therapy

Doxycycline 100 mg b.i.d. for 21 days. If not tolerated, erythromycin and sulfamethoxazole are alternatives.

B. Chancroid

Chancroid is endemic in tropical lands of Africa and Southeast Asia. In Germany it is uncommon; there have been several urban epidemic areas in the USA; it is now considered endemic in New York and South Florida.

■ Clinical Features

Haemophilus ducreyi is a small Gram-negative rod that enters the skin through a minor injury; 3–7 days later a papule appears, which rapidly becomes a pustule and then a painful, foul-smelling undermined ulcer (ulcus molle, because it is soft in contrast to chancre).

Some patients have multiple ulcers. About half develop lymphangitis and then after 1–2 weeks painful lymphadenopathy, which can also break down with discharge and fistula formation.

The simultaneous presence of *Treponema pallidum* and *Haemophilus ducreyi* in the same ulcer is known as ulcus mixtum (mixed ulcer). *Neisseria gonorrhoeae* can also be found in ulcera mollia. Finally ulcera mollia also facilitate the transmission of HIV, as do chancres.

■ Diagnostic Approach

Microscopic examination of a smear reveals Gram-negative rods arranged like "*schools of fish*." Culture is complicated requiring special agars but provides confirmation.

> **Note:** If chancroid is diagnosed, testing should be done for syphilis and HIV, both at the start of therapy and after 6 weeks for syphilis and 3 months for HIV.

■ Therapy

Azithromycin 1.0 g p.o. or ceftriaxone 250 mg i.m., each as a single dose.

C. Granuloma Inguinale

Endemic in the Caribbean and New Guinea, in western countries primarily among homosexuals. *Calymmatobacterium granulomatosis* is a Gram-negative rod with bipolar staining with Giemsa (*safety-pin sign*). Bacteria are seen inside macrophages (*Donovan bodies*).

■ Clinical Features

After a highly variable incubation period, there is an onset of single or multiple nontender papules or subcutaneous nodules, which rapidly break down forming beefy red ulcers. When the nodules develop in the groin they are referred to as *pseudobuboes*, as there is groin swelling without true lymphadenopathy. Later complications are lymphatic obstruction with elephantiasis, and persistent ulcers that may evolve in SCC. Culture is difficult, so diagnosis is usually based on direct examination of a smear to find the characteristic bacteria. PCR can offer confirmation. Once again, mixed infections and HIV should be excluded.

■ Therapy

Azithromycin 1 g p.o. weekly for 3 weeks or ciprofloxacin 750 mg p.o. b.i.d. for 3 weeks.

Other Venereal Diseases

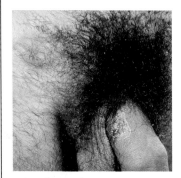

A. Lymphogranuloma Venereum

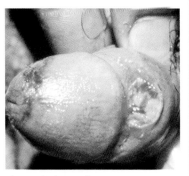

Chancroid: ulcus molle

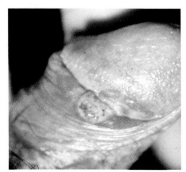

Chancroid: ulcus molle

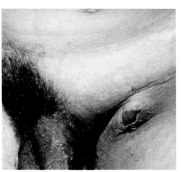

Perforated bubo in chancroid

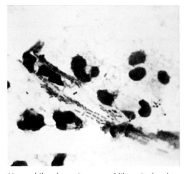

Hemophilus ducreyi arranged like a "school of fish" in Gram stain

B. Chancroid

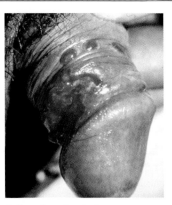

C. Granuloma Inguinale

Infection with the human immunodeficiency virus (HIV) induces an immune deficit primarily involving loss of CD4+ T cells and antigen-presenting dendrite cells. The result is a chronic infection that can progress to acquired immune deficiency syndrome (AIDS) with development of unusual infections, dermatoses, and tumors.

A. Epidemiology

In Africa and Asia, heterosexual transmission of HIV dominates, in contrast to the situation in Western Europe where most patients are homosexual men, prostitutes, or intravenous drug users. In Germany there were around 2000 new infections yearly for some time, but in recent years, around 2600 have been reported. The fear is that homosexual men are being less careful, reassured by therapeutic successes. Worldwide in 2008, an estimated 33 million people had HIV/AIDS; this is 1 in 100 people aged between 15 and 49 years.

B. Pathogenesis

HIV is a retrovirus in the lentivirus family. It has an affinity for CD4+ helper T cells, macrophages, and microglia. HIV can be found in all body fluids. The most important method of transmission is contact of semen or blood with damaged mucosa, especially if genital ulcers (syphilis, herpes) are present; the second main way is via infected blood. While transfusions are so carefully controlled that the risk today is infinitesimal, drug abusers continue to contaminate one another via shared needles. Mother–infant transmission is possible at several levels—intrauterine, intrapartum, and while nursing. It is significantly diminished by antiretroviral therapy.

C. Clinical Classification

Acute HIV infection. Often overlooked or confused with other viral illnesses, this presents with fever, night sweats, maculopapular exanthema, and sometimes oral ulcers 2–8 weeks after transmission of HIV. Later there may be neurological problems such as meningoencephalitis and facial nerve palsy, as well as a period of *generalized lymphadenopathy*.
HIV-associated, non-AIDS-defining illnesses. There are several illnesses that are often seen with HIV infection but are not regarded as AIDS defining; included in this group are bacillary angiomatosis, therapy-resistant oropharyngeal candidiasis, and zoster taking a normal course in a young adult. All suggest the CD4 count is <500/μL.
AIDS. The AIDS-defining illnesses are shown opposite. The Centers for Disease Control and Prevention (CDC) classification combines the clinical features and CD4+ lymphocyte count.

D. Viral Infections

HIV-associated infections often occur in the wrong age group, at an uncommon site, or are unexpectedly severe. Their appearance can help one make the diagnosis of HIV infection. Ulceration, persistence, and dissemination suggest more advanced disease.
Herpes simplex virus. Patients with a CD4 count <200/μL tend to have persistent crusted polycyclic ulcers without spontaneous healing and in atypical sites.
Varicella zoster virus (VZV). Zoster as a segmental reaction of VZV infection can be the first sign of HIV in healthy young adults. Multidermatomal zoster or recurrent varicella suggests a more profound immune deficit. Hemorrhagic or necrotic forms may be associated with central nervous system (CNS) or pulmonary spread. Treatment is with aciclovir 5–10 mg/kg i.v. daily for 5–10 days. Alternatives include famciclovir or valaciclovir.
Cytomegalovirus. This presents as persistent oral or deep, poorly delineated anorectal ulcers. Sometimes there is maculopapular exanthem on the trunk. The main problem is retinitis, usually treated with ganciclovir, sometimes injected into the vitreous body.
Epstein–Barr virus. This causes *oral hairy leukoplakia* with discrete white threads on lateral aspects of the tongue, as well occasionally verrucous mucosal plaques. It is also a factor in Castleman disease and lymphomas, especially pleural.
Human papilloma virus (HPV). Warts tend to be larger and hard to treat. Condylomata acuminata may be very widespread; intraoral lesions are also common. HPV16 and 18 cause cervical and anal carcinoma, which develop rapidly and are aggressive in AIDS patients. Treatment is the same as in non-HIV patients but caution is needed about transmission via laser plume or other destructive measures.
Mollusca contagiosa. There is a close correlation between immune status and clinical findings. Widespread infections or giant lesions, usually on the face, indicate CD4+ count <200/μL.

HIV/AIDS

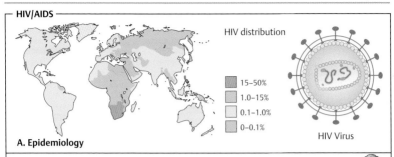

HIV distribution

▨	15–50%
▨	1.0–15%
□	0.1–1.0%
▨	0–0.1%

HIV Virus

A. Epidemiology

Sexual intercourse/body fluids   Injected drugs   Blood products   Mother/child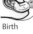

Methods of transmission

B. Pathogenesis

Trans-placental   Birth   Nursing

CD4+ lymphocytes		Clinical stage		
		A	B	C
>500	1	Stage 1		Stage 3
200–499	2			
<200	3	Stage 2		AIDS

A = Asymptomatic, acute retroviral syndrome, lymphadenopathy syndrome
B = HIV-associated but not AIDS-defining illnesses
C = AIDS-defining illnesses

CDC stages

Protozoal infections
• Toxoplasmosis of the brain
• Cryptosporidiosis, chronic gastro-intestinal disease (>1 month)
• Isosporias, chronic intestinal (> 1 month)

Fungal infections
• Candidiasis of the bronchi, trachea, lungs, or esophagus
• *Pneumocystis jiroveci* pneumonia (formerly *Pneumocystis carinii*)
• Coccidiomycosis, disseminated or extra-pulmonary
• Cryptococcosis, extrapulmonary
• Histoplasmosis, disseminated or extra-pulmonary

AIDS-defining illness

C. Clinical Classification

Bacterial infections
• *Mycobacterium avium complex, Mycobacteria,* other species or un-identified, disseminated, or extrapulmonary
• *Mycobacterium tuberculosis:* any site (pulmonary or extrapulmonary)
• Pneumonia, recurrent (> 2/year)
• *Salmonella* septicemia, recurrent

Viral infections
• Cytomegalovirus retinitis and involvement other than the liver, spleen, or lymph nodes
• Herpes simplex virus: chronic ulcers (>1 month); or bronchitis, pneumonitis, or esophagitis
• Progressive multifocal leukoencephalopathy (JC virus)

Others:
• Cervical cancer, invasive • Anal cancer • Encephalopathy: HIV related
• Kaposi sarcoma • Lymphoma: Burkitt, immunoblastic, or CNS
• Wasting syndrome

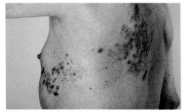

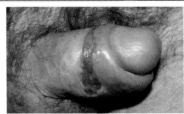

Hemorrhagic zoster   Persistent herpes simplex

D. Viral Infections

E. Fungal Infections

Candidiasis. This is the most common infectious disease among HIV patients with still normal CD4 counts. *Candida albicans* is responsible for >90%. Oral candidiasis is present in 70–80% of HIV patients. If patients have complaints of pain on swallowing or heartburn, gastroscopy is needed to exclude candidal esophagitis. Treat with fluconazole or itraconazole in doses up to 400 mg p.o. daily for 1–2 weeks. Once highly active antiretroviral therapy (HAART) is instituted, the prevalence drops.

Black hairy tongue. Up to 25% of HIV patients have dark-brown hypertrophic papillae on the tongue caused by mixed bacterial and fungal infection. Special tongue brushes are available; they can be combined with isotretinoin solution.

Malassezia-associated dermatoses. Both pityriasis versicolor and *Malassezia* folliculitis with pruritic papulopustules are common and tend to be severe.

F. Bacterial Infections

Pyoderma. Drug abusers tend to have even worse problems with recurrent furuncles, abscesses, and ecthyma. This is not a common feature in homosexuals.

Acute necrotizing ulcerative gingivitis. Chronic mixed infection with fusobacteria and spirochetes is facilitated by immunodeficiency and poor hygiene; it is known as trench mouth. There is inflammation and destruction of the gingival with advancement to bone erosion and tooth loss in AIDS patients.

Mycobacterial infections. Tuberculosis is a major problem worldwide, accounting for many AIDS-associated deaths. Multiresistant strains in debilitated hosts lead only to disasters.

Disseminated infections with *Mycobacterium avium-intracellulare complex* are common in AIDS patients with CD4 counts <100/μL. They typically present with night sweats, weight loss, and lymphadenopathy; skin findings are uncommon but can include disseminated nodules, ulcers, or abscesses. Complicated antibiotic regimens (not routine *M. tuberculosis* regimens) are required; one example is a combination of clarithromycin (500 mg b.i.d.) and ethambutol (15 mg/kg daily) with or without rifabutin (300 mg daily). HAART must also be started, paying careful attention to potential drug interactions.

Bacillary angiomatosis. *Bartonella henselae* and *B. quintana* cause pyogenic granuloma-like vascular tumors, usually when the CD4 count is <200/μL. Tumors can be confused with Kaposi sarcoma. Liver involvement (peliosis) as well as disseminated disease (CNS, lymph nodes, bone) is also possible. Treatment is erythromycin 2.0 g p.o. daily or clarithromycin 1.0 g p.o. daily for 2 months.

Syphilis. HIV infections alter the course of syphilis, while a syphilitic chancre greatly increases the risk of acquiring HIV. Chancres in HIV patients may be multiple, slow to heal, and painfully ulcerated. In secondary syphilis, lues maligna can develop, with ulcerated skin and mucosal lesions as well as a poor general condition. Finally, the disease can progress rapidly to tertiary syphilis and neurosyphilis in just a few years. There are also serological variations: very high VDRL and TPHA titers with false-negative IgM tests, and weakly reactive IgG tests or even seronegativity.

> **Note:** Cerebrospinal fluid (CSF) analysis is mandatory in every HIV patient with syphilis.

Since HIV patients have an increased risk of CNS involvement, some recommend treating all for neurosyphilis (Ch. 36.2), while others still employ benzathine penicillin G 2.4 million IU i.m. weekly for 3 weeks in those with negative CSF serology.

G. Cancers

In HIV/AIDS patients, basal cell carcinoma, squamous cell carcinoma, and melanoma are all not only more common but more aggressive.

Kaposi sarcoma. Caused by HPV8, Kaposi sarcoma occurs in 3% of HIV-positive patients. Clinically, red-brown tumors appear on the skin, starting as subtle oval or ellipsoid macules and papules that follow the skin lines. They evolve into nodules and plaques that are often ulcerated and sometimes resemble pyogenic granulomas. Oral mucosal involvement is common, especially affecting the hard palate; this is not seen with Kaposi sarcoma in HIV-negative patients. The mucocutaneous disease appears more aggressive in African patients. Disseminated disease occurs, especially involving the lungs and gastrointestinal tract.

Regression often occurs when HAART is started. Otherwise, excision, cryotherapy, or radiation therapy (20–30 Gy) is used for individual lesions. Systemic therapy is usually interferon 3 million units thrice weekly, which only appears effective if CD4 >300/μL. In advanced disease, vincristine, vinblastine, or li-

HIV/AIDS

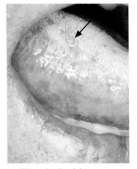

Oral hairy leukoplakia

D. Viral Infections

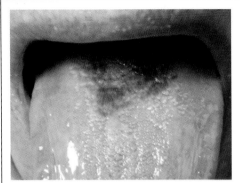

Black hairy tongue

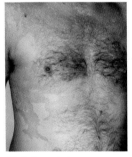

Pityriasis versicolor

E. Fungal Infections

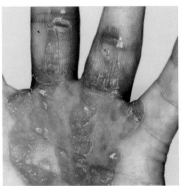

Oral candidiasis

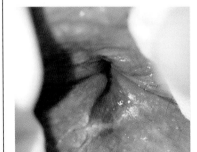

Anal chancre

F. Bacterial Infections

Secondary syphilis

posomal daunorubicin may be given for palliation.

Genital and anal carcinoma. Caused by HPV, usually HPV16 or 18; both are aggressive.

H. Dermatoses

Psoriasis. Rapid appearance of psoriasis or dramatic worsening should suggest HIV infection. Often there are overlaps with reactive arthritis and seborrheic dermatitis.

Drug eruptions. Drug eruptions are some 500-fold more common in HIV patients than the general population. The most common causative agents are *sulfonamides* (usually trimethoprim-sulfamethoxazole), widely used to treat *Pneumocystis jirovecii* pneumonia and toxoplasmosis, antiseizure medications, and proteinase inhibitors. Atypical erythema multiforme progressing to toxic epidermal necrolysis is all too frequent.

Hair disorders. Telogen effluvium may be seen in the early stage following acute infection. Later diffuse chronic loss is a sign of advanced disease. Not uncommonly, patients with low CD4 counts develop trichomegaly, a peculiar unexplained excessive growth of the eyelashes.

Lipodystrophy syndrome. This presents as variable loss of subcutaneous fat of the face and extremities with increased deposits on the nape and abdomen. It is often caused by protease inhibitors but is seen with other regimens (Ch. 18.1).

Eosinophilic folliculitis. This presents with highly pruritic papules and plaques, with pustules favoring the head, neck, arms, and chest. They are rich in eosinophils and it is associated with worsening status; it improves with HAART.

I. Diagnostic Approach

HIV-positive means presence of antibodies against HIV. Direct identification of HIV uses the p24 antigen test or polymerase chain reaction (PCR), while indirect methods to identify antibodies include enzyme-linked immunosorbent assay (ELISA) (screening) and Western blot (confirmation). The Duo test combines p24 antigen and an antibody test. It can be positive 7 days after exposure, and is 99.8% accurate at 28 days after exposure.

Written permission from the patient is required for HIV testing. Only an unequivocal positive test (two positive screening tests, ELISA; and a confirmatory test, western blot) should be reported to the patient. If the initial testing is negative and clinical suspicion persists, testing should be repeated at 6–12 weeks.

Once the diagnosis is made, the viral load and CD4 count are most useful in monitoring the course of the disease.

J. Therapy

Anti-HIV therapy. Anti-HIV or AIDS therapy is often referred to as *HAART*, (highly active antiretroviral therapy) or *cART* (combined antiretroviral therapy) (Ch. 10.11).

Several drugs that attack HIV in different ways are used simultaneously to reduce resistance. Usually two nucleoside reverse transcriptase inhibitors (NRTIs) are combined with a protease inhibitor (PI) or a nonnucleoside reverse transcriptase inhibitor (NNRTI). The choice depends on the clinical status of the patient, the CD4, count and the viral load. The optimal time to initiate therapy in HIV is controversial; general guidelines are shown opposite.

Despite many innovations, resistance and cross-resistance remain major problems. New agents that broaden the spectrum include entry, fusion, and integrase inhibitors.

Primary prophylaxis. If the CD4 is <200/μL, co-trimoxazole is given for prophylaxis against *Pneumocystis jirovecii* and toxoplasmosis.

Check for recommendations on measures to prevent reinfection until immune reconstitution has been achieved.

Treatment of infected mothers. Treatment also reduces the risk of transfer from an infected mother to a newborn child from 30% to around 5%. Measures include antiretroviral therapy during pregnancy, cesarean section, and treatment of the infant for 10–14 days. Mothers should not breast feed.

Emergency measures following HIV exposure. The risk of transmission of HIV from an infected patient to health-care worker following needle injury is 1:200–400. The patient's HIV status should be determined after any needle injury. The wound should be encouraged to bleed for 1–3 minutes and then disinfected.

If the patient is HIV positive, then prophylaxis for the health-care worker should ideally start in the first 2 hours and always before 72 hours. It is usually continued for 28 days. Zidovudine alone has an 80% protective effect. The standard regimen today includes two NRTIs and a PI.

┌─ HIV/AIDS ─

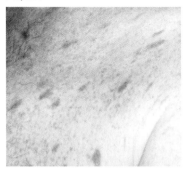
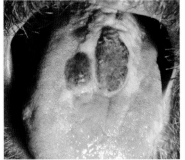

Kaposi sarcoma of the skin and tongue

G. Skin Cancers

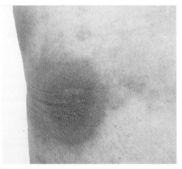
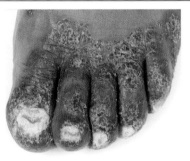

Fixed drug eruption   Hyperkeratotic psoriasis

H. Dermatoses

Clinical stage	CD4+ lymphocytes/μL	HIV RNA/mL (RT-PCR)	Therapy recommendations
AIDS-associated or AIDS-defining illnesses (CDC: B,C)	All values	All values	Definitely
Asymptomatic patients (CDC: A)	<200	All values	Definitely
	201–349	All values	Advisable
	350–500	50 000–100 000 copies	Acceptable
	>500	All values	Generally no
Acute retroviral syndrome	Normal: <500	Very high	Generally no, except in studies

J. Therapy

A. Nutritional Requirements

There is no question that an individual's nutritional status can have major consequence for their skin. Often the interactions can only be appreciated in extreme cases. There are major differences around the globe.

In industrialized countries, adequate nutrition is available to everyone. Malnutrition occurs because of poverty, alcoholism, child or elder abuse, eating disorders, or chronic disease. In less-developed countries, malnutrition is a major problem, but causes so many problems that the skin findings usually assume a secondary role.

B. Malnutrition

The two classic forms of malnutrition are usually described in children but occur at all ages.

■ Marasmus

This is a severe caloric defect, with growth retardation, wasting of subcutaneous fat, and loss of muscle mass, known as starvation in adults. Dry skin, hair and nail growth disturbances, and follicular hyperkeratoses may develop.

■ Kwashiorkor

This is severe protein deficiency but with adequate to low caloric content; there is growth and mental retardation, marked edema, and thickened darkened skin with scales (*flaked paint sign*). Changing bands of light and dark hair color (*flag sign*) reflect varying nutritional levels.

In reality, both overlap so that sometimes the term *marasmic kwashiorkor* is used. Undernourished children may present with edema and flaking skin; similar changes may be seen in adults.

C. Eating Disorders

Failure to ingest adequate amounts of calories or proteins, even though abundant food is available, is an epidemic problem. Most affected individuals are young women, convinced they are overweight, with a disturbance of body image.

■ Anorexia Nervosa

This classic eating disorder is actually quite uncommon; the prevalence is less than 0.5%. It is a potentially fatal disease. Patients refuse to maintain adequate dietary intake. Some are convinced that they are fat; others starve themselves for sports (gymnasts and ballerinas are at special risk). Associated problems include amenorrhea and depression. Skin findings include diffuse alopecia, lanugo hairs, acrocyanosis, pernio and Raynaud syndrome. These individuals often take vitamins, so that carotenemia from excessive vitamin A is not uncommon.

■ Bulimia

This is far more common than anorexia nervosa, affecting up to 5% of young women. It features binge eating followed by purging with laxative abuse or self-induced vomiting. The body weight can be normal or slightly reduced. Symptoms include angular cheilitis in a stretching mouth, knuckle calluses (*Russell sign*), or small scars from incisor-induced trauma, marked caries from repeated exposure to stomach acids, and enlarged salivary glands.

D. Zinc

Zinc is an important cofactor for DNA and protein synthesis, cell division, myelocyte proliferation, and antibody formation; thus it is a key factor in growth, development, and the immune system. Zinc is richest in red meat and poultry. Other good sources include beans, peanuts, whole grains, and dairy products.

■ Zinc Deficiency

Zinc deficiency causes a severe periorificial and acral erosive dermatitis. *Acrodermatitis enteropathica* is a genodermatosis, inherited in an autosomal recessive fashion, with a defect in *ZIP4*, a gene producing a zinc-controlling protein. Affected children have severe acral dermatitis, alopecia, and diarrhea. A similar situation can occur in patients who fail to receive or absorb zinc, such as in inflammatory bowel disease, severe malnutrition, or improper artifical alimentation. These patients all respond within days to oral zinc supplementation.

Note: The differential diagnosis of severe periorificial and acral dermatitis when nutritional problems are suspected includes zinc, biotindependent carboxylases, free fatty acid deficiency, cystic fibrosis, and mixed deficiencies, as well as glucagonoma syndrome

Nutritional Disorders

Daily requirements

Nutritional balance

9 200 kJ
(2 200 kcal)

12 600 kJ
(3 000 kcal)

Proteins
15–20%

Fats 30%

Carbohydrates
50–55%

A. Nutritional Requirements

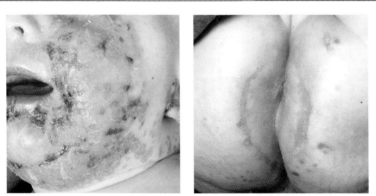

Periorificial erosions and crusts in acrodermatitis enteropathica

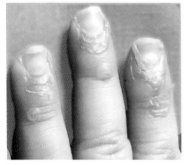

Periungual erythema and blisters

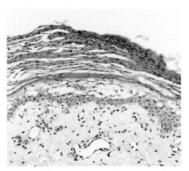

Histopatholgy: marked parakeratosis and vacoluar change

D. Zinc

E. Iron

Iron is part of hemoglobin and also a cofactor for many enzymes.

■ Iron Deficiency

This is the most common cause of anemia. Cracks at corner of mouth *(perlèche)*, glossitis, and diffuse alopecia may result. Two rare findings are:
- koilonychia
- *Plummer–Vinson syndrome*—esophageal webs and dysphagia.

■ Iron Excess

Increased iron absorption and tissue stores result in hemochromatosis (Ch. 27.7).

F. Copper

Copper is another important coenzyme factor.

■ Copper Deficiency

Abnormal intestinal absorption of copper in seen in *Menkes syndrome (kinky hair syndrome)*, inherited in an X-linked recessive fashion and caused by a mutation in the *ATP7A* gene encoding a Cu^{2+}-transporting ATPase. Infants have severe mental retardation, are floppy, and have striking kinky hair.

■ Copper Excess

In *Wilson syndrome*, patients are unable to normally excrete copper, and thus build up high tissue levels, with Kayser–Fleischer corneal ring, blue lunulae, and occasionally pretibial hyperpigmentation. It is treated with penicillamine which often causes *elastosis perforans serpiginosa*, a peculiar dermatosis where abnormal dermal elastic fibers are discharged through the epidermis.

G. Vitamins

Most clinically apparent vitamin deficiencies in adults are mixed, as a result of malnutrition.
- *Vitamin A*—deficiencies are more common in Asia with a predominantly rice diet. Dry skin with follicular prominences (*phrynoderma*) can develop. Common cause of preventable blindness in the Third World. Supplementation programs can reduce overall childhood mortality by 25%.
- *Vitamin B$_1$ (thiamine)*—deficiency causes beriberi with marked edema, cardiac and CNS problems. In western regions, it is primarily a disease of alcoholics.
- *Vitamin B$_2$ (riboflavin)*—deficiency has been shown to cause angular cheilitis, glossitis and seborrheic-dermatitis-like rash.
- *Vitamin B$_3$ (niacin)*—deficiency is known as *pellagra* and is most common in countries where corn is the major staple. Photosensitive dermatitis develops, with thickened dark scales on the neck (*Casal necklace*) and dorsal hands. There is also diarrhea, dementia, and even death. Pellagra was long responsible for putting many patients in mental institutions, especially in the Southern USA in the early part of the 20th century. Excess niacin (used for hyperlipemia) causes flushing.
- *Vitamin B$_6$ (pyridoxine)*—deficiency may cause cheilitis, glossitis, and seborrheic dermatitis.
- *Vitamin B$_{12}$*—the main sign of deficiency is pernicious anemia; a classic physical finding is severe glossitis (Möller–Hunter glossitis). Deficiency is also associated with a vast array of neurological problems.
- *Vitamin C*—deficiency is scurvy, with multiple problems; mucocutaneous signs include gingivitis, bad teeth, and perifollicular hemorrhages with corkscrew hairs. Vitamin C is essential for normal collagen synthesis.
- *Vitamin D*—deficiency in children is rickets, with impeded growth and bone deformities. The ends of the ribs, where they join the costal cartilages, may become enlarged, giving rise to the "rickety rosary." In adults, osteomalacia is the result. Vitamin D$_3$ is synthesized in skin by the action of light on 7-dehydrocholesterol. It is unlikely that sunscreens reduce vitamin D synthesis and thus increase the risk of fractures in the elderly.
- *Vitamin H (biotin)*—this is often prescribed for nail problems, but its exact role is unclear. Lack of biotin-dependent carboxylases may lead to periorificial dermatitis in infants, mimicking zinc deficiency.
- *Vitamin K*—the most common deficiency is iatrogenic, produced by coumarin and leading to bruisability and hemorrhage.

> **Note:** Many vitamins and trace elements can influence skin disorders. Vitamin D analogs are used topically to treat psoriasis, while vitamin A analogs (retinoids) are used both topically and systemically for treating acne, disorders of keratinization, and other problems.

38 Environmental Diseases

Nutritional Disorders

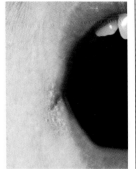

Perlèche with iron deficiency

E. Iron

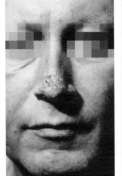

Pellagra

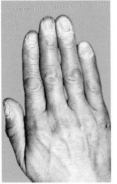

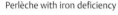

Good nutrition → Vitamin intake adequate

Malnutrition
Unbalanced diet
Antibiotic overuse
Bowel disease

Vitamin supplements

Vitamin toxicity
Vitamin A and D

Hypervitaminosis

Other vitamins

Deficiency diseases ← Hypovita-minoses

Overdosage

Urine

Vitamin balance

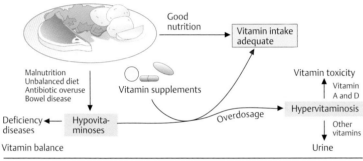

Vitamin	Active form	Needed for
β-Carotene Vegetables, fruit	Retinal Visual pigments	Vision
Vitamin A H_3C CH_3 CH_3 CH_3 CH_2OH CH_3 Retinol 1 mg* Milk, liver, egg yolk	Retinol	Sugar transport
	Retinoic acid Signaling agents	Differentiation
Vitamin B$_1$ H_3C N N NH_2 S CH_3 CH_2—CH_2OH Thiamine 15 mg* Grain, fermented products, pork	TPP Thiamine pyrophosphate	Crucial coenzyme

*daily requirements of adult

Vitamins

G. Vitamins

A. Overview

The sun is the primary energy source for the earth, required for photosynthesis and plant growth, and thus over eons responsible for coal, gas, and oil. Sunlight is needed to ensure adequate vitamin D levels and is also essential to our emotional wellbeing.

The sun puts out energy across a wide spectrum; ultraviolet (UV), visible, and infrared irradiation all reach the earth.

■ Ultraviolet Radiation

UV is the most important part of sunlight from the skin's point of view; it is divided into three classes:

- *UVC* <280 nm; absorbed by the atmosphere and not a factor in sun exposure
- *UVB* 280–320 nm; erythemogenic (causes sunburn) and carcinogenic; only superficial penetration
- *UVA* 320–400 nm; penetrates more deeply, and is most responsible for skin aging; it passes through window glass, causes most photo-induced drug reactions and may promote skin cancers.

Light sources in both the UVB and UVA range are used for phototherapy, demonstrating the therapeutic side of solar radiation (Ch. 11.1).

Protection against UV. The main natural protective agent is melanin. In addition, the stratum corneum provides protection. UVA causes *immediate pigment darkening* by oxidizing existing melanin, while UVB causes an increase in the production of melanin. Appropriate clothing and sunscreens are the best additional protections, along with avoidance.

Sunscreens. Sunscreens can either be blockers, simply reflecting sunlight, or active chemicals that absorb solar radiation. The individual chemical sunscreens tend to be more effective in either the UVA or UVB range, so a combination is usually needed. SPF (solar protection factor) gives a rough guide to the degree of protection; SPF of 20 suggests that someone who can normally stay in the noonday sun for 15 minutes can now stay for 300 minutes.

Protective clothing. Any covering is better than no covering. While special high SPF garments are available, normal clothing protects extremely well against UV.

B. Acute Toxic Effects

Predictable toxic effects are those that occur in every normal individual, just with different thresholds and degree of severity. Some individuals are photosensitive (caused by genetic defects, medications, topical substances) and react in exaggerated fashion.

■ Sunburn

Epidemiology. Everyone develops some degree of erythema after exposure to 10–30 minutes of summer noonday sun. Lack of natural protection (no tan), excessive exposure, reflecting surfaces (water, sand, snow), altitude (degree of filtration of light), and latitude (angle of light) all play a role.

Pathogenesis. The mediators for sunburn are complex. Cytokines, histamine, and DNA damage itself may all participate.

Clinical features. Typically, sunburn is erythematous, sharply delineated, and painful; it runs a crescendo course peaking at 36 hours, before going on to peel. Sunburn may involve just the epidermis, but more often also affects the papillary dermis—these are analogous to 1° and 2° burns.

Histology. The classic feature is individual keratinocyte necrosis (*sunburn cell*).

Differential diagnosis. The only question is if an underlying photosensitivity is present.

Complications. Severe sunburn can lead to fluid loss, electrolyte disturbances, infections, and, rarely, scarring.

Therapy. Cool compresses, topical corticosteroid lotions, and nonsteroidal anti-inflammatory drugs (NSAIDs) are helpful if administered immediately but usually the sunburn is recognized later.

> **Caution:** Avoid topical antihistamines and anesthetics—the main components of most over-the-counter sunburn remedies—because of the risk of sensitization.

C. Chronic Harmful Effects

UV is the single most important environmental hazard for humans. It is responsible for almost all extrinsic aging, DNA damage and elastosis (Ch. 28.3), as well as many skin cancers, although genetic and other environmental factors also play a role. The effects tend to be cumulative over many years.

D. Sunlight-induced Skin Diseases

Some patients react to UV exposure in an abnormal way. A simple classification is given on the next page. The genetic photosensitivity disorders are covered in Ch. 30.2.

Photodermatoses

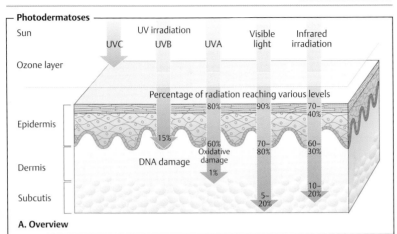

Sun

UV irradiation

UVC UVB UVA Visible light Infrared irradiation

Ozone layer

Percentage of radiation reaching various levels

Epidermis

80% 90% 70–40%

15%

60%
Oxidative damage

70–80% 60–30%

DNA damage

Dermis

1%

Subcutis

5–20% 10–20%

A. Overview

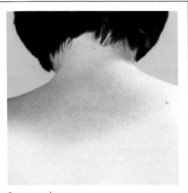

Severe sunburn
B. Acute Toxic Effects

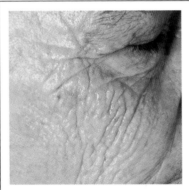

Solar elastosis

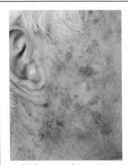

Multiple actinic keratosis
C. Chronic Harmful Effects

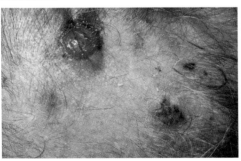

Actinic keratoses and squamous cell carcinoma

E. Phototoxic and Photoallergic Reactions

Many medications can sensitize the skin to UV radiation. A distinction is made between phototoxic and photoallergic reactions; either one can be caused by topical or systemic exposure; almost all are triggered by UVA.

■ Phototoxic Reaction

This is exaggerated sunburn; every patient who takes enough medication and gets enough sun is at risk; a classic example is systemic doxycycline. Many plants, such as giant hogweed, and berloque (coumarin derivative) in perfume, are topical phototoxic agents. Psoralens also cause topical and systemic phototoxicity; PUVA therapy for psoriasis is a "*mini-phototoxic reaction.*" (Ch. 11.1).

■ Photoallergic Reaction

The patient is sensitized to a substance and develops type IV allergy against the substance or its degradation products. Classic examples are systemic phenothiazine, and topical halogenated salicyl anilides in soaps and disinfectants.

Chronic actinic dermatitis is a persistent severe form of dermatitis, initially triggered by a photoallergic reaction but then becoming chronic and therapy resistant even after exposure is stopped

> **Note:** Frequently, the same agent causes toxic and allergic reactions. The challenge is identifying and avoiding the trigger.

F. Idiopathic Disorders

Polymorphic light eruption. This is the most common photosensitivity disorder, affecting 2%–4% of the population. It can appear at any age and typically starts in spring with the first exposure. Lesions may be acneiform, urticarial, erythema multiforme-like, or even blistering. The face and décolletage are most affected.

> **Note:** Polymorphic is a terrible name; lesions are monomorphic in an individual patient, but vary greatly from patient to patient.

Histology shows perivascular lymphocytic infiltrate that is difficult to separate from lupus erythematosus. The best treatment is efficient UVA and UVB protection, gradual exposure to the sun, or hardening with low-dose PUVA. Systemic corticosteroids minimize reaction.

Solar urticaria. Rare patients develop hives (Ch. 17.1) with sun or light exposure; always exclude erythropoietic protoporphyria and photoallergic reactions.

Hydroa vacciniforme. This rare peculiar eruption in children presents with large facial blisters and smallpoxlike scars. In Japan and Mexico it is associated with cutaneous lymphoma.

Actinic prurigo. This is a peculiar photosensitivity among American-Indians; in some tribes (Navaho), up to 20% are light sensitive with dermatitis and cheilitis, worse in spring, and with chronic changes (prurigo). It is surprising that people with millenniums of marked UV exposure have so much photosensitivity—a question for Darwin himself.

G. Photo-aggravated Diseases

Some distinguish between diseases that are almost obligate photosensitive conditions and those that may have a photosensitive component.

■ Obligate Photosensitive Disorders

- *Lupus erythematosus*—those with systemic lupus erythematosus are not only likely to experience exaggerated sunburns but have even developed renal failure following such an event. Sun exposure is a reliable trigger for chronic cutaneous lupus erythematosus.
- *Pemphigus vulgaris and foliaceus*—both are usually very photosensitive; probably mediated by urokinase release.
- *Pellagra*—caused by niacin deficiency; the hallmark is chronic photodermatitis with hyperpigmentation.
- *Porphyria*—many forms, especially erythropoietic porphyria, are extremely photosensitive. Some patients must become "night people."
- *Albinism*—the albinos of the Kuna tribe in the San Blas Islands of Panama are known as "moon children," and revered.

■ Facultative Photosensitive Disorders

Diseases in this group may occasionally flare with sunlight. Examples include psoriasis, atopic dermatitis, lichen planus, and mycosis fungoides; puzzlingly, all usually respond to phototherapy.

Photodermatoses

a) **Genetic diseases** Xeroderma pigmentosum Bloom syndrome Cockayne syndrome Trichothiodystrophy Porphyria (several forms)	c) **Idiopathic diseases** Polymorphic light eruption Solar urticaria Hydroa vacciniforme
	d) **Photo-provoked diseases** Lupus erythematosus Pemphigus Pellagra Porphyria cutanea tarda Albinism
b) **Phototoxic and photoallergic reactions** Mediators include: medications (tetracycline) plants (giant hogweed, meadow grass) chemicals (psoralens, eosin, acridine)	e) **Occasionally photo-provoked diseases** Atopic dermatitis Lichen planus Psoriasis Mycosis fungoides

Classification of photodermatoses
D. Sunlight-induced Skin Diseases

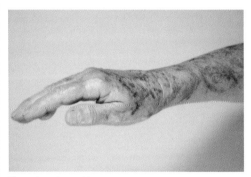

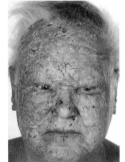

Phytophotodermatiti

Chronic actinic dermatitis

E. Phototoxic and Photoallergic Reactions

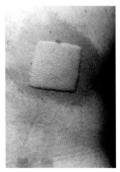

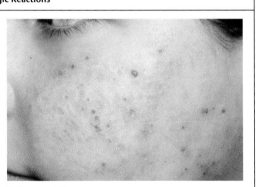

Solar urticaria

Hydroa vacciniforme

F. Idiopathic Disorders

A. Heat

■ Burns

Thermal energy damages the skin causing burns, which are clinically divided based on the depth of damage: 1° affects the epidermis; 2° involve the dermis; and 3° extends deeper. In addition, the extent of body surface is assessed, using the "rule of nines."

Therapy. Immediate measures for minor 1–2° burns include cooling and pain relief. The most common burn seen by dermatologists is sunburn, a classic superficial burn; 1° burns require only a bland dressing; for 2° burns, the blisters should be left intact as a natural dressing for 1–2 days. Nonadherent dressings combined with antiseptics are standard.

Children with > 10% 2° burns, or adults with >15%, are generally admitted. Widespread (>30%) 1–2° burns and all 3° burns are treated in specialized multidisciplinary burn units. Early emphasis is given to fluid replacement and avoiding sepsis, while later both skin grafting and skin substitutes are used.

■ Erythema Ab Igne

Long-term exposure to modest levels of heat produces a reticulated blue-red pattern with pigmentary changes. The typical cause is overuse of a heating pad or sitting in front of a space heater or fireplace for prolonged period. No therapy is available, but the patient should be monitored because of the long-term risk of developing SCC in the injured area.

B. Cold

■ Frostbite

Acute cold injury with skin temperature below 0 °C is frostbite. All cold injuries most often affect the distal extremities. Frostbite requires unprotected exposure to freezing temperatures. Initially it may be underestimated as freezing can reduce pain; as soon as rewarming starts, it is intensely painful.

Therapy. No attempts at rewarming should be made in the field, especially not vigorous rubbing. Once in a warm environment, gentle rewarming with water at 40 °C is recommended. Then burn care should be employed.

■ Immersion Foot

Also known as trench foot, this results from prolonged exposure to low, but nonfreezing temperatures. There is neurovascular damage with pain, mottling, and swelling; later, the limb is very sensitive to cold. Supportive care is needed.

■ Pernio

Also known as chilblain; this is a result of a combination of modest cold injury plus abnormal peripheral vascular reactivity. It presents as blue-red succulent painful papules, usually on the fingers and toes. There is no treatment other than avoidance and rewarming.

> **Note:** Chilblain lupus erythematous and lupus pernio (sarcoidosis) are not cold related but clinically mimic pernio.

■ Other Cold Injuries

Cold may cause panniculitis, such as neonatal subcutaneous fat necrosis from cold delivery tables or "popsicle" panniculitis from cold snacks held in the mouth. Cryoglobulinemia (Ch. 27.4) as well as rare other cryoproteinemias, predispose patients to cold injury.

C. Other Noxious Agents

■ Chemical Injury

This is usually a result of household or industrial accidents. Acids fix the skin, causing sharply delineated areas of necrosis, while bases remain active longer, causing liquefactive necrosis and deeper damage. In an industrial setting, always be sure that proper antidotes are available; treat as burns after thorough rinsing.

■ Electrical Injury

When patients become part of an electrical circuit, there is a burn at the entry site, marked muscle destruction, and a second defect at the exit point, usually the foot. The muscle damage can cause myoglobinemia and renal damage.

■ Lightening Injury

There is a feathery entry site, and high risk of cardiac arrest or CNS damage, as well as muscle damage; it is frequently fatal.

■ Ionizing Radiation

Over years, irradiated skin can evolve into an atrophic mottled telangiectatic scar, which is a fertile ground for cutaneous malignancies.

Heat, Cold, and Other Agents

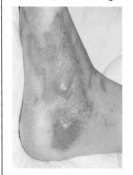
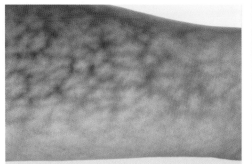

Second-degree burn

Erythema ab igne

A. Heat

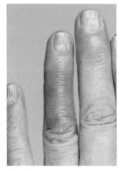
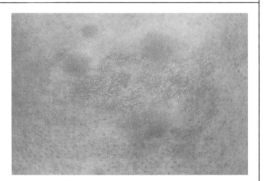

Pernio

Cold panniculitis

B. Cold

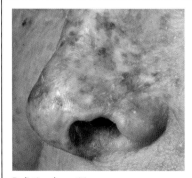
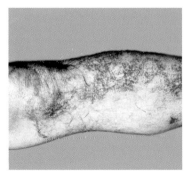

Radiation dermatitis

Chemical cement burn

C. Other Noxious Agents

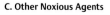

V Appendix

AA	serum amyloid A protein
Ab	antibody
ABC	ATP-binding cassette
ACA	acrodermatitis chronica atrophicans
ACD	allergic contact dermatitis
ACE	angiotensin-converting enzyme
ACR	American College of Rheumatology
ACTH	adrenocorticotropic hormone
ADCC	antibody-dependent cell-mediated cytotoxicity
ADR	adverse drug reaction
Ag	antigen
AI	active ingredient
AIDS	acquired immune deficiency syndrome
AIP	acute intermittent porphyria
AK	actinic keratosis
AK	amyloid from keratin
Akt	serine/threonine protein kinase enzyme (origin of name unclear)
AL	amyloid from immunoglobulin light chain
ALA	aminolevulinic acid
ALM	acrolentiginous melanoma
ANA	antinuclear antibodies
ANCA	antineutrophil cytoplasmic antibodies
APC	antigen-presenting cell
APECED	autoimmune polyendocrinopathy candidiasis ectodermal dystrophy
APL	antiphospholipid
ATRA	all-trans retinoic acid
ATTR	amyloid from transthyretin
AV	atrioventricular
AZT	azathioprine
b.i.d.	twice a day
BALT	bronchus-associated lymphoid tissue
BCC	basal cell carcinoma
BCG	bacille Calmette–Guérin
BCL	B-cell lymphoma
Bcl-2	B-cell lymphoma 2 protein
BL	borderline leprosy
BMZ	basement membrane zone
BP	bullous pemphigoid
BUN	blood urea nitrogen
cAMP	cyclic adenosine monophosphate
cANCA	cytoplasmic antineutrophil cytoplasmic antibodies
cART	combined antiretroviral therapy
CAST	cellular allergen stimulation test
CBC	complete blood count
CBCL	cutaneous B-cell lymphoma
CCR	chemokine receptor
CD	cluster of differentiation
CDC	Centers for Disease Control and Prevention
CDLE	chronic discoid lupus erythematosus
CEA	carcinoembryonic antigen
CFU	colony-forming unit
C_H	constant domain of heavy chain
CHILD	congenital hemidysplasia with ichthyosiform nevus and limb defects
CK	creatine kinase
CK	cytokeration
C_L	constant domain of light chain
CL	cutaneous lymphoma
CMC	chronic mucocutaneous candidiasis
CMV	cytomegalovirus
CNS	central nervous system
COL	collagen
COX	cyclo-oxygenase
CP	cicatricial pemphigoid
CRABP	cellular retinoic-acid-binding protein
CRBP	cellular retinol-binding protein
CREST	calcinosis, Raynaud syndrome, esophageal stenosis, sclerodactyly, telangiectases
CSF	cerebrospinal fluid
CTCL	cutaneous T-cell lymphoma
CTGF	connective tissue growth factor
CTL	cytotoxic T lymphocyte
CVI	chronic venous insufficiency
cw	continuous wave (laser)
CyA	ciclosporin A
DADPS	diaminodiphenyl sulfone (dapsone)
DC	dendritic cell
DEET	diethyl toluamide
DEJ	dermal–epidermal junction
DFSP	dermatofibrosarcoma protuberans
DH	dermatitis herpetiformis
DHF	dihydrofolic acid
DIC	disseminated intravascular coagulation
DIF	direct immunofluorescence
DM	diabetes mellitus
DNA	deoxyribonucleic acid
DOPA	precursor of dopamine
DRESS	drug reaction with eosinophilia and systemic symptoms
dSSc	diffuse cutaneous systemic sclerosis
DT	delayed tanning
DTHR	delayed-type hypersensitivity reaction
DTIC	dimethyl-trizeno-imidazole carboxamide (dacarbazine)
EAC	erythema annulare centrifugum
EB	epidermolysis bullosa
EBA	epidermolysis bullosa acquisita
EBD	epidermolysis bullosa dystrophica

EBJ	epidermolysis bullosa junctionalis
EBS	epidermolysis bullosa simplex
EBV	Epstein–Barr virus
ECG	electrocardiogram
ECHO	enteric cytopathic human orphan (virus)
ECL	enterochromaffin-like
ECM	extracellular matrix protein
ECP	eosinophilic cationic protein
EDS	Ehlers–Danlos syndrome
EGF	epidermal growth factor
EGFR	epidermal growth factor receptor
ELISA	enzyme-linked immunosorbent assay
EM	erythema multiforme
EMA	epithelial membrane antigen
EMLA	eutectic mixture of local anesthetics
EORTC	European Organisation for Research and Treatment of Cancer
ErbB-2	oncogene related to human epidermal growth factor receptor
Er:YAG	erbium: yttrium aluminum garnet (laser)
ESR	erythrocyte sedimentation rate
FEV$_1$	forced expiratory volume in 1 second
FGF	fibroblast growth factor
FGFR	fibroblast growth factor receptor
FOX	Forkhead box
FTA-ABS	fluorescent treponemal antibody-absorption
G6PD	glucose-6-phosphate dehydrogenase
GA	granuloma annulare
GABEB	generalized atrophic bullous epidermolysis bullosa
GAGs	glycosaminoglycans
GALT	gut-associated lymphoid tissue
GDP	guanosine diphosphate
GF	growth factor
GI	gastrointestinal
GNAC	G-protein α subunit
GR	glucocorticoid receptor
GTP	guanosine triphosphate
GVHD	graft versus host disease
Gy	gray
H-chain	heavy chain (immunoglobulin)
H&E	hematoxylin and eosin (stain)
HAART	highly active antiretroviral therapy
HHV	human herpes virus
HIT	heparin-induced thrombocytopenia
HIV	human immunodeficiency virus
HLA	human leukocyte antigen
HPV	human papillomavirus
HSV	herpes simplex virus
HVD	half-value depth
i.m.	intramuscular

ICAM	intercellular adhesion molecule
IF	immunofluorescence
IFN	interferon
Ig	immunoglobulin
IGF	insulinlike growth factor
IIF	indirect immunofluorescence
IL	interleukin
ILVEN	inflammatory linear verrucous epidermal nevus
INR	international normalized ratio
IPD	immediate pigment darkening
IPL	intense pulsed light
IR	irritant reaction
IU	international unit
IUD	intrauterine device
i.v.	intravenous
JAK	Janus kinase
JXG	juvenile xanthogranuloma
Kit	tyrosine kinase (receptor)
KS	Kaposi sarcoma
LAD	linear IgA dermatosis
LASER	light amplification by stimulated emission of radiation
L-chain	light chain (immunoglobulin)
LC	Langerhans cell
LCD	Langerhans cell disease
LE	lupus erythematosus
LFA	lymphocyte function antigen
LL	lepromatous leprosy
LM	lentigo maligna
LMM	lentigo maligna melanoma
LNA	latent nuclear antigen
LP	lichen planus
LSA	lichen sclerosus et atrophicus
lSSc	limited systemic sclerosis
LT	leukotriene
M	molar
MAGP	microfibrillar-associated glycoproteins
MALT	mucosa-associated lymphoid tissue
MCC	Merkel cell carcinoma
MCV	Merkel cell polyomavirus
MED	minimum erythema dose
MEN	multiple endocrine neoplasia
MF	mycosis fungoides
MGUS	monoclonal gammopathy of undetermined significance
MHC	major histocompatibility complex
MIF	migration inhibitory factor
MIFT	microphthalmia-associated transcription factor
MNV	milker's nodule virus
MMF	mycophenolate mofetil
MOP	methoxypsoralen
MPD	minimum phototoxic dose
mRNA	messenger RNA
MRSA	meticillin-resistant Staphylococcus aureus

Abbreviations

389

MTX	methotrexate		**PUVA**	psoralen plus UVA
NBCCS	nevoid basal cell carcinoma syndrome		**q.i.d.**	four times daily
			Qs	quality switch (laser)
Nd:YAG	neodymium-doped yttrium aluminum garnet (laser)		**RA**	retinoic acid
			RAST	radio-allergosorbent test
NEMO	nuclear factor-κB essential modulator		**REM**	reticular erythematous mucinosis
			RhD	rhesus-D antigen
NF	neurofibromatosis		**RICH**	rapidly-involuting congenital hemangioma
NFAT	nuclear factor of activated T cells			
NF-κB	nuclear factor kappa B		**RNA**	ribonucleic acid
NGNCU	nongonococcal nonchlamydial urethritis		**RPR**	rapid plasma reagin
			SALT	skin-associated lymphoid tissue
NICH	noninvoluting congenital hemangioma		**SCC**	squamous cell carcinoma
			SCLE	subacute cutaneous lupus erythematosus
NK	natural killer (cell)			
NL	necrobiosis lipoidica		**SHH**	Sonic hedgehog
NM	nodular melanoma		**SHML**	sinus histiocytosis with massive lymphadenopathy
NMN	Novy–McNeal–Nicolle (medium)			
NNRTI	nonnucleoside reverse transcriptase inhibitor		**SJS**	Stevens–Johnson syndrome
			SLE	systemic lupus erythematosus
NO	nitrous oxide		**SLIT**	sublingual immune therapy
NRTI	nucleoside reverse transcriptase inhibitor		**SLNB**	sentinel lymph node biopsy
			SMOH	Smoothened by hedgehog
NSAID	nonsteroidal anti-inflammatory drug		**SPF**	solar protection factor
			SSc	systemic sclerosis
OAS	oral allergy syndrome		**SSM**	superficial spreading melanoma
OCA	oculocutaneous albinism		**SSR**	severe skin reaction
p.o.	per os (orally)		**SSRI**	selective serotonin reuptake inhibitor
pANCA	perinuclear antineutrophil cytoplasmic antibodies			
			SSSS	staphylococcal scalded skin syndrome
PAS	periodic acid–Schiff (stain)			
PASI	psoriasis area and severity Index		**STAT**	signal transducers and activators of transcription
PCR	polymerase chain reaction			
PCT	porphyria cutanea tarda		**STD**	sexually transmitted disease
PDGF	platelet-derived growth factor		**TB**	tuberculosis
PDGFB	platelet-derived growth factor-β		**t.i.d.**	three times daily
PDGFR	platelet-derived growth factor receptor		T_c	cytotoxic T cell, CD 8+
			TCR	T-cell receptor
PDT	photodynamic therapy		**TD**	tumor depth
PET	positron emission tomography		**TDS**	total dermatoscopy score
PG	prostaglandin		**TEN**	toxic epidermal necrolysis
PG	pyoderma gangrenosum		**TGF**	transforming growth factor
PHACE	posterior fossa Dandy–Walker malformation, segmental hemangioma, arterial anomalies, cardiac anomalies, eye anomalies		T_H	helper T cell, CD4+
			THF	tetrahydrofolic acid
			TL	tuberculoid leprosy
			TLR	toll-like receptor
PI	protease inhibitor		**TMEP**	telangiectasia macularis eruptiva perstans
PLEVA	pityriasis lichenoides et varioliformis acuta			
			TNF	tumor necrosis factor
POEMS	polyneuropathy, organomegaly, endocrinopathy, monoclonal gammopathy, and skin (syndrome)		**TORCH**	toxoplasmosis, other infections, rubella, cytomegalovirus, herpes simplex virus
			TPHA	*Treponema pallidum* hemagglutination assay
PORCN	Porcupine homolog			
PPD-S	purified protein derivative standard		**TPMT**	thiopurine-*S*-methyltransferase
			TPP	thiamine pyrophosphate
PTCH	patched		**TPPA**	*Treponema pallidum* particle agglutination
PTEN	phosphatase and tensin homolog			
PUPPP	pruritic urticarial papules and plaques of pregnancy		T_{reg}	regulatory T cell

TRT	thermal relaxation time	V_L	variable domain of immunoglobulin light chain
TSS	toxic shock syndrome		
UV	ultraviolet	**VZV**	varicella zoster virus
VDRL	Venereal Disease Research Laboratory	**WBC**	white cell count
		WHO	World Health Organization
VEGF	vascular endothelial growth factor	**XP**	xeroderma pigmentosum
vGPCR	viral G-protein-coupled receptor	**YAG**	yttrium aluminum garnet
V_H	variable domain of immunoglobulin heavy chain		

Pages 21, 23, 25, 27, 29, 31, 33, 35, 37, 39, 41, 43, 49, 59, 61, 63, 65, 77, 79, 113, 117, 145, 147, 149, 151, 153, 177, 179, 263

From: Grevers G, Röcken M. Taschenatlas Allergologie. 2nd ed.. Stuttgart: Thieme; 2008.

Pages 9, 107, 379

From: Koolmann J, Röhm K-H. Taschenatlas Biochemie des Menschen. 4th ed. Stuttgart: Thieme; 2009.

Pages 91, 93, 95, 97, 99, 101, 103, 105

From: Lüllmann H, Mohr K, Hein L. Pocket Atlas of Pharmacology. 4th ed. Stuttgart: Thieme; 2010.

Page 45

From: Passarge E. Taschenatlas Humangenetik. 3rd ed. Stuttgart: Thieme; 2008.

The plates from these works were used, sometimes only in part and sometimes with modifications. Any errors are the responsibility of the authors of this book, not of the authors of the original sources.

Page 17

Photograph middle right from: http://www.afrikaansealbinos.nl with kind permission.

Page 131

Photographs with kind permission of the patient. Dr. Claudia Borelli, Munich, Germany, managed treatments A and B, while Dr. Luitgard Wiest, Munich, Germany, was responsible for C.

Page 183

Photograph upper left with kind permission of the patient.

Page 303

Photograph middle right provided by Dr. Christina Ambros-Rudolph, Graz, Austria, with kind permission.

Page 357

Photograph lower right of processionary moth caterpillar, courtesy of Ordnungsamt, Kreis Heinsberg, Heinsberg, Germany, with kind permission.

Page 383

Photograph middle right with kind permission of the patient.

Subject Index